Tribology in Total Hip and Knee Arthroplasty

Karl Knahr
Editor

Tribology in Total Hip and Knee Arthroplasty

Potential Drawbacks and Benefits of Commonly Used Materials

Springer

Editor
Karl Knahr
Orthopaedic Department
Orthopaedic Hospital Vienna-Speising
Vienna
Austria

ISBN 978-3-642-45265-9 ISBN 978-3-642-45266-6 (eBook)
DOI 10.1007/978-3-642-45266-6
Springer Heidelberg New York Dordrecht London

Library of Congress Control Number: 2014934309

Printed on acid-free paper

Springer is part of Springer Science+Business Media (www.springer.com)

Preface

Although great advances have been achieved during the last decades in total hip and knee arthroplasty, we have to accept that not all "improvements" have turned out as real benefit for the success of the implant. This applies especially to modifications in the field of tribology. Many of the evolution steps in the production of wear resistant materials did not bring the expected benefits, on the contrary, some "improvements" turned out to have unexpected drawbacks.

On the traditional tribology day during the 14th EFORT Congress in Istanbul 2013, the invited speakers focussed on these benefits and drawbacks of the commonly used materials for articulation in total hip and knee arthroplasty.

The first part of this book includes chapters on basic principles and clinical data on the most commonly used materials for articulation in total hip arthroplasty – polyethylene, ceramics, metal.

Part II includes chapters focussed on current trends in total knee arthroplasty, e.g. ceramic components or knee implants.

During the last years we realised a hype on ceramic articulations (Part III), mainly caused by introducing the last generation of composite ceramics – allowing larger femoral heads for both primary and revision implants.

Part IV on metal-on-metal articulations was the most discussed topic on this tribology day. Authors expressed many concerns with these materials, but some excellent results were reported as well. Different consensus statements give an – up to date – survey on how to deal with metal articulations referring to femoral head size and resurfacing.

The question of the effectiveness of improvements in cross-linked polyethylene is discussed within the final section of Part V. The main topics of these articles deal with the possible need of antioxidants for further improvements of this material.

This book on tribology comprises a wide range of interesting topics in total hip and knee arthroplasty. I want to thank all the contributing authors for their enormous engagement, and we all hope that we can fulfil the expectations of our readers.

Finally, I want to express my special gratitude to my secretary Mrs. Susanne Bauer. She has gained great experience how to manage all the authors to contribute their article in time and supported me in all the organisational activities when finalising this book.

Vienna, Austria Karl Knahr

Contents

Part I

Basic Principles and Clinical Data on Metal-Ceramic-Polyethylene Articulations

1 Large-Diameter Total Hip Replacement Bearings

Michael M. Morlock, Gerd Huber, and Nick Bishop

1.1 Large Heads in Hip Arthroplasty

The head size in total hip arthroplasty (THA) has always been a topic of controversy. Although it is undisputed that Charnley established the replacement of the hip joint as a standard procedure with his philosophy of "low friction arthroplasty" relying on a small head diameter (22.25 mm) [9], the use of larger heads has never lost its attraction for appealing reasons: greater stability and increased range of motion (Fig. 1.1). At the same time, the disadvantages of increasing the head diameter have always been recognized: higher friction moments and greater wear in hard-soft bearing articulations, which can lead to a higher revision rate. A comparison between the Charnley and Mueller prostheses more than 30 years ago reported better results for the Charnley type, "possibly due to the smaller head" [42]. Nevertheless, as long as the National Joint Replacement Registry of the Australian Orthopaedic Association reports "loosening / lysis and dislocation of prosthesis components" as the two most common reasons for revision (29 and 23 %, respectively [4]), the desire for larger heads will continue (Fig. 1.2). This became very clear by the rapid adoption of larger head sizes in England and Wales between 2003 and 2011: the use of the "traditional" head size of 28 mm decreased by nearly 50 % during this period, while the use of larger diameters increased (Fig. 1.3). This increase was driven by two achievements: the improvement of the wear characteristics of polyethylene (PE) by highly cross-linking (HX-PE) and the renewed popularity of hip resurfacing (HR) with large metal-on-metal (MoM) articulations, initiated by Derek McMinn and Harlan Amstutz [3, 32]. The design surgeons and manufactures were convinced that the problems that had led to failure of large MoM

M.M. Morlock (✉) • G. Huber • N. Bishop
Institute of Biomechanics, TUHH Hamburg University of Technology, Denickestrasse 15, Hamburg 21073, Germany
e-mail: morlock@tuhh.de

K. Knahr (ed.), *Tribology in Total Hip and Knee Arthroplasty*,
DOI 10.1007/978-3-642-45266-6_1, © EFORT 2014

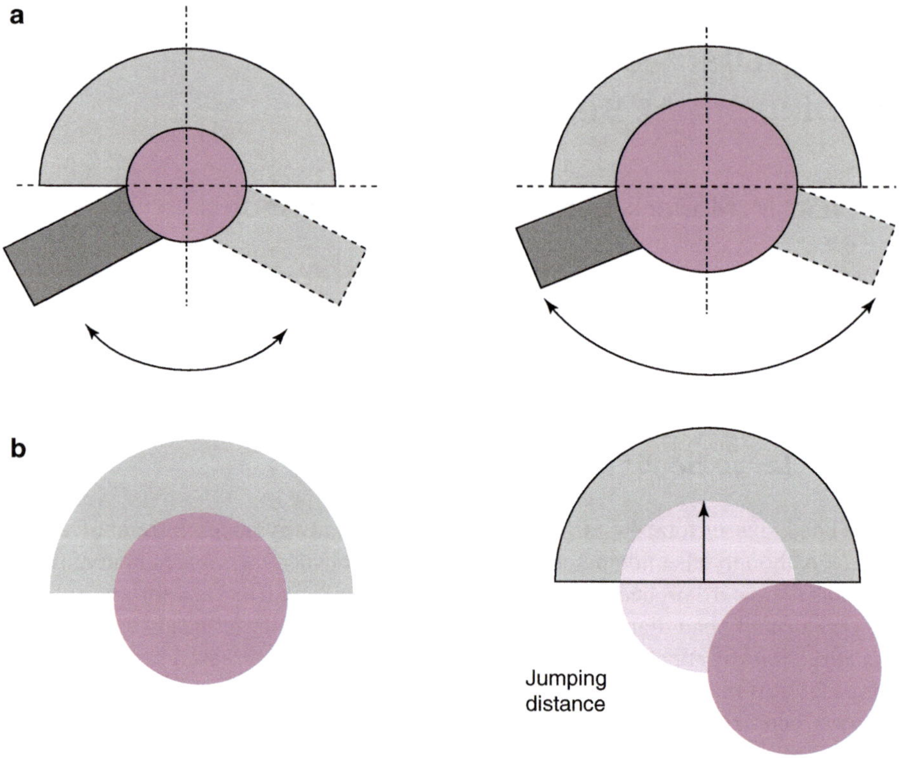

Fig. 1.1 (**a**) Increase in the technical range of motion with larger head sizes. (**b**) Illustration of the "jumping distance," which a ball head has to travel in order to dislocate (half of the diameter)

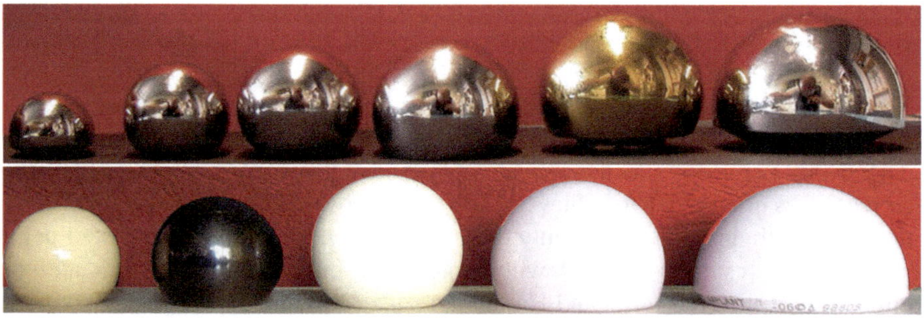

Fig. 1.2 Head sizes available for metal and ceramic head components. The diameters range from 22 mm to above 50 mm in either material

bearings more than 30 years previously had been recognized and resolved with the new designs. Due to the advantages of large heads early postoperatively, many surgeons followed this rapid development. The consequence of this "hype" is now hitting the orthopedic community hard: MoM articulations and HR have nearly

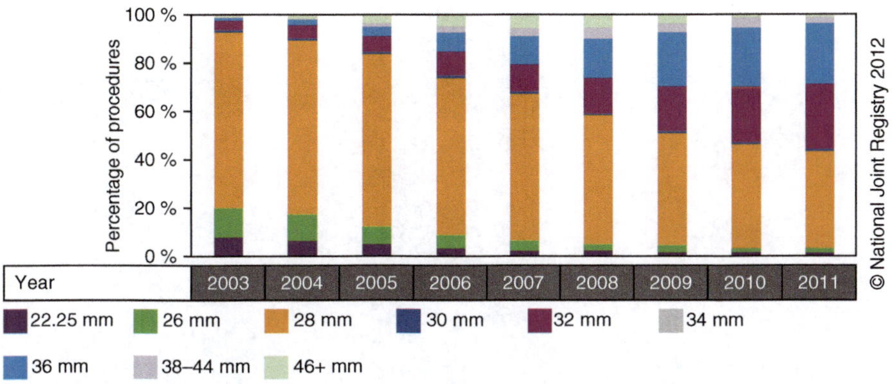

Fig. 1.3 Increase in the use of larger head sizes between 2003 and 2011 as documented in the National Joint Registry Report of England and Wales 2012 [36]

disappeared from the market as a consequence of high revision rates in the registries in comparison with conventional THAs. Adverse responses to metallic debris arising from wear and corrosion, generated either at the bearing articulation and/or the taper interface between head and stem or elevated metal ions in blood or serum, are the dominant reasons for these revisions.

This chapter discusses the potential advantages of large-diameter heads in THA, critically weighing clinical observations with the potential benefits.

1.2 Head Size and Metal-on-Metal Bearing Articulations

Three different prosthesis types can be differentiated for MoM bearings (Fig. 1.4): modular small heads (≤32 mm) THA, modular large heads (≥36 mm), and hip resurfacing arthroplasty. The definition of 36 mm as a cutoff between small and large is somewhat arbitrary and some sources also categorize 36 mm as the largest small head. The three different types show quite different performance in clinical application (Fig. 1.5). The small head modular MoM bearings have been used quite successfully for the last 25 years and show revision rates similar to other conventional bearing articulations. Large head modular MoM bearings demonstrate poor performance, and several authors suggest omitting them completely in the future based on the registry results [44]. A European consensus statement explicitly warns against this type of MoM bearing [18]. Larger modular heads have also been shown to exhibit more fretting and crevice corrosion at the head taper interface [13]. This seems to occur if the head is not sufficiently fixed on the stem taper. This seems to be the origin of the increased serum metal ion concentrations and revision rates observed for large-diameter modular MoM bearings in comparison with large-diameter HR [4, 15]. In the worst case, this can result in fracture of the stem taper, typically close to the open end of the head taper (Fig. 1.6). High friction moments in the joint articulation in adverse lubrication situations may generate micromotions

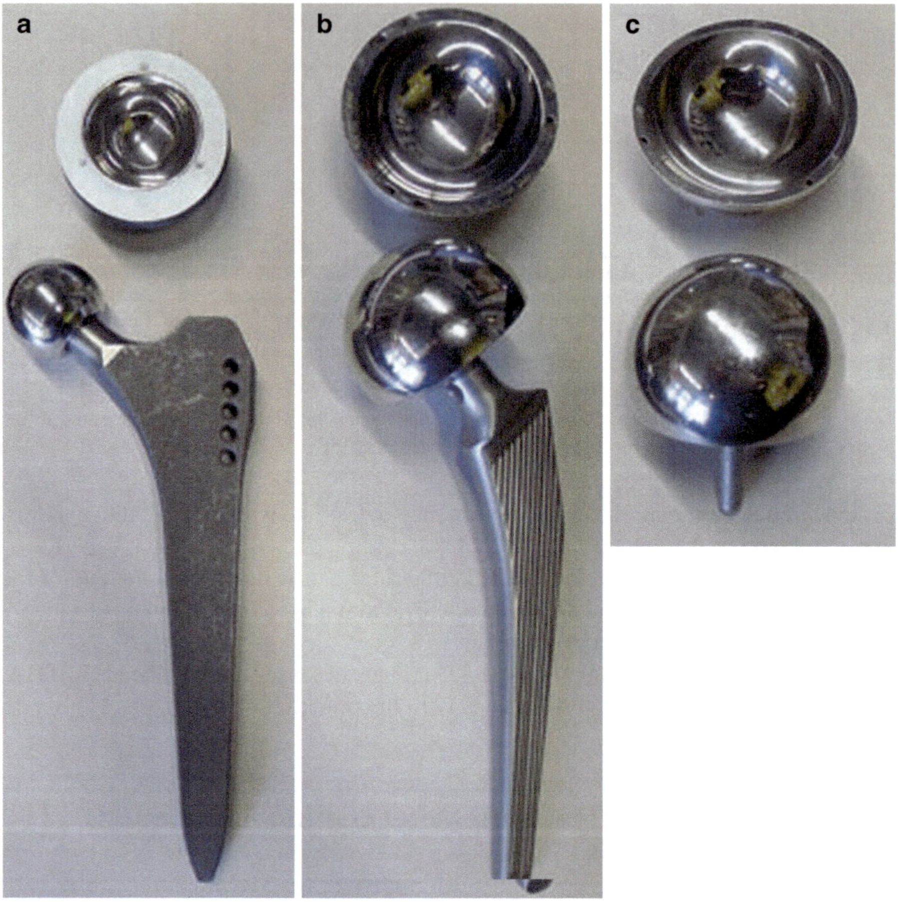

Fig. 1.4 The three different types of MoM THA: (**a**) Modular small-diameter head (≤32 mm). (**b**) Modular large-diameter head (≥36 mm). (**c**) Hip resurfacing arthroplasty (Note: the definition of 36 mm as large is somewhat arbitrary; some sources categorize it as the largest small head)

at the taper junction between head and stem [7] or cup loosening [30, 33]. This friction increase with head diameter is pronounced for MoM and ceramic-on-ceramic (CoC) articulations and further enhanced by the negative effect of resting periods on start-up friction (Fig. 1.7) [7, 8, 35].

In HR, the tendency is the opposite: smaller-diameter resurfacing components show an increased risk for revision [21] and higher blood Co and Cr ion concentrations [38]. Two primary factors are cited to explain the contrasting behavior between HR and large head modular MoM THA: firstly, a smaller angle of coverage for smaller monoblock acetabular cups resulting in a higher risk of edge loading and increased wear [16] and secondly different failure mechanisms in women, who tend to have smaller femoral head diameters [20].

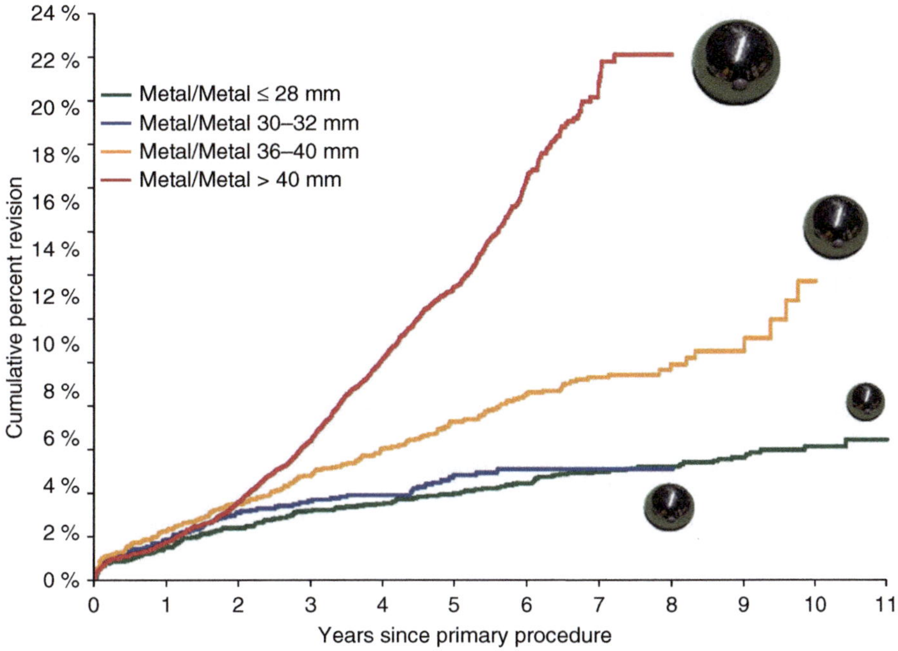

Fig. 1.5 Revision rate for MoM bearings of different head diameters from the Australian Joint Arthroplasty Register [4]

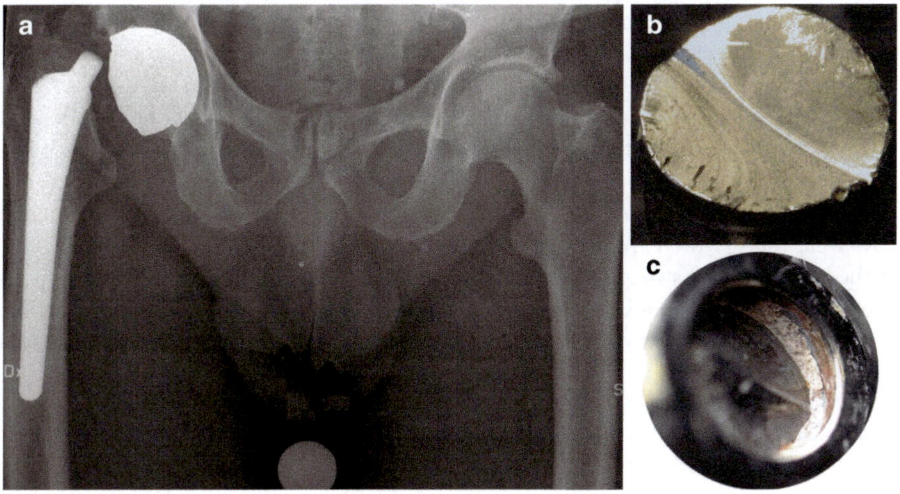

Fig. 1.6 (**a**) Fractured titanium stem taper in a modular large head MoM THA with a titanium adapter sleeve. (**b**) Fracture surface on the stem side. The lines characteristic for fatigue fractures can easily be identified. (**c**) Fracture surface on the broken taper end still sitting inside the female head taper. The white deposits were identified as titanium oxide, characteristic for continuous re-passivation of titanium under fretting or crevice corrosion (Courtesy Ake Hamberg)

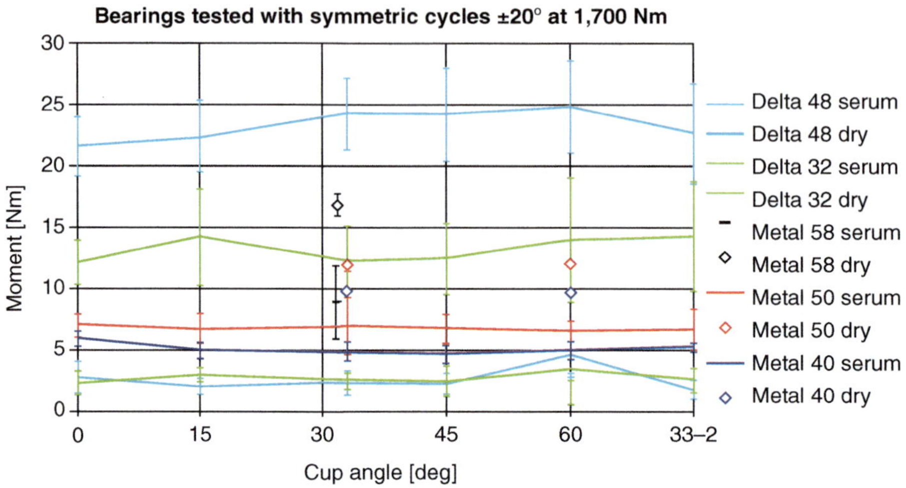

Fig. 1.7 Friction joint moment for different diameters of hard-on-hard articulations in normal (serum) and extremely adverse (dry) conditions (Adopted from Bishop et al. [7]). A cup angle of 33° corresponds to an anatomical cup inclination of 45°

In preclinical testing, larger MoM heads outperformed smaller ones. The resulting design objective was to minimize clearance and increase diameter to optimize wear behavior [12]. The partial success of these HR designs in preclinical testing were misleading, since the overall clinical revision rate for HR is much higher than for small-diameter modular MoM THAs. A recent study voices concerns even for well-functioning HR bearings. Differences in bone and cardiac function between patient groups suggest that chronic exposure to low elevated metal concentrations in patients with well-functioning HR prostheses may have systemic effects [41]. Furthermore, patients with unexplained hip pain leading to revision of a metal-on-metal hip arthroplasty sometimes exhibit satisfactory acetabular cup orientation and low wear rates, which are the factors typically associated with problems [19]. This is the basis for Hart's speculation that patient-specific factors may have been responsible for the failure in a large proportion of these patients. With all these problems, large THA MoM bearings, be they modular or HR, have more or less disappeared from the market.

1.3 Range of Motion

Some of the most commonly claimed reasons for the use of large heads are the improved range of motion (RoM) and function. During normal daily activities, the RoM utilized is quite substantial: flexion/extension can reach up to 124°, abduction/adduction up to 28°, and internal/external rotation up to 33° [23]. During athletic activities such as running, cycling, kick boxing, alpine skiing, wrestling, or free climbing, which are being practiced by some patients with THA (as claimed on the homepages of the respective companies), the RoM is most certainly higher.

The achievable range of motion is limited by impingement between femoral neck and acetabular rim and is determined by prosthesis design as well as component positioning. Head size directly influences this technical RoM. Component positioning determines the "zero" point of the RoM, i.e., how much of the RoM in flexion-extension is actually usable for flexion. Increasing the head size from 28 to 36 mm yields an increase of 13° in the technical RoM (from 123° to 136°). This applies to a hemispherical cup with a modern 12/14 mini taper completely embedded in the head and a slender neck design (proximal neck diameter smaller than the distal diameter of the taper). The technical RoM is not directly related to the active or passive RoM achieved by the patient. The "true" RoM of the patient is heavily influenced by the orientation of the components, the muscular and soft tissue situation. The limit to the RoM is reached, when the neck of the stem impinges on the cup or pelvic bone or when bony impingement occurs somewhere else between femur and pelvis.

Clinically, the theoretical advantage of larger head sizes is not really reflected. Prosthetic design has been shown to be unlikely as a limiting factor to the range of motion, provided that the positioning of the acetabular component is adequate [29]. One year after surgery, increased head size was shown not to improve function [1, 17], and range of motion was not increased at 2 years postoperatively [39]. The benefit of increased RoM of larger heads seems to be limited by the bony anatomy [25]. Extra-large-diameter femoral components may cause iliopsoas impingement, which might be the cause of postoperative pain [10]. These reports demonstrate that the increased technical RoM of larger heads is not directly related to the clinically observed RoM and function and therefore an improved RoM is not a sufficient argument for the use of large heads.

1.4 Dislocation Risk

Nearly all publications document a decrease in the dislocation rate for an increase in head diameter (Fig. 1.8). The absolute numbers, however, are quite different. For heads with a 28 mm diameter (Fig. 1.5), they range over 0.6 % [5], 2.0 % [24], 2.5 % [40], 3.0 % [6], 3.1 % [2], and 3.6 % [37]. For smaller head diameters, the range is even greater: 3.8 % [6] to 18.8 % [37] for a 22 mm head. For larger head diameters, the rates are very low: for heads with 32 mm diameter only 0.5 % [2], and even 0.0 % for 38 mm [40]. This indicates that the head diameter itself is only partly responsible for the dislocation rate. Implant position and soft tissue tension achieved by the surgeon are probably equally, or even more, important: "The theoretical gain in stability obtained by using a large femoral head (above 36 mm) is negligible in cases where there is a high cup abduction angle [43]." Already in 2004, Roy Crowninshield stated that the use of larger femoral heads contributes little to joint stability but elevates the stress within the polyethylene with high abduction acetabular component orientation [11]. The role of combined anteversion [34] and

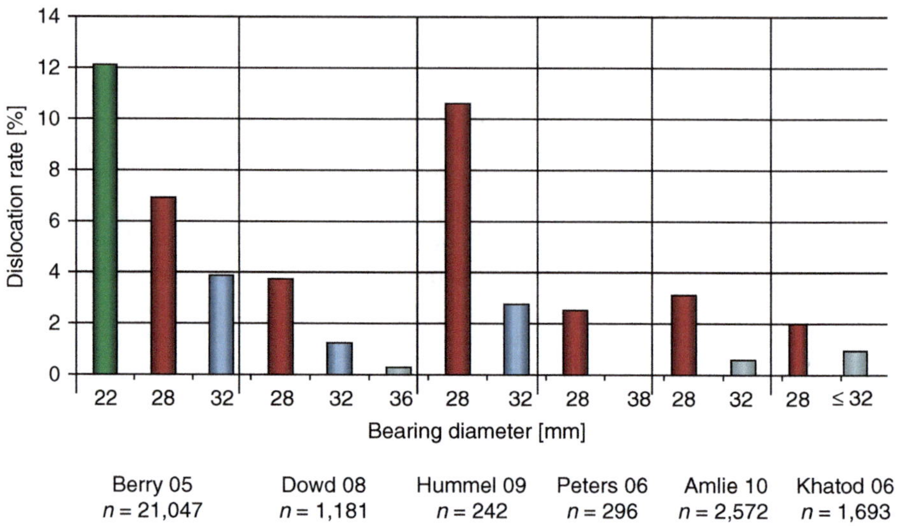

Fig. 1.8 Dislocation ratio vs. head diameter in six different studies [2, 5, 6, 24, 37, 40]

high preoperative range of motion [27] as well as several other factors besides head size was shown to be important for dislocation risk (Paprowsky acetabulum classification, hip abductor deficiency [46]). In excessively obese patients, it was even shown that a reduced cup abduction angle more effectively reduces dislocation risk than head diameter [14].

Considering the advantages and disadvantages of large heads, the important question becomes: How large does it have to be? The 2013 annual joint registry report of the Australian Orthopaedic Association makes a very clear statement in this regard: "Smaller head sizes (less than 32 mm) have the highest rate of revision for dislocation in all age groups. Increasing head size from 32 to 36 mm or larger does not appear to confer any additional protection against revision for dislocation."

1.5 Final Remarks

Considering the pros and cons of large and extra-large heads, it is proposed that the head diameter should be limited to about 36 mm in primary hip arthroplasty – the "36 and under club" founded in 2008 by Carsten Perka from the Charité in Berlin and the first author of this paper is still appropriate; in hard-on-soft bearings utilizing polyethylene, the limit should possibly be 32 mm, since for hard-on-soft bearings wear increases with head diameter. The superior wear characteristics of cross-linked PE reduces but does not remove the increase in wear with increasing head diameter [28]. Larger heads also require thinner inserts, which have shown higher PE wear rates in simulators [22]. In CoC bearings, wear is not influenced by head diameter, but larger heads have been found to generate a greater rate of noises. A recent study of large ceramic-on-ceramic designs reported 21 % squeaking [31].

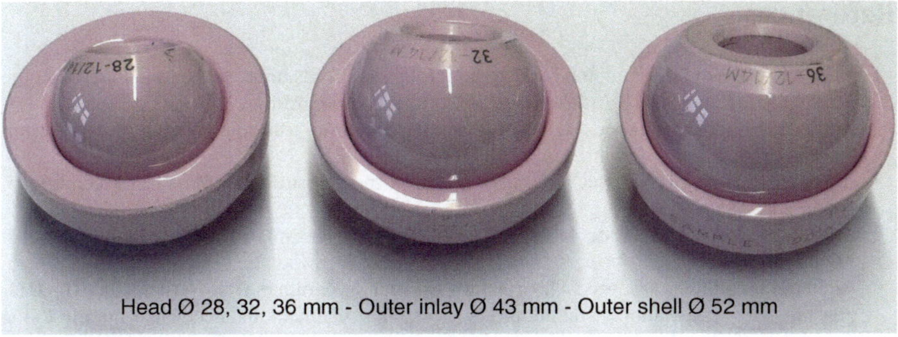

Fig. 1.9 The different head sizes (28, 32, and 36 mm) possible for the same metal back acetabular cup (inner diameter 43 mm, outer diameter 52 mm). The thickness of the inserts (7.5, 5.5, and 3.5 mm) is decreasing with increasing head diameter

Thinner ceramic liners have not been reported to have a higher fracture risk than thicker liners if implanted correctly (Fig. 1.9).

Larger heads reduce the early dislocation rate due to dislocation. However, in the long term, larger heads have been shown to have a greater cumulative revision rate after 9–21 years [45]. An analysis of the Finnish Arthroplasty Register recently showed a reduced risk for dislocation (−90 %) but a higher revision rate (+2 %) after 10 years for head diameters above 36 mm [26].

Total hip arthroplasty is the most successful surgical intervention in the history of orthopedics. The growing number of surgeries performed every year and the success rates in the registries confirm this. From a biomechanical and materials point of view, established prosthesis designs are safe and have the potential to achieve good results in the vast majority of patients over periods in excess of 15 years, as long as patient and surgeon act carefully and responsibly. There is a continuing need to improve implants and utilize newly available materials, but in this process, the risks and side effects of new developments must be carefully considered without focusing purely on the benefits. Continuous surgeon education and training for new implants and procedures is an essential requirement for the introduction of any new development into the clinics. The present problems with large MoM bearings and taper issues have once more demonstrated that successful preclinical testing does not guarantee clinical success but rather comprises a minimal requirement. Novel failure mechanisms, which never appeared in the past, cannot be prevented by preclinical testing, which is based on known problems. The international standards should be extended to include testing of adverse implant conditions rather than considering only the optimal situation. However, even this will not remove the need for a stage-wise clinical introduction of new designs. The challenge in the future will be to differentiate designs that should be categorized as "new."

In summary, there is compelling evidence that larger heads can effectively reduce the early dislocation and revision rates and that smaller heads reduce late revision due to osteolysis and loosening. A sensible choice of the optimum head diameter for the individual patient (as outlined before: not above 32 with X-PE or 36 mm with CoC in primary THA) combined with accurate component positioning will help to further improve the results of total hip arthroplasty.

References

1. Allen CL, Hooper GJ, Frampton CM. Do larger femoral heads improve the functional outcome in total hip arthroplasty? J Arthroplasty. 2013 [Epub before print].
2. Amlie E, Hovik O, Reikeras O. Dislocation after total hip arthroplasty with 28 and 32-mm femoral head. J Orthop Traumatol. 2010;11(2):111–5.
3. Amstutz HC, Le Duff MJ. Background of metal-on-metal resurfacing. Proc Inst Mech Eng H. 2006;220(2):85–94.
4. Australian Orthopaedic Association. National Joint Replacement Registry. Annual Report. Adelaide: AOA; 2012.
5. Archbold HA, Slomczykowski M, Crone M, Eckman K, Jaramaz B, Beverland DE. The relationship of the orientation of the transverse acetabular ligament and acetabular labrum to the suggested safe zones of cup positioning in total hip arthroplasty. Hip Int. 2008;18(1):1–6.
6. Berry DJ, von Knoch M, Schleck CD, Harmsen WS. Effect of femoral head diameter and operative approach on risk of dislocation after primary total hip arthroplasty. J Bone Joint Surg Am. 2005;87(11):2456–63.
7. Bishop NE, Hothan A, Morlock MM. High friction moments in large hard-on-hard hip replacement bearings in conditions of poor lubrication. J Orthop Res. 2013;31(5):807–13.
8. Bishop NE, Waldow F, Morlock MM. Friction moments of large metal-on-metal hip joint bearings and other modern designs. Med Eng Phys. 2008;30(8):1057–64.
9. Charnley J. Low friction arthroplasty of the hip. Berlin: Springer; 1979.
10. Cobb JP, Davda K, Ahmad A, Harris SJ, Masjedi M, Hart AJ. Why large-head metal-on-metal hip replacements are painful: the anatomical basis of psoas impingement on the femoral head-neck junction. J Bone Joint Surg Br. 2011;93(7):881–5.
11. Crowninshield RD, Maloney WJ, Wentz DH, Humphrey SM, Blanchard CR. Biomechanics of large femoral heads: what they do and don't do. Clin Orthop Relat Res. 2004;429:102–7.
12. Dowson D. Tribological principles in metal-on-metal hip joint design. Proc Inst Mech Eng H. 2006;220(2):161–71.
13. Dyrkacz RM, Brandt JM, Ojo OA, Turgeon TR, Wyss UP. The influence of head size on corrosion and fretting behaviour at the head-neck interface of artificial hip joints. J Arthroplasty. 2013;28:1036–40.
14. Elkins JM, Daniel M, Pedersen DR, Singh B, Yack HJ, Callaghan JJ, Brown TD. Morbid obesity may increase dislocation in total hip patients: a biomechanical analysis. Clin Orthop Relat Res. 2013;471(3):971–80.
15. Garbuz DS, Tanzer M, Greidanus NV, Masri BA, Duncan CP. The John Charnley Award: metal-on-metal hip resurfacing versus large-diameter head metal-on-metal total hip arthroplasty: a randomized clinical trial. Clin Orthop Relat Res. 2010;468(2):318–25.
16. Griffin WL, Nanson CJ, Springer BD, Davies MA, Fehring TK. Reduced articular surface of one-piece cups: a cause of runaway wear and early failure. Clin Orthop Relat Res. 2010;468(9):2328–32.
17. Hanna SA, Sewell MD, Sri-Ram K, Miles J, Aston WJ, Pollock RC, Carrington RW, Briggs TW. The effect of femoral head size on functional outcome in primary total hip arthroplasty: a single-blinded randomised controlled trial. Hip Int. 2012;22(6):592–7.
18. Hannemann F, Hartmann A, Schmitt J, Lutzner J, Seidler A, Campbell P, Delaunay CP, Drexler H, Ettema HB, Garcia-Cimbrelo E, Huberti H, Knahr K, Kunze J, Langton DJ, Lauer W, Learmonth I, Lohmann CH, Morlock M, Wimmer MA, Zagra L, Gunther KP. European multidisciplinary consensus statement on the use and monitoring of metal-on-metal bearings for total hip replacement and hip resurfacing. Orthop Traumatol Surg Res. 2013;99:263–71.
19. Hart AJ, Matthies A, Henckel J, Ilo K, Skinner J, Noble PC. Understanding why metal-on-metal hip arthroplasties fail: a comparison between patients with well-functioning and revised birmingham hip resurfacing arthroplasties. AAOS exhibit selection. J Bone Joint Surg Am. 2012;94(4):e22.

20. Hinsch A, Vettorazzi E, Morlock MM, Ruther W, Amling M, Zustin J. Sex differences in the morphological failure patterns following hip resurfacing arthroplasty. BMC Med. 2011; 9:113.
21. Jack CM, Walter WL, Shimmin AJ, Cashman K, de Steiger RN. Large diameter metal on metal articulations. Comparison of total hip arthroplasty and hip resurfacing arthroplasty. J Arthroplasty. 2013;28(4):650–3.
22. Johnson AJ, Loving L, Herrera L, Delanois RE, Wang A, Mont MA. Short-term wear evaluation of thin acetabular liners on 36-mm femoral heads. Clin Orthop Relat Res. 2014;472(2):624–9.
23. Johnston R, Smidt G. Hip motion measurements for selected activities of daily living. Clin Orthop Relat Res. 1970;72:205–15. Ref Type: Journal (Full).
24. Khatod M, Barber T, Paxton E, Namba R, Fithian D. An analysis of the risk of hip dislocation with a contemporary total joint registry. Clin Orthop Relat Res. 2006;447:19–23.
25. Klingenstein GG, Yeager AM, Lipman JD, Westrich GH. Increased range of motion to impingement with large head total hip arthroplasty: point of diminishing returns. Hip Int. 2012;22(3):261–5.
26. Kostensalo I, Junnila M, Virolainen P, Remes V, Matilainen M, Vahlberg T, Pulkkinen P, Eskelinen A, Makela KT. Effect of femoral head size on risk of revision for dislocation after total hip arthroplasty. Acta Orthop. 2013;84(4):342–7.
27. Krenzel BA, Berend ME, Malinzak RA, Faris PM, Keating EM, Meding JB, Ritter MA. High preoperative range of motion is a significant risk factor for dislocation in primary total hip arthroplasty. J Arthroplasty. 2010;25(6 Suppl):31–5.
28. Lachiewicz PF, Heckman DS, Soileau ES, Mangla J, Martell JM. Femoral head size and wear of highly cross-linked polyethylene at 5 to 8 years. Clin Orthop Relat Res. 2009;467(12): 3290–6.
29. Le Duff MJ, Wisk LE, Amstutz HC. Range of motion after stemmed total hip arthroplasty and hip resurfacing – a clinical study. Bull NYU Hosp Jt Dis. 2009;67(2):177–81.
30. Long WT, Dastane M, Harris MJ, Wan Z, Dorr LD. Failure of the Durom Metasul acetabular component. Clin Orthop Relat Res. 2010;468(2):400–5.
31. McDonnell SM, Boyce G, Bare J, Young D, Shimmin AJ. The incidence of noise generation arising from the large-diameter Delta Motion ceramic total hip bearing. Bone Joint J. 2013;95-B(2):160–5.
32. McMinn D, Treacy R, Lin K, Pynsent P. Metal on metal surface replacement of the hip. Experience of the McMinn prothesis. Clin Orthop Relat Res. 1996;(329 Suppl):S89–S98.
33. Morlock MM, Bishop N, Zustin J, Hahn M, Ruther W, Amling M. Modes of implant failure after hip resurfacing: morphological and wear analysis of 267 retrieval specimens. J Bone Joint Surg Am. 2008;90 Suppl 3:89–95.
34. Nakashima Y, Hirata M, Akiyama M, Itokawa T, Yamamoto T, Motomura G, Ohishi M, Hamai S, Iwamoto Y. Combined anteversion technique reduced the dislocation in cementless total hip arthroplasty. Int Orthop. 2014;38(1):27–32.
35. Nassutt R, Wimmer MA, Schneider E, Morlock MM. The influence of resting periods on friction in the artificial hip. Clin Orthop Relat Res. 2003;407:127–38.
36. National Joint Registry. 9th Annual Report for England and Wales; 2012. www.njrcentre.org.uk
37. Padgett DE, Lipman J, Robie B, Nestor BJ. Influence of total hip design on dislocation: a computer model and clinical analysis. Clin Orthop Relat Res. 2006;447:48–52.
38. Parry MC, Eastaugh-Waring S, Bannister GC, Learmonth ID, Case CP, Blom AW. Blood levels of cobalt and chromium are inversely correlated to head size after metal-on-metal resurfacing arthroplasty. Hip Int. 2013;23(6):529–34.
39. Penny JO, Ovesen O, Varmarken JE, Overgaard S. Similar range of motion and function after resurfacing large-head or standard total hip arthroplasty. Acta Orthop. 2013;84(3):246–53.
40. Peters CL, McPherson E, Jackson JD, Erickson JA. Reduction in early dislocation rate with large-diameter femoral heads in primary total hip arthroplasty. J Arthroplasty. 2007;22 (6 Suppl 2):140–4.

41. Prentice JR, Clark MJ, Hoggard N, Morton AC, Tooth C, Paley MN, Stockley I, Hadjivassiliou M, Wilkinson JM. Metal-on-metal hip prostheses and systemic health: a cross-sectional association study 8 years after implantation. PLoS One. 2013;8(6):e66186.
42. Ritter MA, Stringer EA, Littrell DA, Williams JG. Correlation of prosthetic femoral head size and/or design with longevity of total hip arthroplasty. Clin Orthop Relat Res. 1983;176:252–7.
43. Sariali E, Lazennec JY, Khiami F, Catonne Y. Mathematical evaluation of jumping distance in total hip arthroplasty: influence of abduction angle, femoral head offset, and head diameter. Acta Orthop. 2009;80(3):277–82.
44. Smith AJ, Dieppe P, Vernon K, Porter M, Blom AW. Failure rates of stemmed metal-on-metal hip replacements: analysis of data from the National Joint Registry of England and Wales. Lancet. 2012;379(9822):1199–204.
45. Tarasevicius S, Kesteris U, Robertsson O, Wingstrand H. Femoral head diameter affects the revision rate in total hip arthroplasty: an analysis of 1,720 hip replacements with 9–21 years of follow-up. Acta Orthop. 2006;77(5):706–9.
46. Wetters NG, Murray TG, Moric M, Sporer SM, Paprosky WG, la Valle CJ. Risk factors for dislocation after revision total hip arthroplasty. Clin Orthop Relat Res. 2013;471(2):410–6.

Comparing Large-Diameter Metal-on-Metal and Ceramic-on-Ceramic Total Hip Replacement

2

Tiago Barbosa, Frédéric Ramalho, José Ferreira, Tiago Basto, Carlos Vilela, Fernando Lima, and Manuel Mendes

2.1 Introduction

Indications for total hip replacement (THR) have been widened to young active patients with degenerative hip disease, fractures, or avascular necrosis of the femoral head. These patients place greater demands on the prosthetic components, have a longer life expectancy, and probably will need revision surgery [38], therefore the choice of implant, and particularly the bearing surfaces, is of great importance [38].

Regarding the failure of conventional metal-on-polyethylene THR in younger active patients, mainly due to osteolysis [51], new generation hard-on-hard bearings such as ceramic-on-ceramic (CoC) or metal-on-metal (MoM) are promising solutions for the wear problem [18, 27, 31].

The average wear of the polyethylene is low, particularly with highly cross-linked polyethylene (HXLPE) [11, 14, 35, 42]. However, the wear is smaller with MoM and CoC bearings leading to a lower rate of loosening, better survival rates, and fewer potential revisions [7, 17, 22, 38].

T. Barbosa, MD (✉) • F. Ramalho, MD • J. Ferreira, MD • T. Basto, MD • F. Lima, MD
M. Mendes, MD
Department of Orthopaedic Surgery, Centro Hospitalar do Alto Ave,
Rua dos Cutileiros, Creixomil, 4835-044 Guimarães, Portugal
e-mail: atiagobarbosa@gmail.com; fredetal@gmail.com; josefragaferreira@gmail.com; tiago.basto@netcabo.pt; fmlms2009@hotmail.com; pmortopedia@hotmail.pt

C. Vilela, MD
Department of Orthopaedic Surgery, Centro Hospitalar do Alto Ave,
Rua dos Cutileiros, Creixomil, 4835-044 Guimarães, Portugal

Life and Health Sciences Research Institute(ICVS), School of Health Sciences, University of Minho, Braga/Guimarães, Portugal

ICVS/3B's – PT Government Associate Laboratory, Braga/Guimarães, Portugal
e-mail: dr.vilela@sapo.pt

K. Knahr (ed.), *Tribology in Total Hip and Knee Arthroplasty*,
DOI 10.1007/978-3-642-45266-6_2, © EFORT 2014

CoC presents other advantages such as higher fracture strength, biocompatibility, and low friction coefficient [5, 11]; nonetheless fractures and squeaking of ceramic components remain a concern [15, 20, 34, 44].

The use of large-diameter MoM components (≥36) carries the benefits of a low rate of dislocation [10], improved wear properties [45, 56], and a greater range of motion [9]. Unfortunately, in the last years, some complications have been reported, with some catastrophic responses to metal wear products. High failure rates [7], metal hypersensitivity [54], aseptic lymphocyte-dominated vasculitis-associated lesions (ALVAL) [52], adverse reaction to metal debris (ARMD) [29], and pseudotumors [40] are potential complications described. Such problems rapidly alerted the orthopedic community and the rate of implantation of MoM THR decreased [25].

In young and active patients, hard bearings for THR offer potential advantages or superior clinical outcomes. The aim of the study was to evaluate clinical outcomes and complications in such patients, who had undergone a large-diameter MoM THR compared to CoC THR.

2.2 Patients and Methods

Between July 2002 and June 2007, 49 ceramic-on-ceramic (CoC) THRs (37 patients) were implanted in our hospital. In the same center, 27 metal-on-metal (MoM) THRs were implanted in 25 patients during the period of January 2007 to December 2009. A retrospective study was performed, with assessment of clinical and radiological outcomes of CoC THRs in 2011 and MoM THRs in 2012, based on clinical process evaluation and medical appointment of follow-up.

The criteria for inclusion in the study were patients aged between 25 and 70 years undergoing THR for primary or secondary osteoarthritis with a minimum follow-up of 3 years. The following exclusions were applied: patients with acute fractures of the femoral neck, those with bone deficiency requiring the use of bone graft, a history of hip infection, or failure of a previous THR.

In the CoC bearing, we reviewed 32 of 37 patients, corresponding to 42 THRs (CoC group). Five patients were excluded because they did not complete the intended follow-up. There were 23 men and 9 women, with a mean age at surgery of 43.4 years (27–58) and a mean follow-up of 47 months. Ten procedures were bilateral. Concerning the MoM bearing, this comprised 22 THRs (MoM group) implanted in 22 patients. Five patients were excluded because they did not complete the minimum follow-up, 2 of which died of unrelated causes. This group contained 14 men and 8 women, with a mean age at surgery of 55.5 years (39–70) and a mean follow-up of 44.4 months.

2.2.1 Implants

In the CoC group, all patients received uncemented components. Five femoral stems implanted were Profemur® (Wright Medical, Arlington, Tennessee) and 37 Corail® (DePuy, Warsaw, IN). On the acetabular side, five were Procotyl® (Wright Medical,

Arlington, Tennessee), 15 Duraloc® (DePuy, Warsaw, IN), and 17 Pinnacle® (DePuy, Warsaw, IN). The ceramic acetabular liner coupled with a 28- or 32-mm-diameter ceramic head from Biolox® *forte* (15 hips) and Biolox® *delta* (27 hips). The Biolox® *forte* components were used only with Duraloc® system.

Regarding the MoM group, 18 patients received an uncemented femoral component (Corail®; DePuy, Warsaw, IN), with an uncemented acetabular component (ASR XL; DePuy, Warsaw, IN) coupled with a large-diameter metal femoral head. Four patients from this group received another design of uncemented total hip system, manufactured by Wright Medical (Arlington, Tennessee), being in the femoral side Profemur® and the acetabular component Conserve®. With both designs the diameter of femoral head was between 42 and 50 mm.

All 64 THRs were undertaken through a Gibson posterolateral approach.

2.2.2 Clinical, Radiological, and Metal Ion Analysis

The clinical data analyzed included history, level of activity categorized in three levels (light, moderate, or heavy), pre- and postoperative Harris hip score [23], and complication rates. The satisfaction rate related to the final result was also recorded, on a scale of 1–5, where 5 is very satisfied and 1 is not at all satisfied.

Radiological evaluation included an anteroposterior (AP) pelvic radiograph, as well as AP and lateral radiographs of the involved hip. The analysis included radiolucent lines around both the acetabular component and the stem according to DeLee and Charnley [13] and Gruen et al. [19], respectively, periprosthetic osteolysis and component migration.

In the MoM group, blood samples were taken and sent to a certified laboratory for inductively coupled plasma mass spectroscopy analysis of chromium (Cr) and cobalt (Co) concentrations. As suggested by the Medicines and Healthcare Products Regulatory Agency (MHRA), a level above the threshold of 7 μg/l signifies abnormal wear [39].

2.2.3 Statistical Analysis

Kaplan-Meier survival analysis with 95 % confidence intervals was performed. Patients were censored if they underwent revision or were awaiting revision of either the femoral or acetabular components. All data was analyzed statistically using SPSS v17 software (SPSS Inc., Chicago, Illinois) and a p-value <0.05 was considered significant.

2.3 Results

The mean follow-up was 47 months (36–71) in the CoC group and 44.4 months (36–64) in the MoM group. The patient demographics are described in Table 2.1. Although the two groups were comparable concerning gender, mean body mass

Table 2.1 Patient demographics and preoperative diagnoses

	CoC group ($n=42$)	MoM group ($n=22$)	p-value
Mean age (years) (range)	43.4 (27–58)	55.5 (39–70)	<0.0001[a]
Male to female (n, %)	31:11 (74:26)	14:8 (64:36)	0.401[b]
Mean body mass index (kg/m²) (range)	27.88 (21.38–38.02)	27.20 (21.00–44.92)	0.493[b]
Level of activity (n, %)			0.402[b]
Light	18 (42.9)	7 (31.8)	
Moderate	15 (35.7)	9 (40.9)	
Heavy	9 (21.4)	6 (27.3)	
Diagnosis (n)			0.0006[b]
Osteoarthritis	18	17	
Osteonecrosis	14	4	
Developmental dysplasia	0	1	
Autoimmune disease	3	0	
Posttraumatic osteoarthritis	3	0	

[a]*t*-test
[b]Mann-Whitney test

Table 2.2 Preoperative and final review postoperative Harris hip score (HHS) between the two groups

Score	Preoperative	Postoperative	p-value[a]
HHS (range) CoC	44.76 ± 12.0	88.81 ± 13.5	<0.0001
HHS (range) MoM	42.91 ± 13.8	87.59 ± 12.2	<0.0001

CoC ceramic-on-ceramic, *MoM* metal-on-metal
Mean ± standard deviation
[a]Mann-Whitney test

index, and level of activity, there were statistically significant differences regarding the age and surgical indication between them.

Clinical Analysis: Results were assessed with a minimum follow-up of 3 years. All the patients had clinical and radiological evaluation at the last follow-up. Considering each group separately, there was a significant improvement of the HHS compared with preoperative values (Table 2.2). Comparing the pre- and postoperative HHS in MoM and CoC groups, we found that postoperative HHS was significantly better than preoperative HHS in both groups ($p<0.001$, paired sample *t*-test).

A total of 95 % of the patients with CoC bearing were satisfied or very satisfied and all would accept to be operated again, whereas in the MoM group only 82 % were satisfied or very satisfied. However, there were no statistical differences in the rate of satisfaction between the groups ($p=0.677$, Mann-Whitney test).

Radiological Review: Radiological review was performed in both groups. There was no detectable femoral or acetabular osteolysis in the CoC group. We found that in one hip the acetabular component had been improperly positioned with 60° of inclination, thereby outside the safe zone of 40° (±10°) of inclination [32]. However, this patient has remained asymptomatic without complications. Radiological analysis of the MoM group revealed one patient with acetabular osteolysis and no abnormalities concerning the components' position [32].

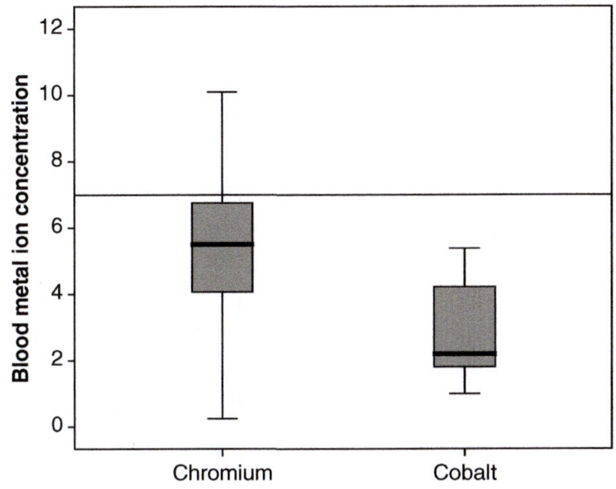

Fig. 2.1 Bar chart showing the distribution of blood metal ion concentrations. *Box lengths* represent the interquartile range and the *horizontal lines* within the boxes the median value. The *black line* represents the threshold of 7 μg/l suggested by the Medicines and Healthcare Products Regulatory Agency

Table 2.3 Data on complications in both groups

	Age/sex	Complication	Procedure
CoC group	58/M	Ceramic head fracture	Cup, head, and liner exchange
	48/M	Squeaking	Close observation
	48/M	Squeaking	Close observation
MoM group	53/M	Septic loosening	Two-stage revision of THR
	52/F	Septic loosening	Two-stage revision of THR
	62/M	Pseudotumor	Surgical excision and acetabular revision
	57/F	Acetabular osteolysis	Awaiting surgery
	50/M	Audible clicking	Close observation

Metal Ion Analysis: A total of 15 patients had returned to give blood samples at the time of the study. The mean blood Cr level was 2.82 μg/l (0.99–5.38) and mean Co level was 5.43 μg/l (0.24–10.10). None of the patients had Cr ion levels outside the normal range. Regarding the Co levels, three patients presented values above 7 μg/l, namely, 8.39, 9.72, and 10.10 (Fig. 2.1). Unfortunately, it was not possible to obtain the preoperative metal ion levels of the patients submitted to revision surgery.

Complications: Analysis of complications did not reveal significant differences between the groups (p:0.111, Mann-Whitney test), although there were a greater number of complications with MoM bearing (Table 2.3).

In the CoC group, one hip (2.4 %) had been revised owing to a femoral head fracture. This complication occurred in a patient that had received a total hip system from DePuy® with Biolox® *forte* ceramic components 3 years after the primary surgery. Two other patients, a man and a woman both aged 48 years, reported an audible squeaking that had started 2 and 3 years postoperatively, respectively. Despite the noise, none of them required revision of their THR.

Considering the large-diameter MoM bearing, the rate of complications was higher, with 4 failures: three hips underwent revision and one was awaiting it.

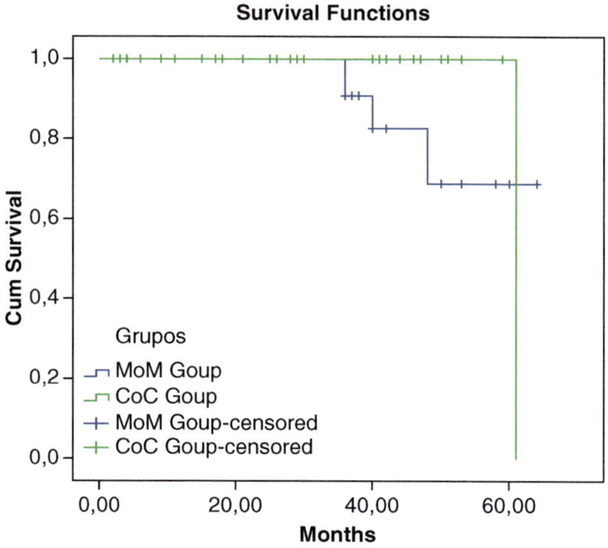

Fig. 2.2 Kaplan-Meier survival curves with 95 % confidence intervals for CoC Group and MoM Group. The survival rate of CoC prostheses was 97.6 % at 47 months postoperative and for MoM was 81.8 % at 44 months postoperative

In fact, one patient developed infection 36 months after the primary surgery and underwent a two-stage revision. Another one, also due to infection, underwent a two-stage revision 4 years after THR. She had another infection 1 year later and required a second revision. A pseudotumor along the THR's scar with macroscopically metallosis was identified in a 62-year-old man, 3 years postoperatively. Her THR was revised with replacement of acetabular component by a press-fit metal-backed cup with bearing surface of cobalt-chrome head with polyethylene liner. The patient who was awaiting revision presented an acetabular osteolysis mainly localized to Charnley and DeLee zone III. Also, one patient with high level of activity reported an audible clicking but did not require revision.

Survival: Considering revision or awaiting revision for any reason as the endpoint, the cumulative survival rate was 97.6 % at 47 months for CoC group and 81.8 % at 44 months for MoM group (95 % confidence interval) (Fig. 2.2).

2.4 Discussion

Both large-diameter MoM THR and CoC THR offer an alternative to standard metal-polyethylene in younger active patients, with their potential advantages. There are few studies comparing large-diameter MoM and CoC THRs.

The purpose of this study was to assess the clinical and radiographical outcomes of these two hard-on-hard bearings. Neither bearing outperformed the other one regarding both clinical and radiographical parameters. However, failures and survivorship for both bearings were different.

We acknowledge the limitations of the study including a limited follow-up, small size sample, and the fact that the evaluation is retrospective. Either rates of wear were not analyzed. The strengths of the study are that the surgeries were performed in a single center by surgeons with large experience with uncemented total hip replacements and the use of validated outcome scales and comparable preoperative parameters between the two groups, with the exception of age and surgical indications. Difference was found in age between the CoC and MoM groups; however, the authors do not consider it a strong limitation because the mean age in the study corresponds to a young population (<56 years). Considering the indication for surgery, there was statistically significant difference between groups. However, primary osteoarthritis and osteonecrosis were the main indications for surgery in CoC and MoM groups, corresponding to 76.2 and 95.5 %, respectively.

Our clinical outcome using HHS, with an average of 88.8 points in the CoC group and 87.59 in the MoM group at final follow-up, corresponded to an increase of 44.05 and 44.68 points, respectively. This is similar to those reported in the literature [3, 38].

Regarding complications, despite different bearing surfaces in both groups, no statistically significant differences were found. However, the high level of failures occurred in the MoM group was alarming.

MoM bearings were presented as a solution for wear and osteolysis [36], using large femoral heads and consequently increasing the stability and range of motion [4, 10, 24, 46]. However, the literature has been showing a high rate of complications requiring revision particularly with ASR XL system [47] which was finally recalled from the market on August 2010. In our study, we found 18.2 % of failures that is in line with others studies of large-diameter MoM bearings [33, 53]. Bernthal et al. [3] reported in a retrospective review of 70 MoM THR with large-diameter femoral heads 17.1 % of failures within 3 years of the primary procedure. Steele et al. [47] showed in a revision of 105 ASR XL, at an average of follow-up of 1.6 years, 15 % of failures. Nonetheless the failure rate for these devices seems to increase with time, reaching to 48.8 % within 6 years [29].

The association between soft tissue lesions and large quantities of particulate debris from accelerated wear of metal prostheses has been suggested in the literature [12, 29, 40]. The sources of metal debris in larger-diameter THR include wear from bearing surface but also the modular taper junctions and corrosion from the exposed non-articulating surface of the hollow femoral head [26]. The design of the implant, smaller diameter of the bearing [30], malposition of the acetabular component, and reduced acetabular cover are factors associated with accelerated wear [12, 28, 41]. One patient in our study with MoM bearing presented with a solid mass interpreted as a pseudotumor. He received a femoral head of 45 mm, and the acetabular component was placed with 48° of inclination and 20° of anteversion. The reason for the development of this adverse soft tissue reaction is unknown, although this lesion may appear in patients with well-positioned MoM THR [30].

We reported one case of radiographically acetabular osteolysis that was waiting revision. A radiographical finding of periprosthetic osteolysis is not common in this type of implant [6], and few studies reported this complication [3, 26]. Randelli et al. [43] found significantly elevated blood metal ion levels in patients with acetabular osteolysis and suggested that patients who present elevated blood metal ion concentrations may be at increased risk for developing radiographically undetectable severe pelvic osteolysis. Our patient had a normal serum Cr ion concentration (5.1 μg/l) and an elevated serum level of Co (9.72 μg/l), however much lower than the mean values reported by Randelli et al. [43] (Cr: 70.1 and Co: 147.0 μg/l).

We found, similar to other studies [16, 28], a disproportionate increase in the concentrations of Co relative to Cr. As the acetabular components had been placed in the safe zone [32], we did not compare the acetabular position with serum metal ion levels.

Comparing with MoM or metal-on-polyethylene, the main complication using CoC bearings is the fracture of the ceramic head and/or liner [21]. The incidence of head fractures ranges from 0.004 to 1.4 % [21] and of liner fractures between 0.01 and 2 % [21]. There has been a significant decrease in ceramic head fractures particularly after the third generation with increased fracture strength [8, 48, 55]. Few papers focused on risk factors for ceramic head fractures, and from data published until today, the only factor that significantly affects the risk of ceramic head fracture is the use of short neck 28 mm heads [48]. It is known the elevation of stress at the taper-bore interface in long neck femoral heads, and some authors hypothesized that long neck designs could facilitate ceramic head fractures [1, 37]. In our study, one case of ceramic head fracture occurred, using Biolox *forte* ceramic components that had been placed with 35° of inclination and 15° of anteversion, with a long femoral neck and a 32 mm head. This patient underwent revision with the use of a ceramic head and polyethylene acetabular liner.

Incidence of squeaking noises in ceramic-on-ceramic bearings ranges from 0.3 to 20.9 % [8]. A rate of 3.9 % of transient squeaking was reported with MoM resurfacing replacements [2]. Walter et al. [50] reported that squeaking may be caused by many factors such as patient-, implant-, and surgical-related factors.

We reported an incidence of squeaking of 4.76 % with CoC bearing. Our two patients were asymptomatic and did not need revision. In both, the acetabular components have been placed within the safe zone [32], and the noise started 2 and 3 years postoperatively. The late presentation of the squeaking was reported in the literature [38, 49, 50], as Mai et al. [34] reported that squeaking often occurred 12–30 months postoperatively.

Another point of interest in our study is that there wasn't any case of osteolysis with CoC bearing which appears to be a good predictor of longer survival expected with this bearing.

Conclusion

The purpose of our study was to compare two hard-on-hard bearings in active patients. We did not find statistically significant differences concerning clinical outcomes and complication rates between the two bearings. However, the high risk and severity of complications associated with large-diameter metal-on-metal THR, with higher rates of failures and a survival rate of 81.8 % at 44 months, does not appear to justify their use despite their potential advantages.

Taking into account the excellent implant survival rates, with no detectable osteolysis at a minimum of 36 months of follow-up, the ceramic-on-ceramic

THR can be an option for young active patients that place greater demands on the prosthetic components.

Acknowledgment We thank Dr. Carla Alves for her support in statistical analysis.

References

1. Aldrian S, Nau T, Gillesberger F, Petras N, Ehall R. Medium-term analysis of modern ceramic-on-ceramic bearing in THA. Hip Int. 2009;19:36–40.
2. Back DL, Dalziel R, Young D, Shimmin A. Early results of primary Birmingham hip resurfacings. An independent prospective study of the first 230 hips. J Bone Joint Surg Br. 2005;87:324–9.
3. Bernthal NM, Celestre PC, Stavrakis AI, Ludington JC, Oakes DA. Disappointing short-term results with the DePuy ASR XL metal-on-metal total hip arthroplasty. J Arthroplasty. 2012;27:539–44.
4. Berry DJ, von Knoch M, Schleck CD, et al. Effect of femoral head diameter and operative approach on risk of dislocation after primary total hip arthroplasty. J Bone Joint Surg Am. 2005;87:2456–63.
5. Bierbaum BE, Nairus J, Kuesis D, Morrison JC, Ward D. Ceramic-on-ceramic bearings in total hip arthroplasty. Clin Orthop Relat Res. 2002;405:158–63.
6. Bizot P, Banallec L, Sedel L, Nizard R. Alumina-on-alumina total hip prosthesis in patients 40 years or younger. Clin Orthop Relat Res. 2000;379:68–76.
7. Bolland BJ, Culliford DJ, Langton DJ, Millington JP, Arden NK, Latham JM. High failure rates with a large-diameter hybrid metal-on-metal total hip replacement: clinical, radiological and retrieval analysis. J Bone Joint Surg Br. 2011;93-B:608–15.
8. Choy WS, Kim KJ, Lee SK, Bae KW, Hwang YS, Park CK. Ceramic-on-ceramic total hip arthroplasty: minimum of six-year follow-up study. Clin Orthop Surg. 2013;5:174–9.
9. Crowninshield RD, Maloney WJ, Wentz DH, Humphrey SM, Blanchard CR. Biomechanics of large femoral heads: what they do and don't do. Clin Orthop. 2004;429:102–7.
10. Cuckler JM, Moore KD, Lombardi Jr AV, McPherson E, Emerson R. Large versus small femoral heads in metal-on-metal total hip arthroplasty. J Arthroplasty. 2004;19(Suppl):41–4.
11. D'Antonio JA, Manley MT, Capello WN, et al. Five-year experience with crossfire highly cross-linked polyethylene. Clin Orthop. 2005;441:143–50.
12. De Haan R, Pattyn C, Gill HS, Murray DW, Campbell PA, De Smet K. Correlation between inclination of the acetabular component and metal ion levels in metal-on-metal hip resurfacing replacement. J Bone Joint Surg Br. 2008;90-B:1291–7.
13. DeLee JG, Charnley J. Radiological demarcation of cemented sockets in total hip replacement. Clin Orthop. 1976;121:20–32.
14. Engh Jr CA, Stepniewski AS, Ginn SD, et al. A randomized prospective evaluation of outcomes after total hip arthroplasty using cross-linked marathon and noncross-linked Enduron polyethylene liners. J Arthroplasty. 2006;21(Suppl):17–25.
15. Fritsch EW, Gleitz M. Ceramic femoral head fractures in total hip arthroplasty. Clin Orthop. 1996;328:129–36.
16. Garbuz DS, Tanzer M, Greidanus NV, Masri BA, Duncan CP. Metal-on-metal hip resurfacing versus large-diameter head metal-on-metal total hip arthroplasty: a randomized clinical trial. Clin Orthop. 2010;468:318–25.
17. Garcia-Rey E, Cruz-Pardos A, Garcia-Cimbrelo E. Alumina-on-alumina total hip arthroplasty in young patients: diagnosis is more important than age. Clin Orthop. 2009;467:2281–9.
18. Girard J, Bocquet D, Autissier G, Fouilleron N, Fron D, Migaud H. Metal-on-metal hip arthroplasty in patients thirty years of age or younger. J Bone Joint Surg Am. 2010;92-A:2419–26.
19. Gruen TA, McNiece GM, Amstutz HC. 'Modes of failure' of cemented stem-type femoral components: a radiographic analysis of loosening. Clin Orthop. 1979;141:17–27.

20. Habermann B, Ewald W, Rauschmann M, Zichner L, Kurth AA. Fracture of ceramic heads in total hip replacement. Arch Orthop Trauma Surg. 2006;126:464–70.
21. Hamilton WG, McAuley JP, Dennis DA, Murphy JA, Blumenfeld TJ, Politi J. THA with delta ceramic on ceramic. Results of a multicenter investigational device exemption trial. Clin Orthop Relat Res. 2010;468:358–66.
22. Hamadouche M, Boutin P, Daussange J, Bolander ME, Sedel L. Alumina-on-alumina total hip arthroplasty: a minimum 18.5-year follow-up study. J Bone Joint Surg Am. 2002;84-A:69–77.
23. Harris WH. Traumatic arthritis of the hip after dislocation and acetabular fractures: treatment by mold arthroplasty: an end-result study using a new method of result evaluation. J Bone Joint Surg Am. 1969;51-A:737–55.
24. Hilton KR, Dorr LD, Wan Z, et al. Contemporary total hip replacement with metal on metal articulation. Clin Orthop Relat Res. 1996;329:S99–105.
25. Holland JP, Langton DJ, Hashmi M. Ten-year clinical, radiological and metal ion analysis of the Birmingham hip resurfacing: from a single, non-designer surgeon. J Bone Joint Surg Br. 2012;94-B:471–6.
26. Jack CM, Walter WL, Shimmin AJ, Cashman K, de Steiger RN. Large diameter metal on metal articulations. Comparison of total hip arthroplasty and hip resurfacing arthroplasty. J Arthroplasty. 2013;28:650–3.
27. Kress AM, Schmidt R, Holzwarth U, Forst R, Mueller LA. Excellent results with cementless total hip arthroplasty and alumina-on-alumina pairing: minimum ten-year follow-up. Int Orthop. 2011;35:195–200.
28. Langton DJ, Jameson SS, Joyce TJ, et al. Accelerating failure rate of the ASR total hip replacement. J Bone Joint Surg Br. 2011;93-B:1011–6.
29. Langton DJ, Jameson SS, Joyce TJ, et al. Early failure of metal-on-metal bearings in hip resurfacing and large-diameter total hip replacement: a consequence of excess wear. J Bone Joint Surg Br. 2010;92-B:38–46.
30. Langton DJ, Jameson SS, Joyce TJ, Webb J, Nargol AVF. The effect of component size and orientation on the concentrations of metal ions after resurfacing arthroplasty of the hip. J Bone Joint Surg Br. 2008;90-B:1143–51.
31. Lee YK, Ha YC, Yoo JJ, Koo KH, Yoon KS, Kim HJ. Alumina-on-alumina total hip arthroplasty: a concise follow-up, at a minimum of ten years, of a previous report. J Bone Joint Surg Am. 2010;92-A:1715–9.
32. Lewinnek GE, Lewis JL, Tarr R, Compere CL, Zimmerman JR. Dislocations after total hip-replacement arthroplasties. J Bone Joint Surg Am. 1978;60-A:217–20.
33. Long WT, Dastane M, Harris MJ, Wan Z, Dorr LD. Failure of the Durom metasul acetabular component. Clin Orthop Relat Res. 2010;468:400–5.
34. Mai K, Verioti C, Ezzet KA, et al. Incidence of 'squeaking' after ceramic-on-ceramic total hip arthroplasty. Clin Orthop. 2010;468:413–7.
35. McCalden RW, MacDonald SJ, Rorabeck CH, Bourne RB, Chess DG, Charron KD. Wear rate of highly cross-linked polyethylene in total hip arthroplasty. A randomized controlled trial. J Bone Joint Surg Am. 2009;91-A:773–82.
36. MacDonald SJ, McAlden RW, Chess DG, et al. Metal-on-metal versus polyethylene in hip arthroplasty: a randomized clinical trial. Clin Orthop Relat Res. 2003;406:282–96.
37. Masonis JL, Bourne RB, Ries MD, McCalden RW, Salehi A, Kelman DC. Zirconia femoral head fractures: a clinical and retrieval analysis. J Arthroplasty. 2004;19:898–905.
38. Nikolaou VS, Edwards MR, Bogoch E, Schemitsch EH, Waddell JP. A prospective randomised controlled trial comparing three alternative bearing surfaces in primary total hip replacement. J Bone Joint Surg Br. 2012;94-B:459–65.
39. No authors listed. Medicines and Healthcare products Regulatory Agency (MHRA).Medical device alert: all metal-on-metal (MoM) hip replacements. 2010 (MDA/2010/033). http://www.mhra.gov.uk/Publications/Safetywarnings/MedicalDeviceAlerts/CON079157. Date last Accessed Dec 2011.
40. Pandit H, Glyn-Jones S, McLardy-Smith P, et al. Pseudotumours associated with metal-on-metal hip resurfacings. J Bone Joint Surg Br. 2008;90-B:847–51.

41. Patil S, Bergula A, Chen PC, Colwell Jr CW, D'Lima DD. Polyethylene wear and acetabular component orientation. J Bone Joint Surg Am. 2003;85-A:56–63.
42. Rajadhyaksha AD, Brotea C, Cheung Y, Kuhn C, Ramakrishnan R, Zelicof SB. Five-year comparative study of highly cross-linked (crossfire) and traditional polyethylene. J Arthroplasty. 2009;24:161–7.
43. Randelli F, Banci L, Favilla S, Maglione D, Aliprandi A. Radiographically undetectable periprosthetic osteolysis with ASR implants the implication of blood metal ions. J Arthroplasty. 2013;28:1259–64.
44. Reinders J, Sonntag R, Heisel C, Reiner T, Vot L, Kretzer JP. Wear performance of ceramic-on-metal hip bearings. PLoS One. 2013;8:e73252.
45. Smith SL, Dowson D, Goldsmith AA. The effect of femoral head diameter upon lubrication and wear of metal-on-metal total hip replacements. Proc Inst Mech Eng H. 2001;215:161–70.
46. Smith TM, Berend KR, Lombardi Jr AV, et al. Metal-on-metal total hip arthroplasty with large heads may prevent early dislocation. Clin Orthop Relat Res. 2005;441:137–42.
47. Steele GD, Fehring TK, Odum SM, Dennos AC, Nadaud MC. Early failure of articular surface replacement XL total hip arthroplasty. J Arthroplasty. 2011;26:14–8.
48. Traina F, De Fine M, DiMartino A, Faldini C. Fracture of ceramic bearing surfaces following total hip replacement: a systematic review. Biomed Res Int. 2013;2013:157247.
49. Walter WL, Kurtz SM, Esposito C, Hozack W, Holley KG, Garino JP, Tuke MA. Retrieval analysis of squeaking alumina ceramic-on-ceramic bearings. J Bone Joint Surg Br. 2011;93-B:1597–601.
50. Walter WL, O'Toole GC, Walter WK, Ellis A, Zicat BA. Squeaking in ceramic-on-ceramic hips: the importance of acetabular component orientation. J Arthroplasty. 2007;22:496–503.
51. Wangen H, Lereim P, Holm I, Gunderson R, Reikeras O. Hip arthroplasty in patients younger than 30 years: excellent ten to 16-year follow-up results with a HA-coated stem. Int Orthop. 2008;32:203–8.
52. Watters TS, Cardona DM, Menon KS, et al. Aseptic lymphocyte-dominated vasculitis-associated lesion: a clinicopathologic review of an underrecognized cause of prosthetic failure. Am J Clin Pathol. 2010;134:886–93.
53. Whitwell GS, Shine A, Young SK. The articular surface replacement implant recall: a United Kingdom district hospital experience. Hip Int. 2012;22:362–70.
54. Willert HG, Buchhorn GH, Fayyazi A, et al. Metal-on-metal bearings and hypersensitivity in patients with artificial hip joints: a clinical and histomorphological study. J Bone Joint Surg Am. 2005;87-A:28–36.
55. Willmann G. Ceramic femoral head retrieval data. Clin Orthop Relat Res. 2000;379:22–8.
56. Wimmer MA, Fischer A, Büscher R, et al. Wear mechanisms in metal-on-metal bearings: the importance of tribochemical reaction layers. J Orthop Res. 2010;28:436–43.

Comparison of Linear Wear Rate According to Femoral Head Sizes in Metal on Conventional UHMWPE Liner

3

Yoon Je Cho, Joo Hyun Lee, and Eun Seong Sagong

3.1 Introduction

Since its initial introduction by Charnley in 1963, polyethylene acetabular liners have been in consistent use for the past 50 years, having been accepted to be safe for use on the human body [1]. Periprosthetic osteolysis and dissociation of articular components owing to polyethylene wear debris have been major causes of total hip arthroplasty failure [2–4]. It is well known that the wear behavior of the hip prosthesis is determined by an interplay of multiple influences including the type of prosthetic implant used along with numerous patient and surgical factors; femoral head size, PE liner thickness, and material characteristics of the bearing surface are some of the factors that fall under the category of prosthetic implant type [5–10].

It has been experimentally proven that UHMWPE wear is affected by the amount of physical stress applied to the articular surface of the prosthesis as well as the motion of the adjoining area. Brown et al. reported that UHMWPE thickness is not an influential parameter as the acetabular cup is thick enough to provide ample protection from high subsurface stresses [5–11]. However, many results suggest that a larger femoral head diameter will increase the sliding area between the liner and the femoral head, hence adding higher stress to the thin liner and resulting in an increased amount of wear [6, 12, 13]. Femoral head size is generally acknowledged to be the most closely related factor to linear wear rate: smaller femoral head size results in a higher linear wear rate, while a larger femoral head results in a higher volumetric wear rate. The aim of this study is to establish polyethylene cup thickness as the more relevant factor contributing to the linear wear rate of conventional UHMWPE acetabular prostheses.

Y.J. Cho (✉) • J.H. Lee • E.S. Sagong
Department of Orthopaedic Surgery, School of Medicine, Kyung Hee University, #1 Hoegi-dong, Dongdaemun-gu, Seoul 130-702, South Korea
e-mail: yjcho@khmc.or.kr

K. Knahr (ed.), *Tribology in Total Hip and Knee Arthroplasty*, DOI 10.1007/978-3-642-45266-6_3, © EFORT 2014

3.2 Study Model

We conducted a retrospective review of patients who had undergone total hip arthroplasty using the cobalt-chromium femoral head and conventional UHMWPE acetabular liner at our institution between July 1992 and December 2002. The patient group was restricted to those for whom follow-up studies were possible. 28 mm femoral heads were used on 128 hips (94 male hips and 34 female hips), and 22 mm heads were used on 102 hips (61 male hips and 41 female hips). In all cases, the Trilogy Acetabular System (HGP II, Zimmer, Warshaw) was used for the acetabular cup, and the conventional UHMWPE (HGP2) liner was used for the liner. The mean age was 45.3 years (range 24–81 years) at the point of operation, and the mean BMI was 24.0 kg/m^2 (range 17.1–32.7 kg/m^2). The mean duration of follow-up was 10.8 years (range 96–144 months). Preoperative and postoperative clinical assessment was performed using the Harris hip scores (HHS), UCLA activity scores, visual analogue scale (VAS), range of motion (ROM), and limb length discrepancy (LLD). Dorr method was incorporated for the radiographic measurement of the wear rate. The amount of wear was determined based on measurements made on enlarged AP radiographs in the standing position, by first subtracting the distance between the upper liner and the femoral head from the distance between the lower liner and the femoral head and then dividing this value by two. The same assessment was made annually at each outpatient follow-up session (Fig. 3.1) [14]. Considering the bedding-in period, the initial checkup for amount of wear was performed 2 years post-op [15, 16]. The differences in wear were compared among different liner thicknesses firstly within each femoral head size group and secondly within male and female groups of each femoral head size group. Statistical analysis

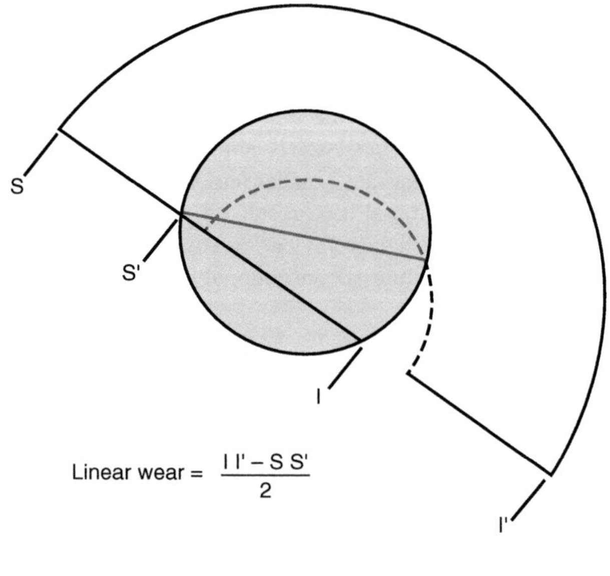

Fig. 3.1 Dorr method to evaluate the linear wear

was performed using bivariate correlation analysis with SPSS ver. 18.0 in order to take into account the influence of gender difference on wear rate.

3.3 Results

3.3.1 Clinical Results

Clinical assessment revealed progression of the preoperative Harris hip score from 60.4 to 95.8 after the operation for the 28 mm femoral head group and 58.4–96.7 for the 22 mm femoral head group. Preoperative UCLA activity scores improved from 4.3 to 8.2 following surgery in the 28 mm group and 4.1–8.8 in the 22 mm femoral head group. VAS assessed prior to the operation also showed improvement from 6.3 to 1.1 following the operation in the 28 mm group and 6.6–0.9 in the 22 mm group. Limb length discrepancy was not observed in either of the two femoral head size groups. Clinical differences according to femoral head size or polyethylene liner thickness were not noted.

3.3.2 Radiologic Results

The mean wear rate was 0.152 and 0.137 mm/year for the 28 and 22 mm femoral head groups, respectively. In both groups, the use of thicker liners resulted in a lower mean wear rate. The differences between polyethylene wear rate according to gender proved to lack statistical significance ($p=0.311$), with mean wear rates observed to be 0.137 mm/year for males and 0.169 mm/year for females in the 28 mm femoral head group and 0.139 mm/year for males and 0.136 mm/year for females in the 22 mm femoral head group. As for the comparison of wear rates between different liner thicknesses, the linear wear rate was seen to decrease in both the 28 and 22 mm femoral head groups as the liner thickness increased: in the 28 mm group, the linear wear rate was 0.223, 0.197, 0.190, 0.182, 0.130, 0.104, 0.095, 0.086, 0.070, 0.064, and 0.059 mm/year for liner thicknesses of 6.2, 7.2, 8.2, 9.2, 10.2, 11.2, 12.2, 13.2, 14.2, 15.2, and 16.2 mm, respectively ($p<0.001$, Table 3.1), and in the 22 mm group, the linear wear rate was 0.172, 0.164, 0.148, 0.139, 0.137, 0.138, 0.123, 0.122, and 0.114 mm/year for liner thicknesses of 6.1, 7.1, 9.1, 10.1, 11.1, 12.1, 13.1, 14.1, and 15.1 mm, respectively ($p<0.001$). Linear wear rate was higher in the 28 mm femoral head group when the polyethylene acetabular lining used was thinner than 10 mm ($p=0.001$), while when the lining was

Table 3.1 Linear wear rate in both groups

	6.2	7.2	8.2	9.2	10.2	11.2	12.2	13.2	14.2	15.2	16.2
28 mm	0.023	0.197	0.109	0.182	0.130	0.104	0.095	0.086	0.070	0.064	0.059
22 mm	0.172	0.164		0.148	0.139	0.137	0.138	0.123	0.122	0.114	

Unit: mm/year

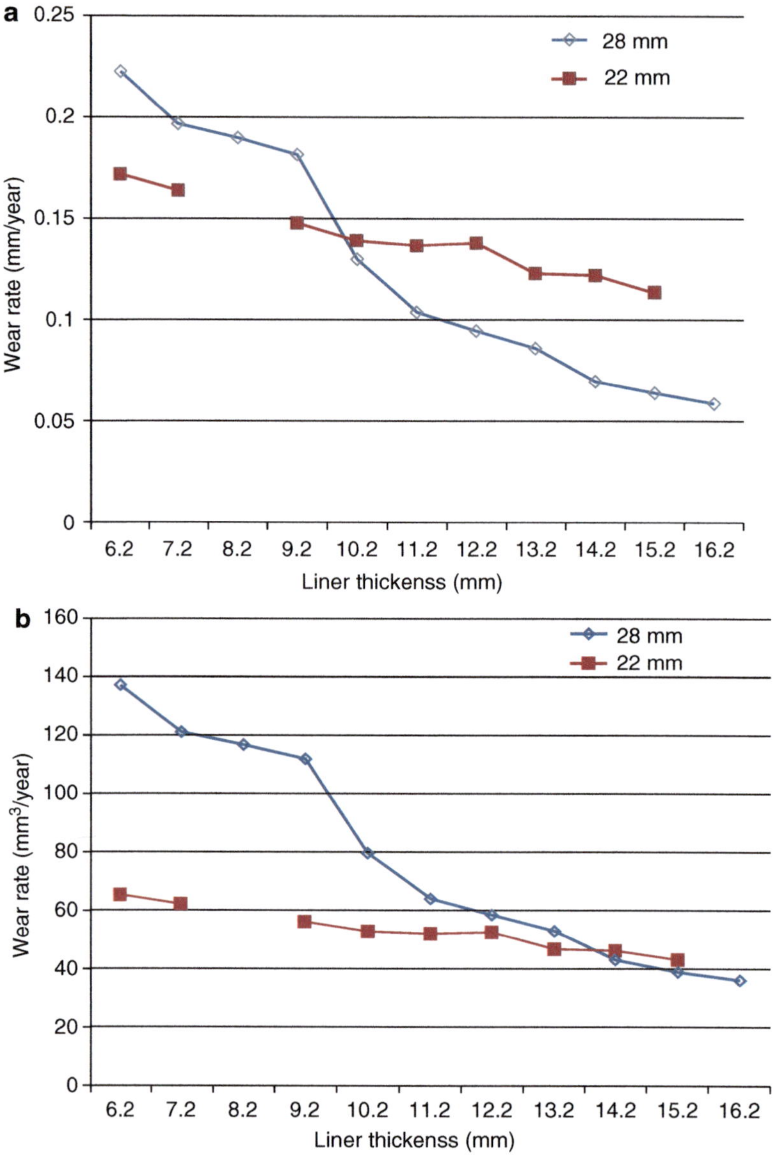

Fig. 3.2 (**a**) Linear wear rate in both groups. (**b**)Volumetric wear rate in both groups

thicker than 10 mm, the linear wear rate was lower in the 28 mm group ($p<0.001$, Fig. 3.2a). Volumetric wear rate was higher in the 28 mm femoral head group than in the 22 mm group when the polyethylene acetabular lining used was thinner than 13 mm, while when the lining was thicker than 13 mm, it was lower in the 28 mm group (Table 3.2, Fig. 3.2b).

Table 3.2 Volumetric wear rate in both groups

	6.2	7.2	8.2	9.2	10.2	11.2	12.2	13.2	14.2	15.2	16.2
28 mm	137.24	121.24	116.93	112.01	80.01	64.01	58.47	52.93	43.08	39.39	36.31
22 mm	65.35	62.31		56.23	52.81	52.05	52.43	46.73	46.35	43.31	

Unit: mm^3/year

3.4 Discussion

Metal-on-polyethylene prostheses have been considered to be harmless for implantation in the human body. Thus, they have been, and still are, the most commonly used prostheses for total hip arthroplasty. Nevertheless, they are not lacking in flaws: periprosthetic osteolysis due to polyethylene wear remains the most frequent postoperative complication, with prostheses completely resistant to wear yet to be developed. Compared to highly cross-linked UHMWPE, which is the most commonly used prostheses in clinical settings today, conventional UHMWPE is more prone to osteolysis by wear debris, leading to higher loosening rates. Impingement between the neck of the metallic stem and the hip socket owing to gradual penetration of the metallic femoral head into the polyethylene acetabulum also contributes to the loosening of the replaced joint [17]. In most studies, wear rate assessment has been based on simple radiography, a two-dimensional analysis for which concerns regarding its accuracy have been suggested. However, Martell et al. reported that there is no significant difference between two-dimensional and three-dimensional methods in the analysis of wear rate, thereby leading to acceptance of two-dimensional analytic results in most recent and ongoing studies [18, 19].

In this study, the annual linear wear rate was assessed by the Dorr method, which is similar to the Livermore method but more useful in that it is simpler [7, 14]. In accordance with previous reports by Sychterz et al., a postoperative 1- to 2-year bedding-in or creep period was allowed before wear rate assessment was performed in this study to enable accurate measurement of polyethylene wear [16]. The annual wear rate for the polyethylene liner was determined to be 0.145 mm, which corresponded with existing study results (0.14 ± 0.09 mm/year for Harris-Galante II acetabular cup reported by Woolson et al., 0.15 mm/year reported by Devane et al.) [20, 21]. Studies have shown the lowest wear rate at which periprosthetic osteolysis begins to occur to be approximately 0.1 mm/year, which explains the high incidence of osteolysis in past total hip arthroplasties where conventional UHMWPE had been used [22]. A number of factors are known to affect the wear rate of conventional UHMWPE, including the positioning of the prosthesis, femoral head size, polyethylene thickness, as well as various patient factors [6, 7, 23]. In a study regarding the relationship between femoral head size and polyethylene wear, Livermore et al. concluded that linear wear was greatest when 28 mm femoral heads were used and least when 22 mm heads were used. Furthermore, the study reported that volumetric wear is greater in hips where larger femoral heads were used [7].

Until now, it has been universally accepted that the definitive factor which influences wear rate is femoral head size, regardless of liner thickness; Woolson et al.

reported that polyethylene liner thickness is irrelevant with its wear rate [20]. However, we have shown in this study that the most wear-prone femoral head size differed between hips with polyethylene liners of different thicknesses, with the highest linear wear rate observed in the 28 mm femoral head group in cases where liners thinner than 10 mm had been used. In addition, the 28 mm femoral head group showed the highest volumetric wear rate when polyethylene liner thickness was less than 13 mm, while it was the 22 mm group with the highest volumetric wear rate when liners thicker than 13 mm were used. In a recent study, Johnson et al. compared the linear wear rates while keeping the femoral head size fixed at 36 mm and altering liner thickness. The study results were in accordance with those of our study: in cases where liners less than 7.9 mm in thickness had been used, the linear wear rate increased as the liner thickness decreased [24]. Currently, highly cross-linked UHMWPE is most commonly used in place of conventional UHMWPE. Based on such existing reports, therefore, it is considered that further research is necessary in order to determine the difference in wear rate according to various liner thicknesses for each femoral head size group for highly cross-linked UHMWPE.

3.5 Summary

With conventional PE liners, thinner (less than 10 mm) liners resulted in higher linear wear rates in the large femoral head (28 mm) group, while thicker (more than 13 mm) liners resulted in higher volumetric wear rates in the small femoral head (22 mm) group. It has been generally accepted that for conventional UHMWPE prostheses, smaller femoral head size leads to increased linear wear rate, and larger femoral head size leads to increased volumetric wear rate. However, the results in this study showed that the linear wear rate is higher in the 28 mm femoral head group for polyethylene prostheses thinner than 10 mm, while the volumetric wear rate is lower in the 28 mm group for prostheses thicker than 14 mm. Conclusively, this study demonstrated that thicker liners result in lower wear rates regardless of femoral head size, thereby identifying the thickness of the polyethylene liner to be the more relevant factor in determining the wear rate of polyethylene prostheses.

References

1. Charnley J, Halley DK. Rate of wear in total hip replacement. Clin Orthop Relat Res. 1975;112:170–9.
2. Dumbleton JH, Manley MT, Edidin AA. A literature review of the association between wear rate and osteolysis in total hip arthroplasty. J Arthroplasty. 2002;17(5):649–61.
3. Harris WH. The problem is osteolysis. Clin Orthop Relat Res. 1995;311:46–53.
4. Sochart DH. Relationship of acetabular wear to osteolysis and loosening in total hip arthroplasty. Clin Orthop Relat Res. 1999;363:135–50.
5. Brown TD, Bartel DL. What design factors influence wear behavior at the bearing surfaces in total joint replacements? J Am Acad Orthop Surg. 2008;16 Suppl 1:S101–6.
6. Maxian TA, Brown TD, Pedersen DR, Callaghan JJ. Adaptive finite element modeling of long-term polyethylene wear in total hip arthroplasty. J Orthop Res. 1996;14(4):668–75.

7. Livermore J, Ilstrup D, Morrey B. Effect of femoral head size on wear of the polyethylene acetabular component. J Bone Joint Surg Am. 1990;72(4):518–28.
8. Pietrabissa R, Raimondi M, Di Martino E. Wear of polyethylene cups in total hip arthroplasty: a parametric mathematical model. Med Eng Phys. 1998;20(3):199–210.
9. Rixrath E, Wendling-Mansuy S, Flecher X, Chabrand P, Argenson JN. Design parameters dependences on contact stress distribution in gait and jogging phases after total hip arthroplasty. J Biomech. 2008;41(5):1137–42.
10. Meding JB, Keating EM, Davis KE. Acetabular UHMWPE survival and wear changes with different manufacturing techniques. Clin Orthop Relat Res. 2011;469(2):405–11.
11. Barbour PS, Barton DC, Fisher J. The influence of stress conditions on the wear of UHMWPE for total joint replacements. J Mater Sci Mater Med. 1997;8(10):603–11.
12. Shen FW, Lu Z, McKellop HA. Wear versus thickness and other features of 5-Mrad crosslinked UHMWPE acetabular liners. Clin Orthop Relat Res. 2011;469(2):395–404.
13. Berry DJ, von Knoch M, Schleck CD, Harmsen WS. Effect of femoral head diameter and operative approach on risk of dislocation after primary total hip arthroplasty. J Bone Joint Surg Am. 2005;87(11):2456–63.
14. Dorr LD, Wan Z. Ten years of experience with porous acetabular components for revision surgery. Clin Orthop Relat Res. 1995;319:191–200.
15. Isaac GH, Dowson D, Wroblewski BM. An investigation into the origins of time-dependent variation in penetration rates with Charnley acetabular cups–wear, creep or degradation? Proc Inst Mech Eng [H]. 1996;210(3):209–16.
16. Sychterz CJ, Engh Jr CA, Yang A, Engh CA. Analysis of temporal wear patterns of porous-coated acetabular components: distinguishing between true wear and so-called bedding-in. J Bone Joint Surg Am. 1999;81(6):821–30.
17. Wroblewski BM. Direction and rate of socket wear in Charnley low-friction arthroplasty. J Bone Joint Surg Br. 1985;67(5):757–61.
18. Sychterz CJ, Yang AM, McAuley JP, Engh CA. Two-dimensional versus three-dimensional radiographic measurements of polyethylene wear. Clin Orthop Relat Res. 1999;365:117–23.
19. Martell JM, Berkson E, Berger R, Jacobs J. Comparison of two and three-dimensional computerized polyethylene wear analysis after total hip arthroplasty. J Bone Joint Surg Am. 2003;85-A(6):1111–7.
20. Woolson ST, Murphy MG. Wear of the polyethylene of Harris-Galante acetabular components inserted without cement. J Bone Joint Surg Am. 1995;77(9):1311–4.
21. Devane PA, Horne JG, Martin K, Coldham G, Krause B. Three-dimensional polyethylene wear of a press-fit titanium prosthesis. Factors influencing generation of polyethylene debris. J Arthroplasty. 1997;12(3):256–66.
22. Dowd JE, Sychterz CJ, Young AM, Engh CA. Characterization of long-term femoral-head-penetration rates. Association with and prediction of osteolysis. J Bone Joint Surg Am. 2000;82-A(8):1102–7.
23. Amstutz HC, Campbell P, Kossovsky N, Clarke IC. Mechanism and clinical significance of wear debris-induced osteolysis. Clin Orthop Relat Res. 1992;276:7–18.
24. Johnson AJ, Loving L, Herrera L, Delanois RE, Wang A, Mont MA. Short-term wear evaluation of thin acetabular liners on 36-mm femoral heads. Clin Orthop Relat Res. 2013;472:624–9.

Part II

Basics and Current Trends on Tribology of Total Knee Arthroplasty

Simulator Testing of Total Knee Replacements

4

Christian Kaddick

4.1 Introduction

The human knee joint is a highly complex system making both the implantation and testing of total knee replacements (TKRs) a very demanding task. The first hydraulic knee simulator was introduced in 1977 [1] followed closely by an ingenious gear-driven mechanical system [2]. Despite the development of TKRs throughout this period, it took another 20 years until the first multi-station wear simulator became available [3]. It is this development that can be regarded as the trigger for standardization and commercialization of TKR wear testing. Unfortunately, there remains an ongoing debate about how best to conduct wear testing of new devices. As a result, there exist two different ISO standards for carrying out wear testing: ISO 14243-1 describes a force-controlled test method, whereas ISO 14243-3 describes a displacement-controlled test method. While both methods accord that the flexion-extension motion of the joint needs to be displacement controlled, the philosophy of anterior-posterior and torsional loads is different: Part 1 of the standard understands anterior-posterior motion of the knee joint as a result of the anterior-posterior load applied, whereas Part 3 describes a predefined anterior-posterior displacement that needs to be generated by the simulator. The same difference between test methods applies to the simulation of torsional motion. Direct comparison to clinical data has revealed an accurate reproduction of the in vivo motions when using the force-controlled test method [4, 5], whereas the displacement-controlled method has yielded certain limitations for constrained implant designs (i.e., tibial post or high conforming designs). However, it is important to note that force-controlled test frames are more complex to design and operate.

C. Kaddick, PhD
EndoLab GmbH, Rosenheim, Germany
e-mail: christian.kaddick@endolab.org

K. Knahr (ed.), *Tribology in Total Hip and Knee Arthroplasty*,
DOI 10.1007/978-3-642-45266-6_4, © EFORT 2014

The attractive option of the force-controlled method is the simulation of soft tissue constraints. As with any patient, the test frame requires sufficient ligament stiffness to avoid instability of the knee joint. An extensive discussion about the "correct" ligament stiffness has led to a revision of ISO 14243-1 in 2009. The test standard now defines much weaker soft tissue and also includes a small zone where no ligament forces are acting at all. As a result, both the anterior-posterior and torsional displacement increases when compared to the previous version of the test standard. This can be regarded as one step towards more realistic simulation of typical patient behavior. An excellent, in depth discussion of the aforementioned topics can be found in [6].

4.2 Benefits of Current Improvements in Standardized TKR Wear Testing

At the time of writing, our database (EndoLab®) hosts a total of 195 knee wear test series representing over 600 tested specimens. Approximately 30 % of those specimens were tested according to the most recent test standard (ISO 14243-1:2009) simulating a reduced ligament stiffness.

When comparing the test results of one design of a fixed-bearing type implant, the wear rate increased approximately 67 % from 20.21 mg per million cycles (StdDev 2.37) measured according to the old standard to 33.91 mg per million cycles (StdDev 1.95) measured to the new standard. As shown in Fig. 4.1, the complete group of fixed-bearing type implants tested did not show a statistically significant difference. However, it is assumed that this behavior is mainly related to improvement of the wear rates seen in the last decade. That is, the general trend indicating increased wear rates associated with testing according to ISO 14243-1:2009 (i.e., less rigid ligament structures) is somewhat diminished due to the improved wear characteristics of next-generation TKR designs and materials.

The most profound difference in wear rates was found for posterior-stabilized (PS) fixed-bearing knees. A median wear rate of 5.60 mg per million cycles was found for the old (high ligament stiffness) test standard, whereas 11.26 mg per million cycles were measured for the new standard. This statistically significant difference (student t-test, $p=0.020$) is macroscopically related to the contact of the tibial post (see Fig. 4.1) which was not present for most tests performed according to the old test standard.

4.3 Benefits of Upcoming Improvements to Standardized TKR Wear Testing

The apparent discrepancy between wear features seen in retrievals (i.e., delamination) and the adhesive/abrasive wear seen in simulator studies requires further improvements of the existing test standards. One approach, currently adopted by the ASTM expert group, is simulation of daily living activities such as stair assent/decent, sit to stand, stand to sit, squatting, and kneeling. These heavy-duty activities require further development of test equipment which is typically limited to level walking cycles.

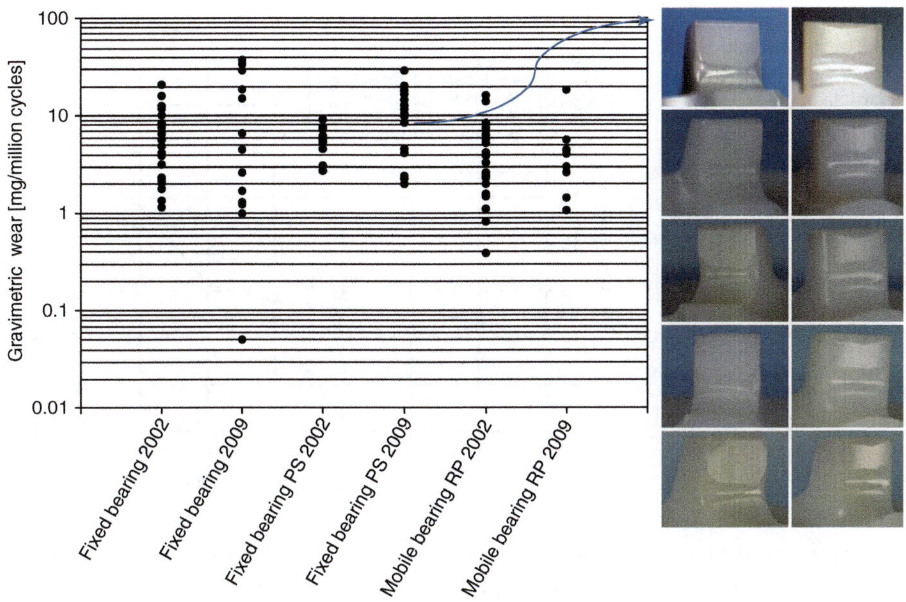

Fig. 4.1 Direct comparison of wear rates measured for ISO 14243-1:2002 and ISO 14243-1:2009 (*left*) and macroscopic appearance of the tibial posts after testing according to ISO 14243-1:2009 (*right*)

In parallel, material degradation by oxidation effects are still in the focus of ongoing research [7]. Up to now, there is no established method that allows for real-time aging of components.

It is also of great importance to note that whereas knee implants tested under laboratory conditions are isolated from contaminants, third-body particles may be generated in vivo by bone cement (PMMA) or interlocking metal-metal interfaces. As shown in Fig. 4.2, the addition of PMMA particles increases wear rates significantly. As such, including oxidation effects and third-body contaminants in future test standards may more closely reflect physiological conditions, thereby simulating actual in vivo performance of TKRs.

Generally speaking, the trend of future test standards is to consider in vivo worst-case scenarios rather than level walking of a light-weight patient wearing a perfectly implanted TKR under absolutely clean conditions [8, 9].

4.4 Summary and Conclusion

Standardized wear testing has become a successful tool in the development of total knee replacements. However, the increase in number of implantations, including more active patients, has expanded the subpopulation deviating from the standardized loading conditions. Heavy-duty daily living activities, nonideal implantation, third-body contamination, low soft tissue constraint, and other factors are known to

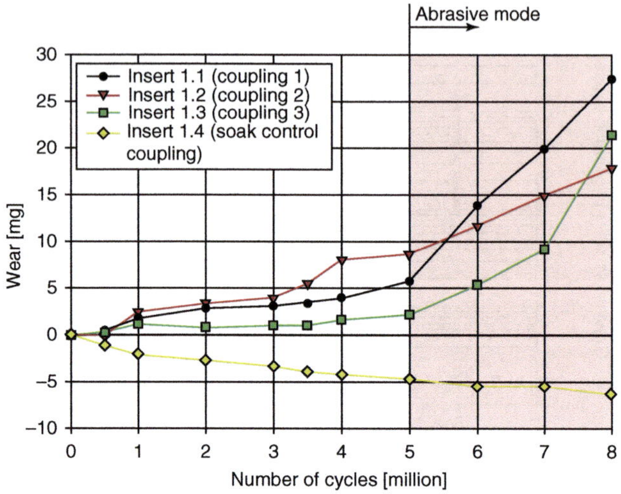

Fig. 4.2 Increased wear due to contamination of the test fluid with PMMA particles

trigger discrepancies between in vitro and in vivo wear of TKRs. Fortunately, recent research results and continuing improvements in simulator design are offering enhanced test methods for the next generation of high-endurance devices.

References

1. Dowson D, Jobbins B, ÓKelly J, Wright V. Chapter 7. A knee joint simulator. In: Evaluation of artificial hip joints. Biological Engineering Society: London; 1977. p. 79–90.
2. Stallforth H, Ungethuem M. Entwicklung eines Kniegelenksimulators. Arch Orthop Unfall-Chir. 1977;90:343–53.
3. Walker PS, Blunn GW, Broome DR, Perry J, Watkins A, Sathasivam S, Dewar ME, Paul JP. A knee simulating machine for performance evaluation of total knee replacements. J Biomech. 1997;30:83–9.
4. DesJardins JD, Banks SA, Benson LC, Pace T, LaBerge M. A direct comparison of patient and force-controlled simulator total knee replacement kinematics. J Biomech. 2007;40:3458–66.
5. Ngai V, Schwenke T, Wimmer MA. In-vivo kinematics of knee prostheses patients during level walking compared with the ISO force-controlled simulator standard. Proc Inst Mech Eng H. 2009;223:889–96.
6. Haider H. Tribological assessment of UHMWPE in the knee. In: Kurtz S, editor. UHMWPE biomaterials handbook. Amsterdam: Elsevier; 2009.
7. Oral E, Ghali BW, Neils A, Muratoglu OK. A new mechanism of oxidation in ultrahigh molecular weight polyethylene caused by squalene absorption. J Biomed Mater Res. 2012;100B: 742–51.
8. Papoola O, Yao JQ, Johnson TS, Blanchard CR. Wear, delamination, and fatigue resistance of melt-annealed highly crosslinked UHMWPE cruciate-retaining knee inserts under activities of daily living. J Orthop Res. 2010;28(9):1120–6.
9. Schwiesau J, Schilling C, Kaddick C, Utzschneider S, Jansson V, Fritz B, Blömer W, Grupp TM. Definition and evaluation of testing scenarios for knee wear simulation under conditions of highly demanding daily activities. Med Eng Phys. 2013;35:591–600.

5 Total Knee Replacement with Ceramic Components: Evaluation, Material Characteristics and Clinical Performance

Philipp Bergschmidt, Rainer Bader, Daniel Kluess, Carmen Zietz, and Wolfram Mittelmeier

5.1 Introduction

Total knee replacement (TKR) has developed to a safe and reliable procedure in orthopaedic surgery [1–3]. However, wear particles are able to trigger the well-known cascade of osteolysis inducing aseptic implant loosening. Furthermore, hypersensitivity to allergens such as chromium, cobalt and nickel may lead to implant failure. These facts cause a rising interest in research for alternative implant materials in TKR [3, 4].

The use of ceramics in total hip replacement is based on excellent tribology and corrosion resistance based on a high level of oxidation. Therefore, alumina was the first ceramic material being applied in total hip replacement (THR) (1970) [5] and in partial knee replacement (1972) [6].

However, ceramics in total joint replacement may also provide disadvantages. The brittleness and lower tensile strength of ceramics compared to ductile metal components results in a lower fracture toughness. Kircher et al. [7] published a series of ceramic cup and head fractures in THR underlining these risks. Moreover, metallic components can provide roughened surfaces, whereas ceramic femoral components exhibit smooth surfaces in general. Early implant loosening was often connected to the ceramic-bone interface and the insufficient osseous integration of smooth ceramic materials [8]. Therefore, fixation of ceramic components without cement is not recommended so far [9]. Nevertheless, in reports of cemented ceramic cups, a spontaneous debonding of the acetabular cups from the bone cement has been observed [8, 10].

P. Bergschmidt, Dr. med (✉) • R. Bader • D. Kluess • C. Zietz • W. Mittelmeier
Department of Orthopaedics, University Medicine Rostock,
Doberaner Strasse 142, Rostock 18057, Germany
e-mail: philipp.bergschmidt@med.uni-rostock.de

K. Knahr (ed.), *Tribology in Total Hip and Knee Arthroplasty*,
DOI 10.1007/978-3-642-45266-6_5, © EFORT 2014

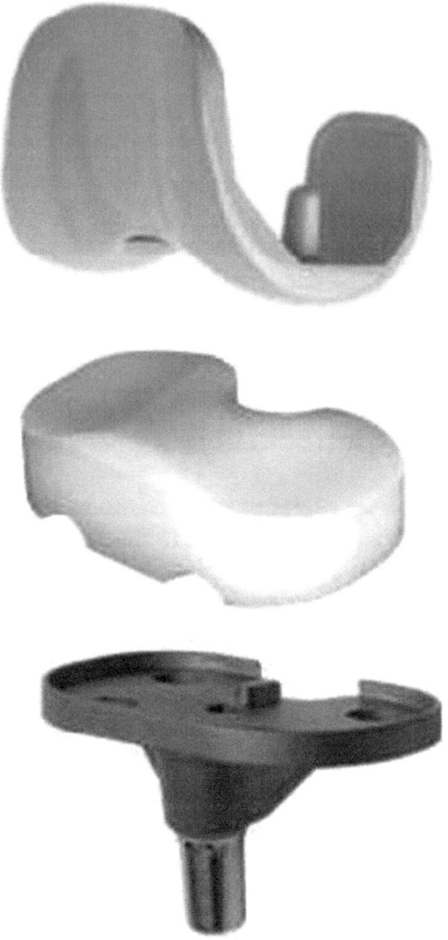

Fig. 5.1 Multigen Plus Knee with BIOLOX®delta ceramic femoral component

Since the first clinical use of ceramics, the material properties, manufacturing methods and implant design have been improved, and the fracture risk is reduced to a lower probability. Hence, the development of a TKR system with a monobloc composite ceramic femoral component made of BIOLOX®delta (CeramTec AG, Plochingen, Germany) was encouraged (Fig. 5.1). However, ahead of clinical implementation, a series of preclinical testings under standard and worst-case conditions was claimed in order to provide a high level of implant safety.

5.1.1 Ceramic Materials in TKR

Oxide ceramics used for total joint replacement can be divided into alumina (Al_2O_3), zirconia (ZrO_2) and composite ceramics and provide different mechanical properties. The first ceramic TKR system (KOM-1, Kyocera, Kyoto, Japan) was based on cementless fixed alumina femoral components combined with ultra-high molecular weight polyethylene (UHMWPE) [11]. Femoral components of zirconia have also been used for TKA (Bi-surface, Kyocera, Kyoto, Japan) [12]. Whereas alumina has the longest history of clinical application in orthopaedic surgery, zirconia was established in total joint arthroplasty in the 1985 [13].

Alumina consists of a polycrystalline monophasic structure and is characterized by chemical inertness and corrosion resistance as well as stability against aging. Its high hardness provides a surface resistance against damages and wear but also a lower flexural strength and fracture toughness compared to other ceramics, e.g. zirconia and composite ceramics. Zirconia consists of a polycrystalline tetragonal and monoclinic structure, which leads to the risk of phase transformation during aging but can be stabilized with yttrium (yttrium-stabilized zirconia). However, a specific series of zirconia femoral heads for THR were recalled [13] and limited results [14] reduced the confidence in the ceramic material.

Because of these disadvantages, composite ceramics are favoured. Composite ceramics used in orthopaedics are zirconia-toughened alumina (Al_2O_3 with approx. 25 % ZrO_2), alumina-toughened zirconia (ZrO_2 stabilized with Y_2O_3 with approx. 20 % Al_2O_3) and alumina matrix composite (AMC) which is based on the zirconia-toughened alumina composition with the additives strontium aluminate and chromium oxide. The combination reduces phase transformation of zirconia, improves hardness of alumina and provides an additional crack stopper by interposed strontium aluminate in the alumina matrix [15].

The new TKR system used in our experimental and numerical investigations consists of an alumina composite ceramic (AMC) femoral component (BIOLOX®delta) and is based on the same design as the metallic femoral component of the Multigen Plus Knee system (Lima Corporate, San Daniele, Italy) (Fig. 5.1).

5.1.2 Numerical and Experimental Analyses of Mechanical and Wear Behaviour of the Composite Ceramic Femoral Component

We developed several finite-element models to analyse different standard and worst-case conditions like in situ loading, intraoperative impaction behaviour and the influence of distal femur preparation. The finite-element-analysis (FEA) of the in situ situation considering different cement layer thicknesses, slightly tilted implant position and in conditions like stumbling showed up to 12.6 times higher stress in the ceramic femoral component in comparison to normal gait (Fig. 5.2). However, maximum calculated stresses did not reach the critical stress limit for BIOLOX®delta ceramic [16].

A dynamic FEA of intraoperative impaction determined stresses in the ceramic femoral component while the implant was hit using a hammer and an impactor. Comparison of ceramic and cobalt-chromium components showed higher stresses in the ceramic material, but values were beneath the critical values for implant failure [17]. However, intraoperative observations showed a high press-fit of the cemented femoral component, which can be due to inadequate preparation of the distal femur involving the anterior and

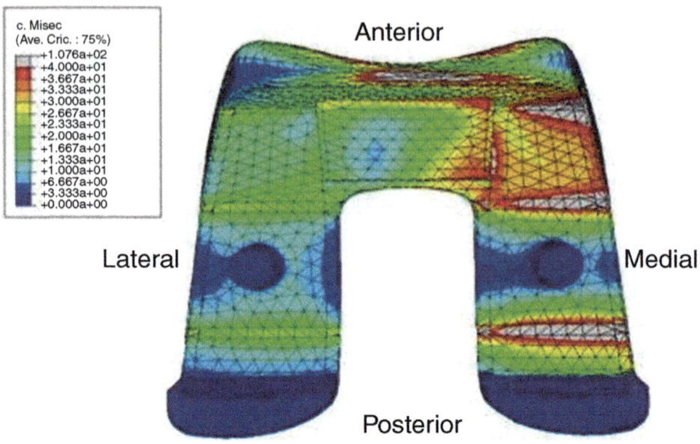

Fig. 5.2 Finite-element-analysis of the ceramic femoral component considering a tilted implant position. High stresses at the medial side of the component were seen. However, maximum stresses did not reach the critical stress limit for BIOLOX®delta ceramic

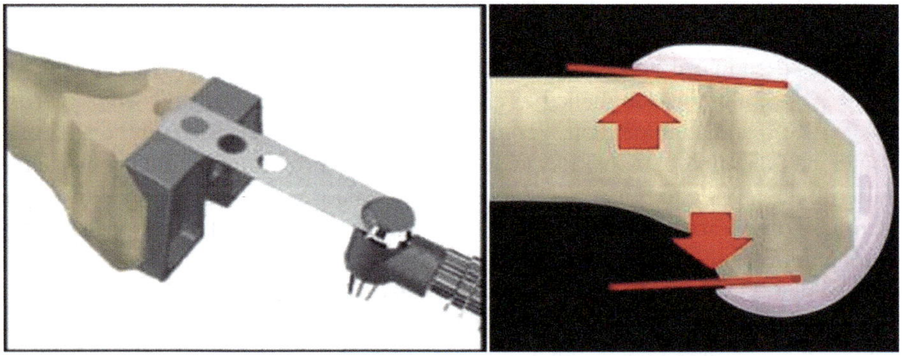

Fig. 5.3 Inadequate preparation of the bone stock with a total deflection of only 4° in the anterior and posterior cut caused by deflection of the sawblade results in a high wedge load (*red arrows*) that reaches critical stress limits of the BIOLOX®delta ceramic

posterior resection. This might lead to bending of the femoral component, the so-called wedge load, amplifying the load caused by impaction. In order to prove this hypothesis, an additional finite-element-analysis was performed to clarify the influence of the distal femur resection angle [18]. In this context, inadequate preparation occurs from deflection of the sawblades from the guided direction of the guiding block, especially in cases with sclerotic bone (Fig. 5.3). Preliminary results showed that the ceramic femoral component may be sensitive to an insufficient prepared distal femur since bending causes high stresses. Critical stresses for the ceramic material were determined in cases with total deflection of only 4° in the anterior and posterior cut. Furthermore, an anterior deflection showed a higher influence than a posterior deflection. In particular, the anterior resection is more prone for sawblade deflection due to the tangential cutting direction through the hard anterior cortical bone. Therefore, preparation of the distal femur should be carried out very carefully, at best using an additional resection template for an accurate anterior and posterior resection. Furthermore, the usage of a silicone damper can lead to a significant decrease in stress peaks [9, 17, 18].

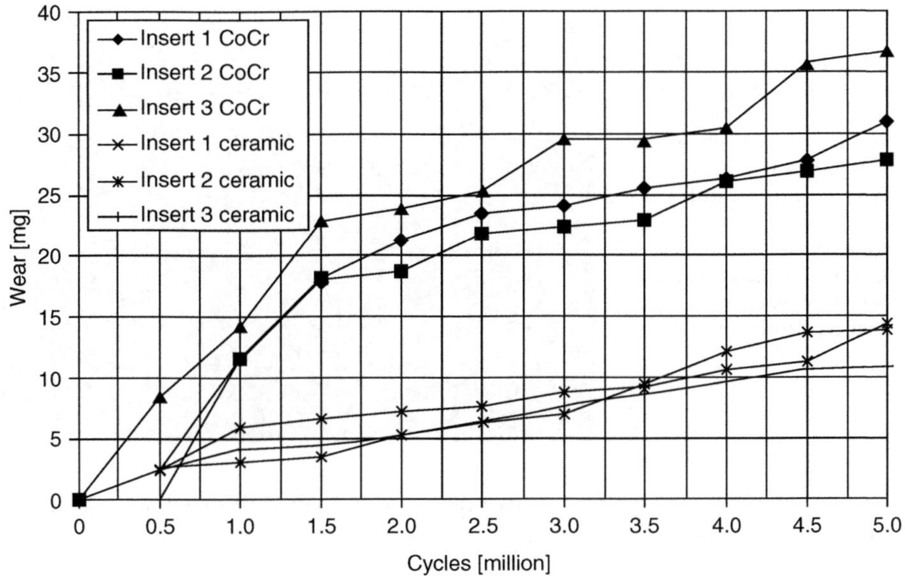

Fig. 5.4 Gravimetrical wear at the UHMWPE tibial inserts of the Multigen Plus Knee made of BIOLOX®delta ceramic and CoCrMo over five million cycles with the presence of third-body particles (bone cement). Gravimetrical wear of polyethylene inserts in combination with ceramic femoral components is in average four to five times lower than with metallic components

Several experimental and clinical studies showed reduced abrasive wear of ceramic-on-polyethylene bearings in TKR in comparison to metal-on-polyethylene bearings due to the low friction of ceramic surfaces [19–22]. During the surgical procedure, bone cement particles can be generated and may be left inside the knee joint. Those particles may be able to serve as third-body wear particles in between the articulating surfaces. The importance of third-body wear is increased by the fact that 42 % of the debris left in situ after primary cemented TKR were found to be bone cement particles, which are able to damage the surfaces of the implants accelerating the wear process [23]. Fracture of the cement mantle, relative movements between bone and cement or implant and cement and aging of the cement can further lead to increased release of bone cement particles.

To determine the effect of third-body particles, a comparative wear testing study using standard UHMWPE inserts and femoral components of identical design but different materials (ceramic vs. cobalt-chromium) was performed in a multi-station knee simulator (EndoLab GmbH) under standard ISO 14243 conditions including additional application of bone cement particles to the test chambers. The results showed a significantly higher gravimetrical wear at the tibial inserts in combination with metallic femoral components in comparison to tibial inserts in combination with ceramic femoral components under third-body wear conditions (Fig. 5.4) [24]. Gravimetrical wear of polyethylene inserts in combination with ceramic femoral

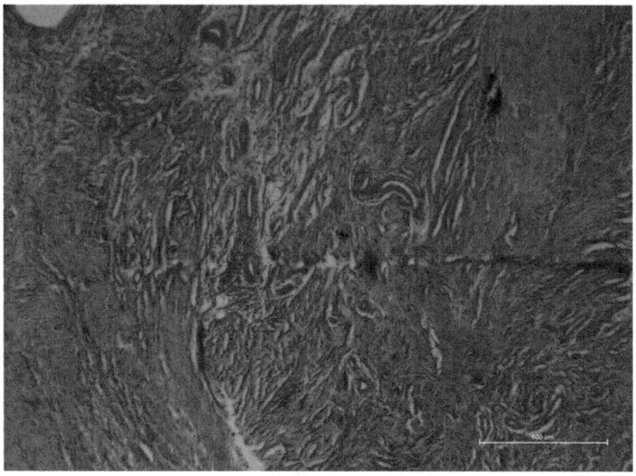

Fig. 5.5 Biopsy histology of the adhesion tissue at proximal recess taken during arthroscopy 4 weeks after primary metallic TKA showing a lymphoplasmacellular fibrous tissue (SLIM Type I) consistent with a type IV allergic reaction, haematoxylin eosine (Courtesy of the Department of Pathology, University Medicine Rostock)

components is in average four to five times lower than with metallic components and under third-body wear condition as low as for metallic components without third-body particles [19–22, 24, 25].

5.2 Implant Allergy

The biological effect of wear particles depends on the material, the quantity of wear, the surface structure of the particles and their size [3]. Metal ions, which are released into the tissue, can lead to periprosthetic tissue reactions with the development of granuloma [26]. In addition, in cases of specific sensitization to metallic debris and ions, hypersensitivity reactions may occur. The effect of metallic wear particles on metal-on-metal articulations has been observed in total hip replacement (THR) with the presence of pseudotumor-like periprosthetic tissue reactions. These have been histologically described as an aseptic lymphocyte-dominated vasculitis-associated lesion (ALVAL) or 'lymphocyte-dominated immunological answer' (LYDIA) [26, 27]. In accordance to the consensus classification by Krenn [28], the histological tissue pattern is defined as lymphoplasmacellular fibrous infiltration in a type I or IV SLIM (synovial-like interface membrane) with the presence of wear debris. However, the histological tissue pattern cannot show clear differences between primary toxic and immunologic reaction on the wear debris (Fig. 5.5).

Cobalt, chromium and nickel have the highest potential to trigger hypersensitivity reactions. The rate of contact allergy of the skin among the general population is on average 13.1 % for nickel, 3 % for cobalt and 1 % for chromium [29]. In this context, a different reaction of the skin and the periprosthetic tissue has to be considered, and a positive allergometry on metal ions does not consequently lead to reactions in the joint [30]. Therefore, allergometry and other tests like the lymphocyte transformation test (LTT) can provide additional information, but the clear diagnosis of an implant allergy reaction can only be set in combination of dermatology testing devices, histological tissue pattern, clinical examination and anamnesis [31].

On apparent allergy against metallic implant components, different alternative solutions to standard endoprostheses next to ceramics should be taken into account for primary implantation or revision of total knee replacement, e.g. the use of non-allergic metallic implants, such as ZrNb alloys, or potential allergy-inducing metallic materials after masking the implant surface using a suitable coating, e.g. Ti(Nb) N-coated implants [32].

Titanium is not suitable for the articulating surface in total knee replacement due to its wear characteristics. Surface modifications, e.g. by TiN, show superior results in comparison to standard metallic implants regarding wear in knee simulator studies [32], but own clinical data presented slightly lower clinical outcome score values with the use of coated implants in TKR [33]. Furthermore, in clinical observations, partial failures of such thin surface modifications at femoral heads were seen, especially under the presence of third-body particles [34].

Therefore, ceramics may be a promising solution as alternative material in case of metal allergy. A case of revision of a total knee replacement with a metal femoral component using a ceramic implant due to metal hypersensitivity showed a satisfactory outcome in 12-months follow-up [35].

5.3 Clinical Results of Composite Ceramic Implants in TKR

First clinical implantation of the BIOLOX®delta femoral component of the Multigen Plus Knee was realized in our hospital in 2006. A prospective international multicentre study was started to evaluate the clinical and radiological outcomes ($n = 110$) [9]. In addition, a prospective comparative study with the ceramic and metallic Multigen Plus Knee as well as another standard metallic implant was initiated in our clinic [36].

Complications related to the ceramic material were not seen so far. Radiological results were unremarkable (Fig. 5.6). Preliminary functional outcome measurement with the use of three evaluation scores (HSS-, WOMAC- and SF-36-score) showed significant improvements from preoperative to the postoperative evaluations for the ceramic implant. HSS score amounted 85.7 ± 11.7 points and range of motion was $112.6° \pm 15.0°$ after 24 months of evaluation in the multicentre study. Studies with metallic implants have reported a mean postoperative HSS score between 85.0 and 93.0 points [37, 38]. Earlier evaluations with ceramic knee components have exhibited HSS score values of 86 points and a range of motion between 113° and 124° at a follow-up period between one and 10 years [39–41].

The ceramic implant was comparable with other TKR systems. This was also proven by comparable functional and radiological outcomes of the standard metallic implants in the comparative study. Clinical experience underlines the fact that precise intraoperative preparation of the bone stock and use of an additional resection template for an extended anterior and posterior resection are required to avoid stress concentration by reducing wedge loading during impaction.

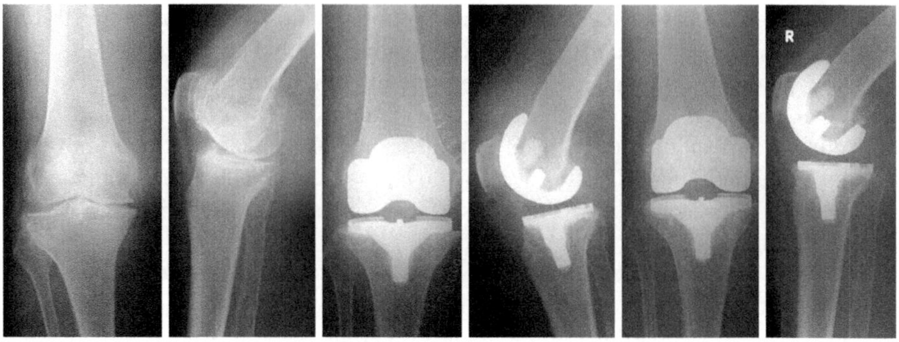

Fig. 5.6 X-rays of a study patient preoperative, 5 days and 24 months after the implantation of a Multigen Plus Knee with BIOLOX®delta ceramic femoral component

5.4 Future Applications

At this point, preliminary clinical results indicate a successful implementation of the Multigen Plus Knee with BIOLOX®delta ceramic femoral component. The clinical and radiological results are encouraging for a long-term survival of the composite ceramic femoral component. Therefore, ceramic implants could be a promising solution not only for patients with allergies against metallic implant materials but also for the 'normal' osteoarthritic patients. Long-term clinical follow-up is necessary to draw conclusions regarding the superiority of the ceramic knee implants concerning wear, especially under third-body wear conditions, and long-term survivorship.

Regarding the brittleness of the ceramic material, an extensive preclinical testing of new ceramic implants is necessary. Those tests must involve next to standard ISO test methods worst-case situations as described in order to provide a high implant safety.

In total joint replacement, the focus is increasing on hypersensitivity reactions to implant materials. In this context, the objective is to find valid methods for diagnosing an implant allergy as well as optimum solutions in the case of sensitization to specific implant materials [30, 31].

At this point, fixation of ceramic components is recommended with cement [8, 9]. Furthermore, own investigations showed that BIOLOX®delta ceramic has improved characteristics in third-body wear [24]. This may be an advantage in septic TKR loosening treated by two-stage revisions using temporary cement spacers with zirconia particle ingredients. Hence, remaining in situ ceramic particles bear the risk of increasing wear on the metal and polyethylene surfaces.

Concerning an 'all-ceramic knee', the tibial tray requires components with sufficient mechanical stability in case of bone loss and malpositioning. Future efforts should be focused on finding solutions for a cement-free fixation of ceramic knee implants for patients with hypersensitivity to bone cement components and a revision system with ceramic femoral components.

References

1. Bergschmidt P, Bader R, Finze S, Ansorge S, Kundt G, Mittelmeier W. Bicondylar knee arthroplasty – influence of preoperative functional restriction on early functional postoperative outcome. Z Orthop Unfall. 2008;146:344–51.
2. Bader R, Mittelmeier W, Steinhauser E. Failure analysis of total knee replacement. Basics and methodological aspects of the damage analysis. Orthopade. 2006;35:896–903.
3. Kircher J, Bergschmidt P, Bader R, Kluess D, Besser-Mahuzir E, Leder A, Mittelmeier W. The importance of wear couples for younger endoprosthesis patients. Orthopade. 2007;36: 337–46.
4. Thomas P. Allergologische Aspekte der Bioverträglichkeit von Titanbasisimplantaten. Biomaterialien. 2001;2:35–44.
5. Boutin P. Total arthroplasty of the hip by fritted aluminum prosthesis. Experimental study and 1st clinical applications. Rev Chir Orthop Reparatrice Appar Mot. 1972;58:229–46.
6. Langer G. Ceramic tibial plateau of the 70s ceramics for total knee replacement: status and options. In: Garino JP, Willmann G, editors. Bioceramics in joint arthroplasty. New York/ Stuttgart: Thieme; 2002.
7. Kircher J, Bader R, Schroeder B, Mittelmeier W. Extremely high fracture rate of a modular acetabular component with a sandwich polyethylene ceramic insertion for THA: a preliminary report. Arch Orthop Trauma Surg. 2009;129(9):1145–50.
8. Hannouche D, Hamadouche M, Nizard R, Bizot P, Meunier A, Sedel L. Ceramics in total hip replacement. Clin Orthop Relat Res. 2005;430:62–71.
9. Bergschmidt P, Bader R, Ganzer D, Hauzeur C, Lohmann CH, Rüther W, Tigani D, Rani N, Lopez Prats F, Zorzi C, Madonna V, Rigotti S, Benazzo F, Rossi SMP, Kundt G, Bloch HR, Mittelmeier W. Ceramic femoral components in total knee arthroplasty – two year follow-up results of an International Prospective Multi-Centre Study. Open Orthop J. 2012;6:176–82.
10. Hamadouche M, Boutin P, Daussange J, Bolander ME, Sedel L. Alumina-on-alumina total hip arthroplasty: a minimum 18.5-year follow-up study. J Bone Joint Surg Am. 2002;84-A:69–77.
11. Heimke G, Leyen S, Willmann G. Knee arthroplasty: recently developed ceramics offer new solutions. Biomaterials. 2002;23(7):1539–51.
12. Nakamura T, Akagi M, Yasuda T, Nakagawa Y, Shimizu M. A new knee prosthesis with bisurface femoral component made of zirconia-ceramic. Key Eng Mater. 2002;218–220:563–6.
13. U.S. Food and Drug Administration, MedWatch Safety Alerts for Human Medical Products. St. Gobain Desmarquest Zirconia Ceramic Femoral Head. 2001. http://www.fda.gov/Safety/MedWatch/SafetyInformation/SafetyAlertsforHumanMedicalProducts/ucm172706.htm. Accessed 29 June 2011.
14. Hernigou P, Bahrami T. Zirconia and alumina ceramics in comparison with stainless-steel heads. J Bone Joint Surg Br. 2003;85(4):504–9.
15. Piconi C, Maccauro G, Muratori F, Brach Del Prever E. Alumina and zirconia ceramics in joint replacements. J Appl Biomater Biomech. 2003;1(1):19–32.
16. Schultze C, Kluess D, Martin H, Hingst V, Mittelmeier W, Schmitz KP, Bader R. Finite element analysis of a cemented ceramic femoral component for the real assembly situation in total knee arthroplasty. Biomed Tech. 2007;52:301–7.
17. Kluess D, Mittelmeier W, Bader R. Intraoperative impaction of total knee replacements: an explicit finite-element-analysis of principal stresses in ceramic vs. cobalt-chromium femoral components. Clin Biomech (Bristol, Avon). 2010;25:1018–24.
18. Kluess D, Bergschmidt P, Mueller I, Mittelmeier W, Bader R. Influence of the distal femoral resection angle on the principal stresses in ceramic total knee components. Knee. 2012;19(6):846–50.
19. Bal BS, Garino J, Ries M, Oonishi H. Ceramic bearings in total knee arthroplasty. J Knee Surg. 2007;20:261–70.
20. Oonishi H, Kim SC, Kyomoto M, Masuda S, Asano T, Clarke IC. Change in UHMWPE properties of retrieved ceramic total knee prosthesis in clinical use for 23 years. J Biomed Mater Res B Appl Biomater. 2005;74:754–9.

21. Oonishi H, Ueno M, Kim SC, Oonishi H, Iwamoto M, Kyomoto M. Ceramic versus cobalt-chrome femoral components; wear of polyethylene insert in total knee prosthesis. J Arthroplasty. 2009;24:374–82.
22. Minoda Y, Kobayashi A, Iwaki H, Iwakiri K, Inori F, Sugama R, Ikebuchi M, Kadoya Y, Takaoka K. In vivo analysis of polyethylene wear particles after total knee arthroplasty: the influence of improved materials and designs. J Bone Joint Surg Am. 2009;91 Suppl 6:67–73.
23. DeBaets T, Waelput W, Bellemans J. Analysis of third body particles generated during total knee arthroplasty: is metal debris an issue? Knee. 2008;15:95–7.
24. Zietz C, Bergschmidt P, Lange R, Mittelmeier W, Bader R. Third-body abrasive wear of tibial polyethylene inserts combined with metallic and ceramic femoral components in a knee simulator study. Int J Artif Organs. 2013;36(1):47–55.
25. Affatato S, Cristofolini L, Leardini W, Erani P, Zavalloni M, Tigani D, Viceconti M. A new method of in vitro wear assessment of the UHMWPE tibial insert in total knee replacement. Artif Organs. 2008;32:942–8.
26. Willert HG. Reactions of the articular capsule to wear products of artificial joint prostheses. J Biomed Mater Res. 1977;11(2):157–64.
27. Willert HG, Buchhorn GH, Fayyazi A, Flury R, Windler M, Köster G, Lohmann CH. Metal-on-metal bearings and hypersensitivity in patients with artificial hip joints. A clinical and histomorphological study. J Bone Joint Surg Am. 2005;87(1):28–36.
28. Krenn V, Poremba C, Schneider J, Kendoff D, Gehrke T, Kretzer JP, Thomsen M, Huber M. Histopathologische Differenzialdiagnostik bei gelenkimplantatallergischen Fragestellungen. Orthopade. 2013;42:614–21.
29. Eben R, Walk R, Summer B, et al. Implant allergy register – a first report. Orthopade. 2009;38:557–62.
30. Thomsen M, Rozak M, Thomas P. Verwendung von Allergieimplantaten in Deutschland-Ergebnisse einer Umfrage. Orthopade. 2013;42:597–601.
31. Thomas P, Summer B, Krenn V, Thomsen M. Allergiediagnostik bei Verdacht auf Metallimplantatunverträglichkeit. Orthopade. 2013;42:602–6.
32. Bader R, Bergschmidt P, Fritsche A, Ansorge S, Thomas P, Mittelmeier W. Alternative Werkstoffe und Lösungen in der Knieendoprothetik für Patienten mit Metallallergie. Orthopade. 2008;37:136–42.
33. Bergschmidt P, Bader R, Finze S, Schulze C, Kundt G, Mittelmeier W. Comparative study of clinical and radiological outcomes of unconstrained bicondylar total knee endoprostheses with anti-allergic coating. Open Orthop J. 2011;5:354–60.
34. Raimondi MT, Pietrabissa R. The in-vivo wear performance of prosthetic femoral heads with titanium nitride coating. Biomaterials. 2000;21:907–13.
35. Bergschmidt P, Bader R, Mittelmeier W. Metal hypersensitivity in total knee arthroplasty: revision surgery using a ceramic femoral component – a case report. Knee. 2012;19(2):144–7.
36. Bergschmidt P, Bader R, Kluess D, Zietz C, Schwemmer S, Kundt G, Mittelmeier W. Total knee replacement system with a ceramic femoral component versus two traditional metallic designs: a prospective short-term study. J Orthop Surg. 2013;21(3):294–9.
37. Ersozlu S, Akkaya T, Ozgur AF, Sahin O, Senturk I, Tandogan R. Bilateral staged total knee arthroplasty in obese patients. Arch Orthop Trauma Surg. 2008;128(2):143–8.
38. Bin SI, Nam TS. Early results of high-flex total knee arthroplasty: comparison study at 1 year after surgery. Knee Surg Sports Traumatol Arthrosc. 2007;15:350–5.
39. Kim YH, Sohn KS, Kim JS. Range of motion of standard and high-flexion posterior stabilized total knee prostheses. A prospective, randomized study. J Bone Joint Surg Am. 2005;87:1470–5.
40. Yasuda K. Long-term clinical results of cruciate-retaining total knee arthroplasty using the alumina ceramic condylar prosthesis [abstract]. Scientific Exhibit No. SE035, AAOS Meeting, San Francisco; 2004.
41. Akagi M, Nakamura T, Matsusue Y, Ueo T, Nishijyo K, Ohnishi E. The bisurface total knee replacement: a unique design for flexion: four-to-nine-year follow-up study. J Bone Joint Surg Am. 2000;82:1626–33.

In Vivo Wear of Highly Crosslinked Polyethylene in Total Knee Arthroplasty

6

Pedro Hinarejos Gomez and Ignasi Pinol Jurado

6.1 The Polyethylene Problem: The Wear

The main causes for knee arthroplasty revision later than 5 years in the study by Sharkey et al. [42] were polyethylene wear and aseptic loosening. Polyethylene wear has become a concern in total knee arthroplasty (TKA), because it has been stated as the main cause for osteolysis [1]. The presence of polyethylene particles in the joint, which are phagocytised by macrophages and giant cells [2], causes the release of many proinflammatory interleukins, which activate the osteoclasts, the main responsible cells for osteolysis [4, 22, 24].

In order to decrease the number of polyethylene particles, many strategies have been developed in the last decades:

- Improvements in alignment instruments, and navigation, because misalignment is one of the causes that has been related to increased polyethylene wear [44]
- Improvements in the femoral surfaces, as the use of oxidised zirconium [17, 45]
- Improvements in the sterilisation techniques of polyethylene [5]
- Improvements in the polyethylene by adding antioxidant agents as vitamin E [38]
- Improvements in the polyethylene by increasing the crosslinking

6.2 Polyethylene Evolution

The manufacturers have developed some evolutive changes from the historical polyethylene, which was used more than three decades ago, to the contemporary polyethylene. More recently, two generations of highly crosslinked polyethylene (HXLPE) have been developed.

P.H. Gomez (✉) • I.P. Jurado
Orthopedic Surgery Department, Parc de Salut Mar, Universitat Autonoma Barcelona, Barcelona, Spain
e-mail: 92292@parcdesalutmar.cat; 98390@parcdesalutmar.cat

K. Knahr (ed.), *Tribology in Total Hip and Knee Arthroplasty*,
DOI 10.1007/978-3-642-45266-6_6, © EFORT 2014

6.2.1 Historical Polyethylene

The so-called historical polyethylene was sterilised with gamma radiation in air, and many free radicals were produced during this process. That polyethylene had less resistance against wear. Moreover, the ageing of that polyethylene began after manufacturing, and a phenomenon called shelf or storage oxidation was developed [3]. Obviously, the "historical polyethylene" suffered a severe delamination process.

6.2.2 Contemporary Polyethylene

The next step in the polyethylene evolution was the so-called contemporary polyethylene that was sterilised with gamma radiation but without oxygen, in inert conditions: in nitrogen, in argon or in vacuum [3]. Other systems for sterilisation were also used (ethylene oxide or gas plasma). This contemporary polyethylene has no shelf oxidation, and the delamination is less frequent and severe than with the historical one.

6.2.3 First Generation of Highly Crosslinked Polyethylene (HXLPE)

Some decades ago, Grobbelaar et al. described that the use of higher doses of gamma radiation to the polyethylene causes the remotion of hydrogen atoms, shortening the length of the chain of polyethylene, and covalent unions between different chains, the so-called crosslinking phenomenon, which causes a decrease in the wear rate [14]. In this process of crosslinking, however, many free radicals are originated causing an increase in the oxidation. It seems that there is no additional benefit in the wear rate with radiation doses greater than 15 Mrads [33].

The use of the first generation of HXLPE, as well as avoiding the shelf storing oxidation, improves the wear resistance because of the changes in the mechanical properties. On the other hand, increasing the dose of gamma radiation significantly reduces the resistance against fractures.

HXLPE has been widely used in hip arthroplasty for more than 10 years, and it has been proved in vivo that it shows less wear than the conventional polyethylene, analysing both linear and volumetric wear rates [6, 27, 32, 37]. Moreover, a reduction in the incidence of osteolysis in vivo has been demonstrated in hip arthroplasty [31].

In knee arthroplasty, however, the use of the first generation of HXLPE caused some concerns, because it was related to the possibility of tibial post fracture in the posterior-stabilised knees, caused by the reduction in the resistance against fractures [43].

6.2.4 Second Generation of HXLPE

Trying to better balance the three aspects for a better polyethylene (a wear reduction, with a better oxidative resistance, but with improvements in the fracture resistance), a second generation of crosslinked polyethylene has been developed.

In this new generation of HXLPE, radiation doses higher than 100 cGy have been avoided, and new techniques in the manufacturing process have been introduced as the adding of vitamin E to reduce the presence of free radicals [38] or the sequential irradiation used in the X3 polyethylene by Stryker [47].

The evidence for the use of HXLPE in knee arthroplasty, however, is mainly based upon in vitro studies using knee simulators [36, 43, 46–48].

6.3 HXLPE Performance "In Vitro" in TKA

Several studies have compared the polyethylene wear in a knee simulator between a TKA with a conventional poly and a HXLPE: Tsukamoto et al. [45] found a five- to eight-fold reduction in wear with HXLPE after a 5.5 million cycle test. Wang et al. [47] found a wear reduction greater than 60 % with the HXLPE X3 by Stryker®, both in cruciate retaining and cruciate substituting TKA. Popoola et al. [40] found a wear reduction of 72–85 % with a HXLPE NexGen® (Zimmer, Warsaw, Ind, USA).

6.4 HXLPE Performance "In Vivo" in TKA

6.4.1 Studies of Wear in Retrieved Implants

In a study with revised total hip arthroplasties, the retrieved inserts with HXLPE evidenced similar wear than those inserts with conventional one [41].

In a recent study, MacDonald et al. [30] found that retrieved remelted HXLPE inserts exhibited lower oxidation indices compared to conventional inserts, but this should be proved in the longer follow-up period.

6.4.2 Studies of Polyethylene Particles in the Synovial Fluid In Vivo

As it was demonstrated by Kim et al. [26], the performance in vivo of a TKA between theoretical better surfaces does not necessarily cause an improvement in the polyethylene wear. They found no advantages when using an oxidised zirconium (OxZr) femoral component over a conventional cobalt-chrome (CoCr) one in the characteristics of the polyethylene particles in the synovial fluid in the 6–8 years follow-up period.

We only know two studies that have evaluated the polyethylene wear in vivo in TKA with HXLPE [18, 23].

Iwakiri et al. [23], in a study with a very small number of patients analysed, found a reduction in the polyethylene number of particles if a HXLPE was used.

Nevertheless, they only compared three cases in one group and four cases in the other one, and the study was retrospective.

Hinarejos et al. [18] reported the results of a randomised trial in 34 patients using the same implant and comparing a conventional contemporary polyethylene with a

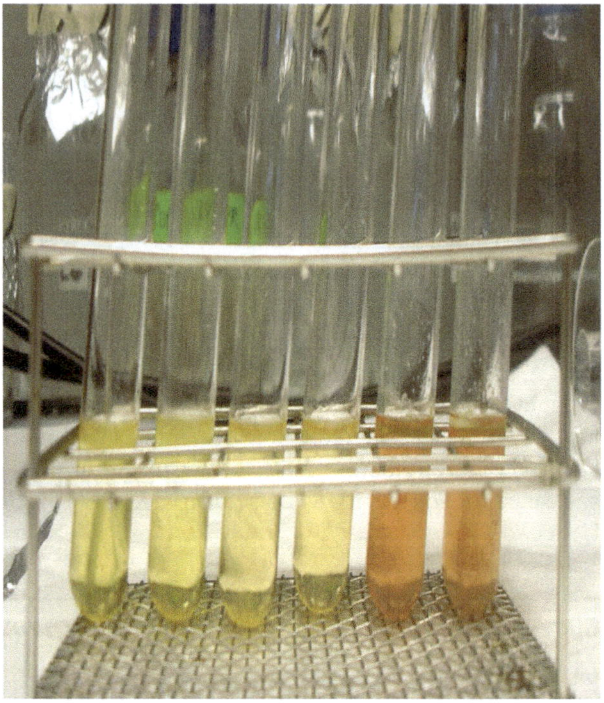

Fig. 6.1 Three millilitre of synovial fluid of each sample was processed according to the technique described by Minoda et al. [35]

HXLPE treated with three cycles of sequential irradiation and annealing process. They analysed the polyethylene particles in the synovial fluid 1 year after surgery following the technique described by Minoda et al. [35] (Fig. 6.1), and with the scanning electron microscope analysis (Figs. 6.2 and 6.3), they could not find significant differences in the concentration of polyethylene or in the total number of particles between both groups with different types of polyethylene (Figs. 6.4, 6.5, 6.6 and 6.7). Moreover, the size and the shape of polyethylene particles were similar in both groups. The only factor that they found to correlate with the concentration of polyethylene particles in the synovial fluid was the size of the prosthetic components. In this study, Hinarejos et al. have found a high variability in the concentration of polyethylene particles in the synovial fluid, much greater than the variability found with the knee simulator studies. This high variability suggests that in vivo there are many factors that can influence in the polyethylene wear as the activity of the patients [39], their weight, the alignment of the arthroplasty, the tension and balance of the ligaments, the size of the components, the design geometry of the implant [8] and probably many others. Probably, the type of polyethylene is not the most significant factor in the polyethylene wear in vivo.

The adverse biological reactions that cause osteolysis are not only dependent on the concentration but also on the size of the polyethylene particles [9], because particles >10 μm have fewer inflammatory effects because they cannot be phagocytised [13, 16]. The first generation of HXLPE generated smaller particles, which had

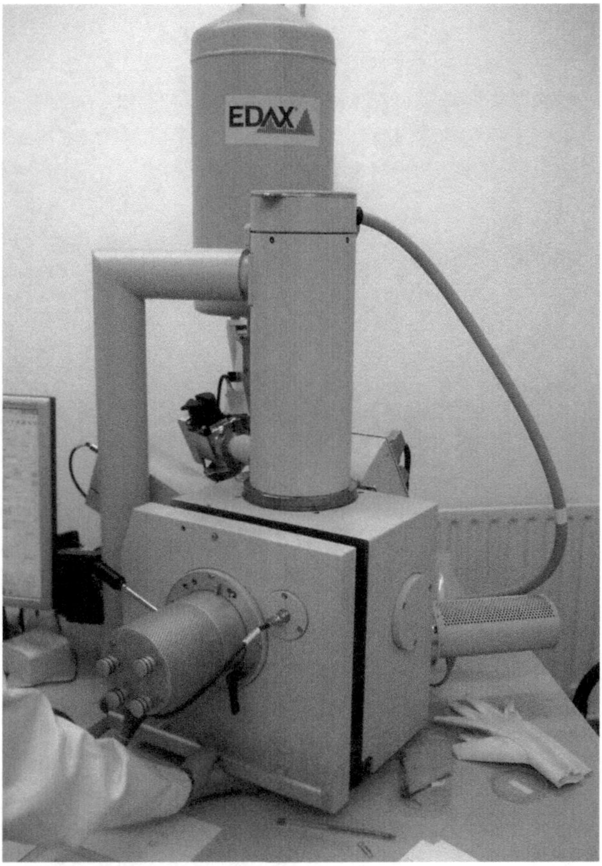

Fig. 6.2 Scanning electron microscopy Quanta 200

been previously related with more osteolysis [20], but more recent studies with newer HXLPE have not found differences in the size of the particles [7, 10, 11, 18].

It has also been stated that elongated particles are more proinflammatory than round ones [16], but no significant differences in the shape of the polyethylene particles with the use of HXLPE have been found [18].

Poly wear in vivo using HXLPE with longer follow-up should be studied, because the wear of different types of polyethylene could be different as the polyethylene ages, as it has been reported in some in vitro studies [15, 29, 34, 43].

6.4.3 Studies of Implant Survival

Gioe et al. [12] analysed in a register study a group of "premium" implants, which include HXLPE, and they could not find an increase in the survival rate up to 7 years with these implants, even when they are causing an increasing cost in the implant.

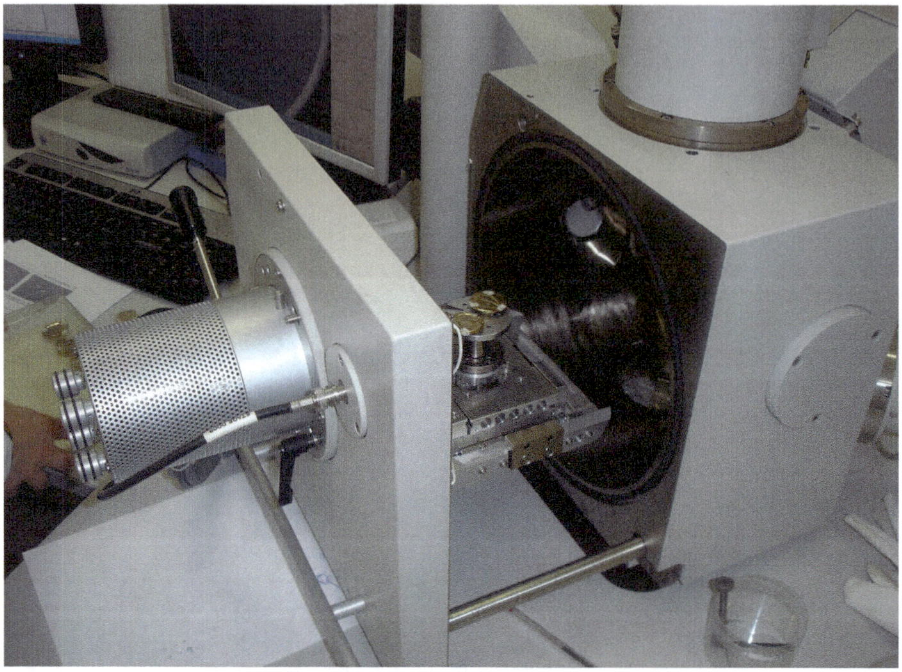

Fig. 6.3 The filter after synovial fluid processing was coated with a 40 nm gold layer and analysed in the scanning electron microscopy

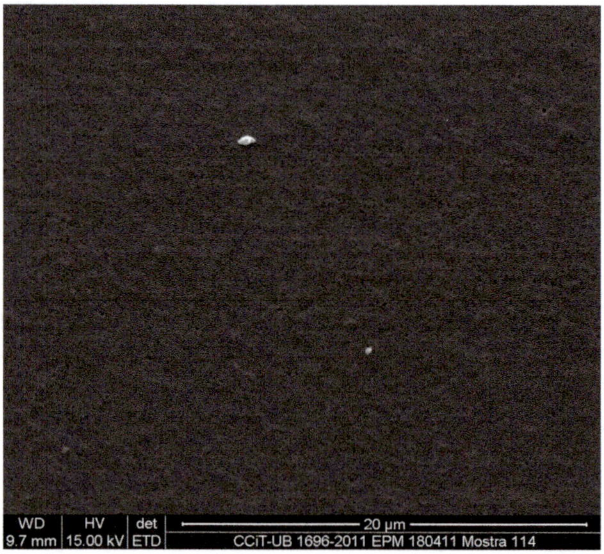

Fig. 6.4 Scanning electron microscopy of a sample of conventional polyethylene: some round polyethylene particles <1 μm are shown

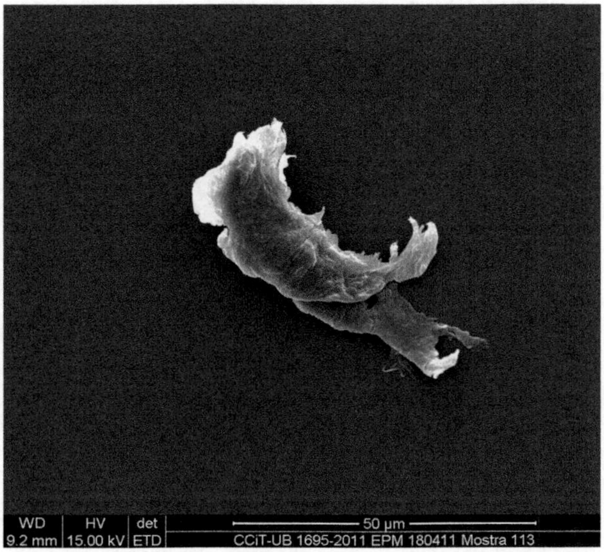

Fig. 6.5 Scanning electron microscopy of a sample of conventional polyethylene shows a big sheet of polyethylene

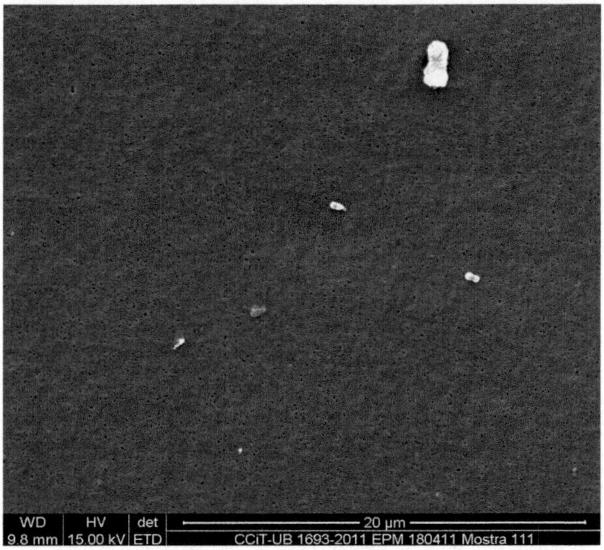

Fig. 6.6 Scanning electron microscopy of a sample of crosslinked polyethylene shows polyethylene particles of different sizes and shapes

In the same way, in another register study, Inacio et al. [21] found a similar survival rate of the 62.177 analysed implants using a contemporary polyethylene or a HXLPE up to 5 years.

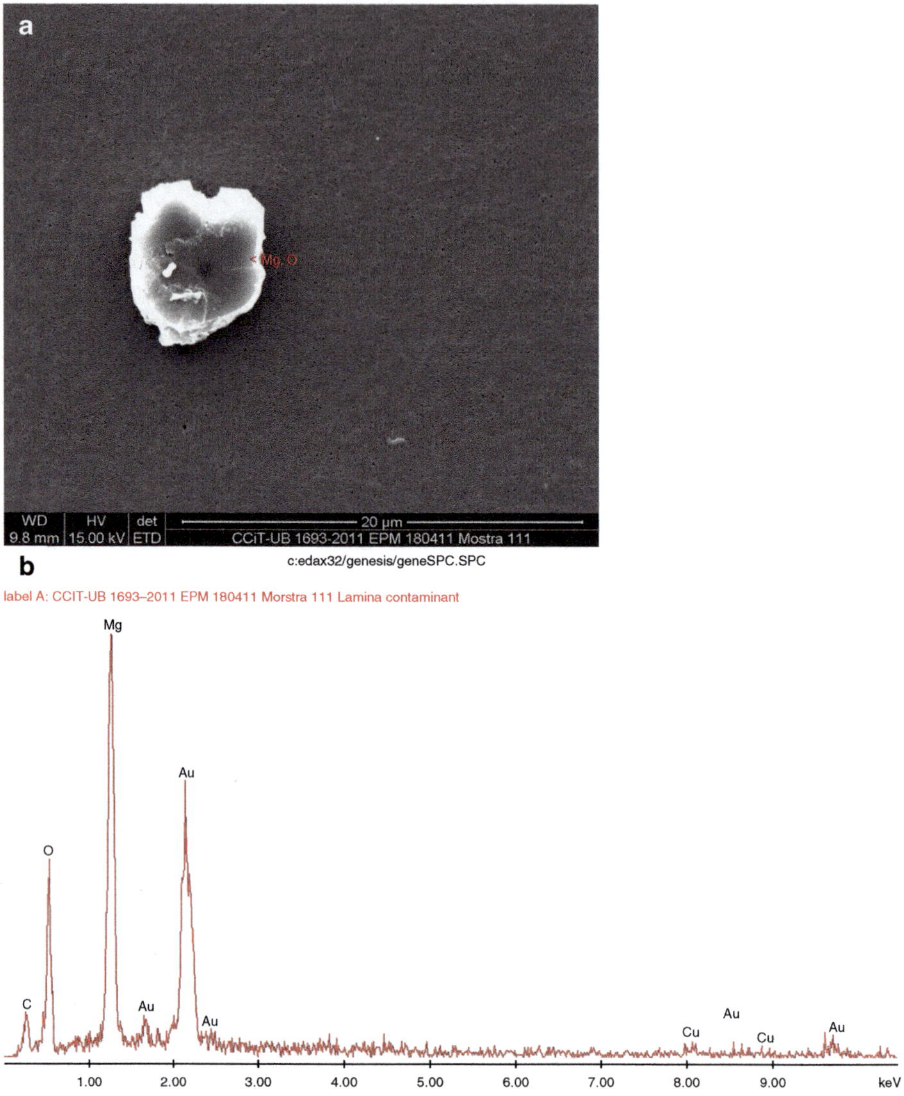

Fig. 6.7 (**a**, **b**) Scanning electron microscopy of a contaminant particle composition is confirmed by spectrophotometry analysis

Conclusions

In a review article, Lachievickz and Geyer [28] balanced pros and cons of HXLPE in the knee, and they think that the advantages have not been fully proved, so they recommend a cautious use of crosslinked polyethylene in the knee until the advantages have been clearly demonstrated.

Moreover, the use of HXLPE in TKA has been associated with some complications related to a reduced fracture strength [19], such as fractures of the posterior-stabilised tibial post [25] or the patellar pegs, so more research is needed to prove the theoretical advantages of HXLPE and some cost-benefit studies should be done before its widespread use in TKA can be advised.

References

1. Atkins GJ, Haynes DR, Howie DW, Findlay DM. Role of polyethylene particles in periprosthetic osteolysis: a review. World J Orthop. 2011;2:93–101.
2. Baxter RM, Freeman TA, Kurtz SM, Steinbeck MJ. Do tissues from THA revision of highly crosslinked UHMWPE liners contain wear debris and associated inflammation? Clin Orthop Relat Res. 2011;469:2308–17.
3. Berry DJ, Currier BH, Mayor MB, Collier JP. Gamma-irradiation sterilization in an inert environment: a partial solution. Clin Orthop Relat Res. 2012;470:1805–13.
4. Chiba J, Rubash HE. A biochemical, histologic, and immunohistologic analysis of membranes obtained from failed cemented and cementless total knee arthroplasty. Clin Orthop Relat Res. 1994;309:278.
5. Crowninshield RD, Muratoglu OK. How have new sterilization techniques and new forms of polyethylene influenced wear in total joint replacement). J Am Acad Orthop Surg. 2008;16 Suppl 1:S80–5.
6. Dorr LD, Wan Z, Shahrdar C, Sirianni L, Boutary M, Yun A. Clinical performance of a Durasul highly cross-linked polyethylene acetabular liner for total hip arthroplasty at five years. J Bone Joint Surg Am. 2005;87:1816–21.
7. Dumbleton JH, D'Antonio JA, Manley MT, Capello WN, Wang A. The basis for a second-generation highly cross-linked UHMWPE. Clin Orthop Relat Res. 2006;453:265–71.
8. Essner A, Herrera L, Hughes P, Kester M. The influence of material and design on total knee replacement wear. J Knee Surg. 2011;24:9–17.
9. Fisher J, Bell J, Barbour PS, Tipper JL, Matthews JB, Besong AA, et al. A novel method for the prediction of functional biological activity of polyethylene wear debris. Proc Inst Mech Eng H. 2001;215:127–32.
10. Galvin AL, Jennings LM, Tipper JL, Ingham E, Fisher J. Wear and creep of highly crosslinked polyethylene against cobalt chrome and ceramic femoral heads. Proc Inst Mech Eng H. 2010;224:1175–83.
11. Galvin AL, Tipper JL, Jennings LM, Stone MH, Jin ZM, Ingham E, et al. Wear and biological activity of highly crosslinked polyethylene in the hip under low serum protein concentrations. Proc Inst Mech Eng H. 2007;221:1–10.
12. Gioe TJ, Sharma A, Tatman P, Mehle S. Do "premium" joint implants add value?: analysis of high cost joint implants in a community registry. Clin Orthop Relat Res. 2011;469:48–54.
13. Green TR, Fisher J, Stone M, Wroblewski BM, Ingham E. Polyethylene particles of a 'critical size' are necessary for the induction of cytokines by macrophages in vitro. Biomaterials. 1998;19:2297–302.
14. Grobbelaar CJ, du Plessis TA, Marais F. The radiation improvement of polyethylene prostheses. A preliminary study. J Bone Joint Surg Br. 1978;60-B:370–4.
15. Haider H, Weisenburger JN, Kurtz SM, Rimnac CM, Freedman J, Schroeder DW, et al. Does vitamin E-stabilized ultrahigh-molecular-weight polyethylene address concerns of cross-linked polyethylene in total knee arthroplasty? J Arthroplasty. 2012;27:461–9.
16. Hallab NJ, Jacobs JJ. Biologic effects of implant debris. Bull NYU Hosp Jt Dis. 2009;67:182–8.
17. Heyse TJ, Chen DX, Kelly N, Boettner F, Wright TM, Haas SB. Matched-pair total knee arthroplasty retrieval analysis: oxidized zirconium vs CoCrMo. Knee. 2011;18:448–52.

18. Hinarejos P, Piñol I, Torres A, Prats E, Gil-Gomez G, Puig-Verdie L. Highly crosslinked polyethylene does not reduce the wear in total knee arthroplasty: in vivo study of particles in synovial fluid. J Arthroplasty. 2013;28:1333–7.
19. Huot JC, Van Citters DW, Currier JH, Collier JP. The effect of radiation dose on the tensile and impact toughness of highly cross-linked and remelted ultrahigh-molecular weight polyethylenes. J Biomed Mater Res B Appl Biomater. 2011;97:327–33.
20. Illgen 2nd RL, Forsythe TM, Pike JW, Laurent MP, Blanchard CR. Highly crosslinked vs conventional polyethylene particles–an in vitro comparison of biologic activities. J Arthroplasty. 2008;23:721–31.
21. Inacio MC, Cafri G, Paxton EW, Kurtz SM, Namba RS. Alternative bearings in total knee arthroplasty: risk of early revision compared to traditional bearings: an analysis of 62,177 primary cases. Acta Orthop. 2013;84:145–52.
22. Ingham E, Fisher J. The role of macrophages in osteolysis of total joint replacement. Biomaterials. 2005;26:1271–86.
23. Iwakiri K, Minoda Y, Kobayashi A, Sugama R, Iwaki H, Inori F, et al. In vivo comparison of wear particles between highly crosslinked polyethylene and conventional polyethylene in the same design of total knee arthroplasties. J Biomed Mater Res B Appl Biomater. 2009;91: 799–804.
24. Jacobs JJ, Roebuck KA, Archibeck M, Hallab NJ, Glant TT. Osteolysis: basic science. Clin Orthop Relat Res. 2001;393:71–7.
25. Jung KA, Lee SC, Hwang SH, Kim SM. Fractured of a second-generation highly cross-linked UHMWPE tibial post in a posterior-stabilized scorpio knee system. Orthopedics. 2008;31:1137.
26. Kim YH, Park JW, Kim JS. Comparison of the Genesis II total knee replacement with oxidised zirconium and cobalt-chromium femoral components in the same patients: a prospective, double-blind, randomised controlled study. J Bone Joint Surg Br. 2012;94:1221–7.
27. Kurtz SM, Gawel HA, Patel JD. History and systematic review of wear and osteolysis outcomes for first-generation highly crosslinked polyethylene. Clin Orthop Relat Res. 2011;469:2262–77.
28. Lachiewicz PF, Geyer MR. The use of highly cross-linked polyethylene in total knee arthroplasty. J Am Acad Orthop Surg. 2011;19:143–51.
29. MacDonald D, Sakona A, Ianuzzi A, Rimnac CM, Kurtz SM. Do first-generation highly crosslinked polyethylenes oxidize in vivo? Clin Orthop Relat Res. 2011;469:2278–85.
30. MacDonald DW, Higgs G, Parvizi J, Klein G, Hartzbrand M, Levine H, et al. Oxidative properties and surface damage mechanisms of remelted highly crosslinked polyethylenes in total knee arthroplasty. Int Orthop. 2013;37:611–5.
31. Mall NA, Nunley RM, Zhu JJ, Maloney WJ, Barrack RL, Clohisy JC. The incidence of acetabular osteolysis in young patients with conventional versus highly crosslinked polyethylene. Clin Orthop Relat Res. 2011;469:372–81.
32. Manning DW, Chiang PP, Martell JM, Galante JO, Harris WH. In vivo comparative wear study of traditional and highly cross-linked polyethylene in total hip arthroplasty. J Arthroplasty. 2005;20:880–6.
33. McKellop H, Shen FW, Lu B, Campbell P, Salovey R. Development of an extremely wear-resistant ultra high molecular weight polyethylene for total hip replacements. J Orthop Res. 1999;17:157–67.
34. Micheli BR, Wannomae KK, Lozynsky AJ, Christensen SD, Muratoglu OK. Knee simulator wear of vitamin E stabilized irradiated ultrahigh molecular weight polyethylene. J Arthroplasty. 2012;27:95–104.
35. Minoda Y, Kobayashi A, Iwaki H, Miyaguchi M, Kadoya Y, Ohashi H, et al. Polyethylene wear particles in synovial fluid after total knee arthroplasty. Clin Orthop Relat Res. 2003; 410:165–72.
36. Muratoglu OK, Bragdon CR, Jasty M, O'Connor DO, Von Knoch RS, Harris WH. Knee-simulator testing of conventional and cross-linked polyethylene tibial inserts. J Arthroplasty. 2004;19:887–97.

37. Mutimer J, Devane PA, Adams K, Horne JG. Highly crosslinked polyethylene reduces wear in total hip arthroplasty at 5 years. Clin Orthop Relat Res. 2010;468:3228–33.
38. Oral E, Muratoglu OK. Vitamin E diffused, highly crosslinked UHMWPE: a review. Int Orthop. 2011;35:215–23.
39. Naudie DD, Ammeen DJ, Engh GA, Rorabeck CH. Wear and osteolysis around total knee arthroplasty. J Am Acad Orthop Surg. 2007;15:53–64.
40. Popoola OO, Yao JQ, Johnson TS, Blanchard CR. Wear, delamination, and fatigue resistance of melt-annealed highly crosslinked UHMWPE cruciate-retaining knee inserts under activities of daily living. J Orthop Res. 2010;28:1120–6.
41. Schroder DT, Kelly NH, Wright TM, Parks ML. Retrieved highly crosslinked UHMWPE acetabular liners have similar wear damage as conventional UHMWPE. Clin Orthop Relat Res. 2011;469:387–94.
42. Sharkey PF, Hozack WJ, Rothman RH, Shastri S, Jacoby SM. Insall Award paper. Why are total knee arthroplasties failing today? Clin Orthop Relat Res. 2002;404:7–13.
43. Stoller AP, Johnson TS, Popoola OO, Humphrey SM, Blanchard CR. Highly crosslinked polyethylene in posterior-stabilized total knee arthroplasty: in vitro performance evaluation of wear, delamination, and tibial post durability. J Arthroplasty. 2011;26:483–91.
44. Thienpont E, Fennema P, Price A. Can technology improve alignment during knee arthroplasty. Knee. 2013;20 Suppl 1:S21–8.
45. Tsukamoto R, Chen S, Assano T, Ogino M, Shoji H, Nakamura T, Clarke IC. Improved wear performed with crosslinked UHMWPE and zirconia implants in knee simulation. Acta Orthop. 2006;77:505–11.
46. Utzschneider S, Harrasser N, Sadoghi P, Weber P, Schroder C, Pietschmann MF, et al. Crosslinked polyethylene in knee arthroplasty: a simulator study evaluating the positive influence on the tribocontact area in the fixed-bearing knee. Arch Orthop Trauma Surg. 2010; 130:1419–24.
47. Wang A, Yau SS, Essner A, Herrera L, Manley M, Dumbleton J. A highly crosslinked UHMWPE for CR and PS total knee arthroplasties. J Arthroplasty. 2008;23:559–66.
48. Williams PA, Brown CM, Tsukamoto R, Clarke IC. Polyethylene wear debris produced in a knee simulator model: effect of crosslinking and counterface material. J Biomed Mater Res B Appl Biomater. 2010;92:78–85.

Part III

The Hype of Ceramic – Will It Continue?

Ceramic Articulations: (Much) More Benefits than Concerns

7

Roberto Binazzi

Total hip arthroplasty (THA) probably is the orthopaedic surgical procedure most frequently performed in the world, and we can certainly affirm that it has improved dramatically the life quality of many people that in the past were condemned to the life of an invalid.

In recent years THA has made enormous progress in surgical technique, design and quality of materials. Nevertheless, there are still many issues that are under debate, as to the type and the level of fixation (cement or not cement? metaphyseal or meta-diaphyseal?), the size of the articular components (large or small heads?) and, more recently, the type of bearing (polyethylene or alternative bearings, i.e. metal-on-metal or ceramic-on-ceramic?).

The original metal-on-PE joint has functioned well for many years and is still the most frequently used type of articulation. However, the widening of indications to operate on more and more young people and the great increase of activity level in all patients have determined an increase of wear of the components, with many cases of aseptic loosening. This is particularly true in patients with anatomically small acetabula, when we are obliged to implant small cups (46–48 mm maximum) with PE liners of minimal thickness, just few millimetres.

In 2011 Kjærsgaard-Andersen presented a very interesting search about the bearings used in many countries. Norway, Sweden and Denmark were among the most "traditional" countries, with a rate of metal-on-PE ranging between 95 % (Denmark and Norway) and 98 % (Sweden). It was even more interesting to notice that the PE that was mostly used in these countries was not the more modern X-linked (4 % in Norway, 7 % in Sweden) but the "old" ultra-high-molecular-weight polyethylene (UHMWPE), 91 % in both these countries. Canada represented a step forward "alternative bearings", with 78 % of metal-on-PE, 11 % of Met-Met and 9 % of

R. Binazzi
Department of Orthopedics and Hip Surgery, Villa Erbosa Hospital, Bologna, Italy
e-mail: binazzi@gmail.com

K. Knahr (ed.), *Tribology in Total Hip and Knee Arthroplasty*,
DOI 10.1007/978-3-642-45266-6_7, © EFORT 2014

Cer-Cer. In this country there is also a clear preference for X-linked PE (59 %) against the old UHMWPE (19 %). Australia showed a 32 % of alternative bearings (20 % of Cer-Cer and 12 % Met-Met), Italy 39 % (29 % Cer-Cer and 10 % Met-Met) and the USA 43 % of alternative bearings, but mostly due to Met-Met of surface replacements (37 %), with 6 % of Cer-Cer.

***

All three bearings have given good clinical results and, as we have seen, are used widely all over the world.

However, for each of them, doubts and concerns have been raised, producing a substantial lack of certainty among the less experienced orthopaedic surgeons.

7.1 Metal-on-Metal

Starting from the 1990s, the so-called second-generation metal-on-metal has experienced a sort of second youth, especially with the wide diffusion of surface replacement. Early clinical results have been good, but recently some problems have started to raise doubts about the opportunity of using this type of articulation.

Some patients, in fact, showed an early, progressive, severe osteolysis, almost exclusively localised in the proximal femur and usually associated with high levels of circulating cobalt and chromium ions. This syndrome was called ALVAL (aseptic lymphocytic vasculitis-associated lesions). Patients necessitated an early revision, even in the absence of important clinical symptoms, in order to avoid a progressive, severe osteolysis.

Moreover, a number of patients showed a periarticular soft-tissue mass, progressively expanding, that was called "pseudotumour". These masses have been described in a rate of up to 39 % [1] and required surgical removal.

The chronic high level of circulating cobalt and chromium ions led many researchers to hypothesise also that, in some way, they could be responsible of a genotoxicity with development of tumours. This has never been demonstrated, but it cannot be ruled out with certainty.

In addition, all these issues have caught the attention of many lawyers with, as a result, a number of requests of compensation.

In conclusion, we can say that today metal-on-metal technology is progressively disappearing, even for the surface replacement. In fact, more and more surgeons are abandoning it for the fear of possible requests of compensation.

7.2 Metal/Ceramic-PE

As we have seen, a PE liner or an all-PE cup are the most frequently used ones in the world. There are many reasons for that, including the good performance in terms of wear of modern PE, the large availability and, last but not least, the reduced cost.

However, since it was introduced, PE has raised some concerns about its wear products, the debris, able to activate an immunological reaction, leading to osteolysis and loosening.

Thus, the research has been addressed to produce a type of PE that could show a long-lasting wear resistance and, at the same time, an excellent mechanical strength. Then, ultra-high-molecular-weight PE (UHMWPE) was introduced in the 1970s since in tribological experimental tests it had shown a superior wear performance compared to standard PE. UHMWPE has represented the most popular type of PE, implanted widely all over the world, in times when alternative bearings were not available, at least in large scale. However, some concerns were still existing regarding the mechanical properties of the new PE. This was particularly important in case of scratched or damaged metal heads, producing a severe increase of wear.

Thus in the 1990s, the notable improvement of alternative bearings and, at the same time, the appearance of several reports about the osteolysis induced by UHMWPE wear products convinced many researchers that it was necessary to improve the quality of UHMWPE, in particular wear resistance.

The solution was found by irradiating PE in order to produce the so-called cross-linking that is promoting bonds that link one polymer chain to another. The concept was excellent, and the result was an important reduction of wear compared to conventional PE.

Highly cross-linked and thermally treated polyethylene (XLPE) was then introduced at the end of the 1990s and was hailed as the definitive solution to reduce wear when compared to conventional polyethylene.

Early and midterm clinical results were clearly better and XLPE started to be adopted all over the world, although many surgeons continued to use UHMWPE. Wear of the plastic liner decreased from 0.1 to 0.03–0.05 mm/year with a metal-on-PE articulation and from 0.05 to 0.02 mm/year for a ceramic-on-PE articulation [2, 3]. The difference between a metallic and a ceramic head is important. Hendrich et al. [4] and Meftah et al. [5] both showed a significant reduction of wear rate for XLPE when using a ceramic head.

However, as it had happened for UHMWPE, XLPE raised important concerns when it, about 10 years after its clinical introduction, started showing some cases of delamination and rim fracture [6]. These liners were examined and presented evidence of measurable oxidation at the bearing surface. Again, we had to think of a process that could eliminate the decrease of mechanical strength consecutive to oxidation. Vitamin E is a well-known antioxidant compound, and it was thought that adding it to the XLPE would reduce oxidation to a minimum. Thus, the first liners were produced through a postirradiation "diffusion" process. It seemed the invention of the wheel and the companies rapidly declared that finally the perfect PE had been created. Unfortunately, nobody had thought that the "diffusion" of vitamin E inside XLPE was obtained with a thermal treatment.

Thus, it was necessary to introduce a modification in the production process of XLPE-vitamin E. Consequently, the powder of PE and vitamin E were mixed in a preliminary phase, before consolidation and irradiation, in order to eliminate the necessity of any thermal process. Obviously, again it has been said, the "perfect PE" has finally been created! However, this is not the only "problem" related to the use of this type of plastic liner. In fact, we know that the debris of XLPE is much more active as a starter of the immunological chain leading to osteolysis and loosening. We all remember what happened when Hylamer was advertised some years ago as the "eternal PE". As a result, all patients with this type of liners had to be revised at producer's expenses within a few years for severe osteolysis.

Finally, we have to think that most patients operated with THA all around the world require cups of minimal dimensions for ethnical (Chinese, Indian, Mediterranean and South American patients) or pathological reasons (for instance, dysplastic acetabula are always hypoplastic). In a small cup, ranging from 40 to 46–48 mm, the PE liner shows a thickness of few millimetres that, in a young and active subject, does not seem trustworthy.

7.3 Ceramic-on-Ceramic

Cer-Cer has shown by far the best performance in terms of wear. In fact, Bitsch et al. [2] and Olyslaegers et al. [3] have reported that the amount of wear of a Cer-Cer implant ranges between 0.002 and 0.005 mm/year against 0.02 mm/year of a ceramic-XLPE and 0.03–0.05 mm/year of a metal-on-XLPE.

Nevertheless, ceramic has raised some concerns too. The first question mark regards the ceramic alleged brittleness. There is a sort of legend about fractures in ceramic implants which determines a quite big fear and distrust among orthopaedic surgeons. However, the evidence coming from the literature is clearly showing that, on the contrary, ceramic articulations break in a negligible number of cases. D'Antonio in 2007, at the 35th Meeting of the Hip Society in San Diego, reported an analysis of an impressive series of 52,000 (!!) ceramic THA of a single company with a 0.008 % fracture rate of the liners and a 0.017 % head fracture. More recently, the RIPO (register of implants in Emilia-Romagna region, Italy), very precisely updated by Aldo Toni and co-workers at the Rizzoli Institute in Bologna, shows a series of about 14,000 delta ceramic-on-ceramic THA implanted between 2004 and 2012, with 0 (0 %) ball head fractures and 0.09 % liner fractures. It has to be said that the improvement of surgical technique, with correct placement and impaction of the ceramic liner, was very important in reducing the fracture rate. In this regard, the use of a new inserter that is still under clinical trial is very promising, and already showing excellent results in terms of exact insertion angle and perfect cleanliness and dryness of the ceramic outer taper.

Another concern about ceramic implants was due to the limited availability of sizes. Until 10 years ago, effectively, the smallest ceramic liner could be inserted into a cup as big as 52 mm, which means in a small percentage of cases. The introduction of Biolox delta ceramic allowed the use of a cup as small as 42 mm with a 28 mm head and 44 mm with a head of 32 mm.

Finally, we cannot omit what is probably the most important concern about ceramic-on-ceramic implants that is the emission of a large number of noises, the so-called squeaking. This is still a largely unexplained phenomenon; however we can list some clear points:

1. The emission of articulation noise is not exclusive of Cer-Cer bearings, but it is common in all mechanical devices and a THA is a mechanical device.
2. The prevalence of squeaking is widely variable, ranging between 0.2 % [7] and an incredible 20.9 % [8].
3. There is a large series of different explanations reported in the literature: wear debris from metallic components of the Cer-Cer implant [7, 9], disruption of the fluid film lubrication with stripe wear [10], edge loading due to acetabular component malpositioning [11], microseparation and subluxation of the femoral head [10], use of short necks [8] and metal contamination of the ball head [12]. The number and the variety of hypothesis probably mean that nobody is totally correct and squeaking is a multifactorial, quite limited phenomenon. In fact, most authors report a prevalence around 1.8–2 %.
4. Up to now, there is *no* evidence that squeaking has a clinical relevance or that it compromises the mechanical integrity and/or the clinical longevity of the implant. Chevillotte et al. [13] studied a series of 100 ceramic-on-ceramic THA at 10 years and concluded that squeaking is an isolated phenomenon without any clinical consequence. Walter WL (personal communication, 2013) has reported the incidence of revision THA for squeaking according to the Australian Register: in 55,417 Cer-Cer THA, it was 0.03 %.
5. Recent studies have reported that the noise can disappear with the time [14].

Conclusion

Three different bearings are today available on the market, metal/ceramic-PE, ceramic-on-ceramic and metal-on-metal. Considering the negligible wear rate and thus the possibility of being used even with minimal thickness, ceramic-on-ceramic is the gold standard for young, active and small patients (cup smaller than 50 mm, as in dysplastic patients). Ceramic showed also an excellent biocompatibility. Ceramic-on-XLPE can be used in patients older than 70 years or inside big cups (>52 mm). Metal-on-metal represents a big question mark, for the suspect of genotoxicity and for the legal problems that it is causing, and thus has been progressively abandoned.

References

1. Bosker BH, Ettema HB, Boomsma MF, Kollen BJ, Maas M, Verheyen CC. High incidence of pseudotumour formation after large-diameter metal-on-metal total hip replacement: a prospective cohort study. J Bone Joint Surg Br. 2012;94(6):755–61.
2. Bitsch RG, Loidolt T, Heisel C, Ball S, Schmalzried TP. Reduction of osteolysis with use of Marathon cross-linked polyethylene. A concise follow-up, at a minimum of five years, of a previous report. J Bone Joint Surg Am. 2008;90(7):1487–91.
3. Olyslaegers C, Defoort K, Simon JP, Vandenberghe L. Wear in conventional and highly cross-linked polyethylene cups: a 5-year follow-up study. J Arthroplasty. 2008;23(4):489–94.

4. Hendrich C, Wollmerstedt N, Ince A, Mahlmeister F, Gobel S, Noth U. Highly cross-linked ultra high molecular weight polyethylene acetabular liners in combination with 28mm Biolox heads. In: Bioceramics in alternative bearings in joint arthroplasty, 10th biolox symposium proceedings. Darmstadt: Steinkopff Verlag; 2006. p. 181–4.
5. Meftah M, Ebrahinpour PB, He C, Ranawat AS, Ranawat CS. Preliminary clinical and radiographic results of large ceramic heads on highly cross-linked polyethylene. Orthopedics. 2011;34(6):133.
6. Duffy GP, Wannomae KK, Rowell SL, Muratoglu OK. Fracture of a cross-linked polyethylene liner due to impingement. J Arthroplasty. 2009;24:158–9.
7. Murphy SB, Ecker TM, Tannast M. Two- to 9-year clinical results of alumina ceramic-on-ceramic THA. Clin Orthop Relat Res. 2006;453:97–102.
8. Keurentjes JC, Kuipers RM, Wever DJ, Schreurs BW. High incidence of squeaking in THAs with alumina ceramic-on-ceramic bearings. Clin Orthop Relat Res. 2008;466(6):1438–43.
9. Rodriguez JA. The squeaking hip is a multifactorial concern. Orthop Today. 2008;28(92).
10. Ranawat AS, Ranawat CS. The squeaking hip: a cause for concern-agrees. Orthopedics. 2007;30(9):738.
11. Walter WL, O'Toole GC, Walter WK, Ellis A, Zicat BA. Squeaking in ceramic-on-ceramic hips: the importance of acetabular component orientation. J Arthroplasty. 2007;22(4):496–503.
12. Chevillotte C, Trousdale RT, Chen Q, Guyen O, An KN. "Hip squeaking": a biomechanical study of ceramic-on-ceramic bearing surfaces. Clin Orthop Relat Res. 2010;468(2):345–50.
13. Chevillotte C, Pibarot V, Carret JP, Bejui-Hughes J, Guyen O. Hip squeaking: a 10-year follow-up. J Arthroplasty. 2012;27(6):1008–13.
14. Komistek R, et al. ISTA presentation. 2009.

Medium- to Long-Term Results of Ceramic-on-Ceramic Bearings in Total Hip Arthroplasty

8

Alexandra Pokorny-Olsen and Karl Knahr

8.1 History of Ceramic-on-Ceramic Bearings

The use of ceramics in total hip arthroplasty dates back to the 1970s. The wear and consequent osteolysis associated with polyethylene bearings leading to prosthetic failure resulted in the search for new bearing materials.

Boutin in France and Mittelmeier in Germany introduced this material to total hip arthroplasty [1, 2]. But initial results were discouraging. High rates of loosening of the components and ceramic fracture were encountered. This was caused by a combination of material, design and surgeon related factors. The first generation of ceramics featured low purity and density and large grain size distribution. Unfavourable designs like skirt or mushroom head attributed to failure. Mittelmeier tried to improve the design by using a threaded ceramic cup guaranteeing better primary stability. Although this modification reduced the fracture rate to some extent, fracture rates of up to 13.4 % were still reported [3]. Furthermore, the design still showed high failure rates for aseptic loosening due to missing bony ingrowth [4]. Monobloc designs associated with loosening were soon abandoned. With the advances in ceramic technology, the relatively brittle ceramic material of the first designs became more durable. Improvements in the production process and quality management like hot isostatic pressing and laser etching as well as proof testing of all components resulted in a significant increase in mechanical strength. The third generation of ceramics was introduced under the trade name BIOLOX®forte (CeramTec TM, Plochingen) (Fig. 8.1). According to its manufacturer it is the most widely used ceramic material for total hip arthroplasty in the world. It is produced from synthetic, fine-grained, high-purity alumina with minor amounts of sintering aids. The resulting higher-quality alumina featured decreases grain size, inclusions and grain boundaries and has a significantly greater burst strength than previous ceramics.

A. Pokorny-Olsen (✉) • K. Knahr
Orthopädisches Spital Wien-Speising GmbH, Speisinger Strasse 109, 1130 Vienna, Austria
e-mail: alexandra.pokorny-olsen@oss.at

K. Knahr (ed.), *Tribology in Total Hip and Knee Arthroplasty*,
DOI 10.1007/978-3-642-45266-6_8, © EFORT 2014

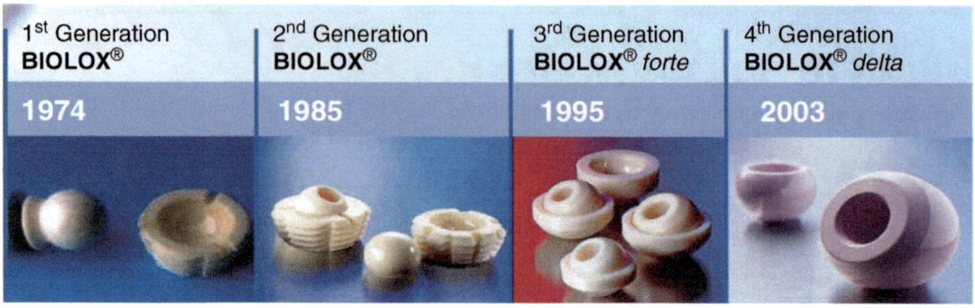

Fig. 8.1 History of ceramic bearings (*Source*: CeramTec TM)

Aiming at further improvement of tribological qualities and at reduction of the risk of ceramic fracture, the fourth generation of ceramics was created. This marked the introduction of new materials to the alumina. The BIOLOX®delta (CeramTec TM) is an alumina matrix composite ceramic consisting of approximately 82 vol% alumina (Al_2O_3), 17 vol% zirconia (ZrO_2) as well as 0.5 vol% chromium oxide and 0.3 vol% strontium. By adding these materials, crack energy is diffused and subsequently the risk of fracture is reduced. It also shows superior wear rates in simulator conditions. Recently, another type of ceramics, the alumina-toughened zirconia (ATZ®, Mathys TM), showed even lower in vivo wear rates under adverse conditions [5].

8.2 Tribological Properties

Ceramic bearings show superior tribological properties compared to other bearings. The most important is the significantly lowest wear rate and friction [6–8]. To date, the main reason for revision surgery in total hip arthroplasty remains aseptic loosening due to wear [9, 10]. Volumetric wear for alumina-on-alumina bearings has been reported to be 2,000–5,000 times less than for metal-on-polyethylene bearings. In in vitro testing, volumetric wear is highest during the run-in period and usually reaches 0.1–0.2 mm^3 per million cycles. During the steady-state phase, low values of less than 0.01 mm^3 per million cycles are measured [11]. However, results obtained in vivo have shown different results than the laboratory findings with sometimes extreme wear rates. To simulate in vivo use of bearings, adverse conditions like microseparation have been investigated in the laboratory. Under those extreme conditions, an increased wear rate of 1.24 mm^3 per million cycles was observed [12].

But newer generations of ceramics like BIOLOX®delta (CeramTec TM) or ZTA® (Mathys TM) show extremely low wear rates even under adverse conditions. These range around 0.13 mm^3 per million cycles. Alumina-toughened zirconia (ATZ®, Mathys TM) has a reported mean wear rate of 0.06 mm^3 per million cycles [5].

Contrary to polyethylene wear, ceramic wear particles are bioinert. They do not trigger immune reactions leading to osteolysis. Alumina particles undergo phagocytosis process by macrophages. Only in the presence of a large amount of wear particles, a foreign body reaction is found. Alumina ceramic is highly oxidized and therefore resistant to corrosion. For all those reasons, it has the highest biocompatibility of all bearing materials.

Furthermore, ceramic is a hydrophilic material featuring superior lubrication conditions due to the high wettability.

8.3 Ceramic Fracture (Figs. 8.2 and 8.3)

Ceramic is one of the hardest materials. On the downside though, this allows no way to deform without breakage. Therefore accurate positioning of the acetabular component is crucial. Other factors like impingement, contact of head and rim during repositioning as well as change of position of the liner after initial improper insertion have been identified as risk factors for failure [13]. With regard to the ceramic head, damage to or debris on the taper, mismatch between head and taper as well as manufacturing problems like autoclave and shock cooling have been identified as reasons for fracture [14, 15]. The introduction of zirconia-toughened alumina has significantly increased crack resistance. Literature review shows excellent results for newer generation ceramic bearings [16].

The longest documented analysis of 5,500 ceramic hip replacements reported only 13 cases of fracture over 25 years, including eight of the femoral head and five of the acetabular components [16].

Another long-term retrospective analysis of 109 hips by Petsatodis et al. over 20 years showed no revision due to fracture [17]. The same result was found in

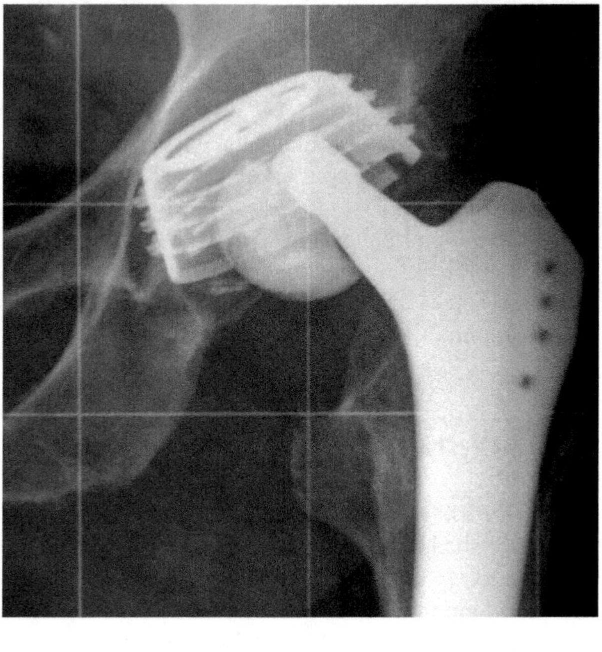

Fig. 8.2 Fracture of ceramic head

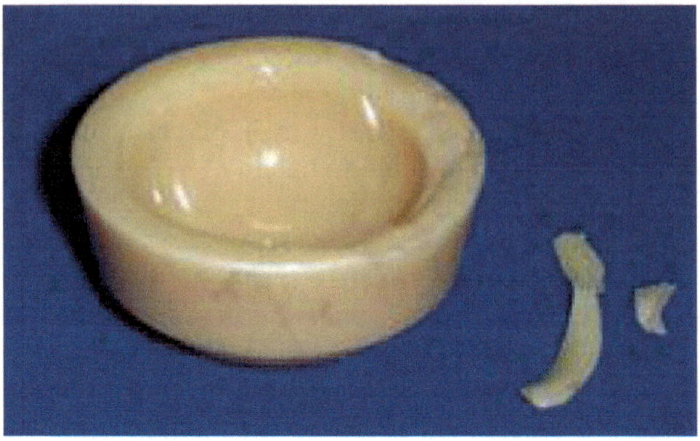

Fig. 8.3 Fracture of ceramic liner

Table 8.1 Overview of mid- to long-term results of ceramic bearings [18, 20, 23–29]

Author	Mean follow-up (years)	Number of hips	Survivorship % revision for any cause	Survivorship % revision bearing related
Park et al. [23]	9.6	112	95.3	98
Chevilotte et al. [24]	8.8	100	96	n.a.
Lewis et al. [25]	8.1	56	96	100
Lusty et al. [35]	6.5	301	96	99.4
Lee et al. [26]	10.9	88	99	99
Kress et al. [27]	10.5	75	97	100
Molloy et al. [28]	10	301	98	100
Sollarino et al. [29]	13	68	97	100
Kim et al. [20]	11.1	93	100	100
Petsatodis et al. [18]	20.8	109	84.4	n.a.

another long-term study by Toni et al. in a consecutive series of 147 patients [18]. No ceramic fracture was detected at 17-year follow-up. Similar findings were published by Kim et al. for young patients and dysplastic hips [19]. The largest study including 52,000 ceramic implants used since 2003 reported a fracture rate of 0.008 % for ceramic inserts and 0.017 % for femoral heads [20]. In a multicenter study by Murphy et al., 1,709 hips were evaluated and a fracture rate of 0.27 % for ceramic liners was found [21]. Therefore Hannouche et al. concluded that ceramic liner fracture caused by impact force during normal life is likely to occur in vivo [16]. Around the 10-year mark, ceramic bearings all show survivorships between 95 and 100 % (Table 8.1).

8.4 Hip Noise

Starting in 2006, reports on audible phenomena in association with ceramic bearings were published. Patients complained of episodes of squeaking, clicking, grating or grinding, often associated with a special positioning, e.g. deep flexion. The aetiology is still not fully investigated and thought to be multifactorial. Friction caused by diminished lubrication [30], which originates from the bearing, leads to the generation of vibration which is thought to be transmitted through the prosthesis. If the frequency is within the range audible to humans, a noise is registered. The development of hip noise is associated with microseparation of the bearing materials, which can generate edge loading and areas of increased wear – stripe wear. Another factor seems to be the prosthetic material used as well as prosthetic design. Some designs featuring an ensleeved cup can lead to neck-rim impingement and third-body wear [31]. Specific alloys like titanium-molybdenum-zirconium alloy and various stem designs have been linked to higher rates of squeaking noises [32, 33]. Incidences are variable, with reports from 0.3 to 10.7 % [34, 35].

8.5 Material and Method

The Alloclassic® hip system (Zimmer TM) was introduced in 1979 and has shown reliable long-term results. After some modifications, the Alloclassic Variall® system was presented. It has been in use at our institution since 1998. The stem is made of Protasul titanium alloy TiAlNb. Its rectangular, cementless design creates a diaphyseal press fit. Secondary stability is achieved by bony ingrowth onto the grit-blasted surface. Primary stability is achieved by the acetabular "screwlike" design, which is threaded into the bone. The rough titanium surface of the conical acetabular component guarantees its long-term stability (Fig. 8.4).

We used a 28 mm alumina-on-alumina ceramic Cerasul® head in combination with this system. Cerasul® is a third-generation alumina oxide introduced by Sulzer Orthopedics TM in Europe in 1998. It is a hot isostatic-pressed ceramic available in three head sizes: small, medium and large.

As bearing partner, the Cerasul® liners (Zimmer, TM) were used. Until today, no fracture of Cerasul gamma liners has been reported to the manufacturer. The fracture rate for Cerasul heads ranges around 0.01 % (Source: Zimmer TM).

Between 1998 and 2003 a series of 337 patients (346 hips) had been treated with the Alloclassic Variall/Cerasul combination at our institution. We retrospectively reviewed this series, which guaranteed a minimum 9-year follow-up.

Of these patients, 48 were deceased and 61 patients could not be contacted due to change of address or refused to participate in the study. This left a total of 237 patients for analysis.

Seven surgeons performed the procedure using a standard lateral transgluteal (Bauer) approach.

Patients were invited to a clinical exam and radiographic evaluation and the HHS was assessed.

8.6 Results

Two hundred and thirty-seven hips (224 patients) were included in the study. The mean age at surgery was 61 years (range 40–84 years). The majority of patients were female (66 % vs. 34 %). The mean follow-up was 10.6 years, ranging from 8.9 to 13.9 years. The mean BMI was 28.4 (±3.7).

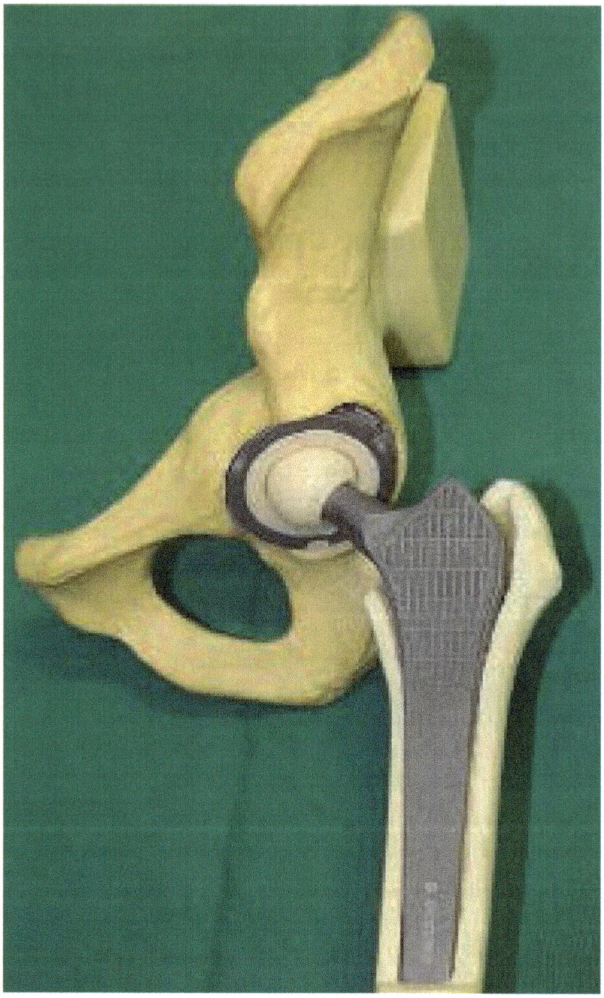

Fig. 8.4 Alloclassic Variall® hip system (Zimmer TM)

Table 8.2 Reason for revision

Reason for revision surgery	Number of cases (total $n=9$)
Pelvic fracture	$n=4$
Hip noise	$n=3$
Recurrent instability	$n=1$
Aseptic loosening of stem	$n=1$

Osteoarthritis was the main reason for surgery ($n=214$), followed by avascular necrosis ($n=10$), revision surgery ($n=6$), rheumatoid arthritis ($n=4$) and posttraumatic cases ($n=3$).

Mean HHS at follow-up was 92 points (Table 8.2).

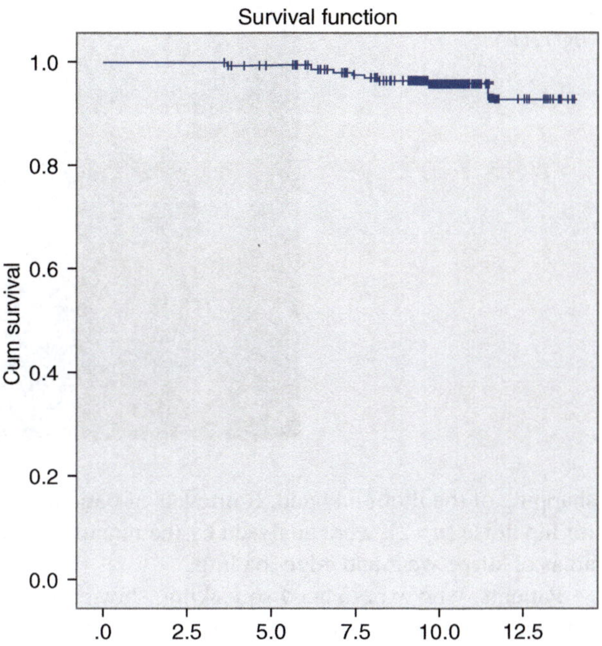

Fig. 8.5 Kaplan-Meier Survival Analysis

All surviving implants had radiographic evidence of stable bony ingrowth.

Nine patients (4.02 %) required revision surgery at a mean of 95 months (range 0.5–138 months). Four cases were due to traumatic reasons. All had experienced acetabular fracture leading to replacement of the acetabular cup by revision prosthesis (Burch-Schneider). Three patients reported a disturbing acoustic phenomenon starting around eight years after surgery (mean 96 months). One patient experienced an intermittent "squeaking" noise on deep flexion, which could not be reproduced in clinical setting. Two female patients were revised for a "clicking" noise associated with increasing pain. One patient showed recurrent instability, requiring revision surgery only 2 weeks after the initial surgical intervention. This patient had been treated with a pelvic Chiari osteotomy 20 years priorly and showed an increased BMI of 37. One patient experienced aseptic loosening of the stem 99 months after surgery.

Overall no aseptic loosening of the cup could be documented. Therefore we found a survival rate of 100 % for aseptic loosening of the cup and 99.6 % for aseptic loosening of the stem as end point. The survival rate for revision for any cause was 96.2 % (Fig. 8.5).

The occurrence of noisy hips was assessed via questionnaire. If a squeaking hip was encountered, demographics and body characteristics as well as onset of symptoms and possible triggers were analysed (Figs. 8.6 and 8.7).

Nine patients (3.8 %) experienced a noisy hip. One patient reported transient squeaking, which could not be found in clinical exam or audiography. Four (1.7 %) patients reported clicking and three (1.3 %) patients a grinding noise. One (0.4 %) patient felt a snapping sensation associated with noise, which could be identified as

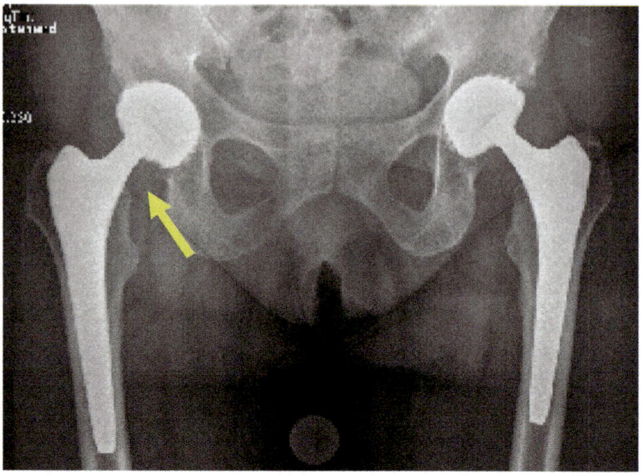

Fig. 8.6 X-ray of noisy hip (*right side*)

snapping of the iliotibial band. Retrievals of patients, who received revision surgery for hip noise ($n=2$), were analysed by the manufacturer. They all showed increased areas of stripe wear and edge loading.

Patients, who experienced squeaking, showed no significant differences in age, BMI or activity level when compared to silent hips.

8.7 Discussion

Reports on failures of ceramic bearings due to fracture still make surgeons anxious to use this kind of bearing. The reputation as a brittle, unreliable and sensitive material dates back to the first and second generation of ceramic bearings, which sported fracture rates of up to 13.4 % [17]. However, even then most reports of these early designs featured low fracture rates of 0–6.9 %. The reported fracture rate plummeted with the introduction of third-generation ceramics to 0.02 % and fourth generation shows fracture rates of 0.002 % [14]. The new fourth-generation ceramic shows supreme wear rates with a reported wear rate of 0.13 mm^3/million cycles for the BIOLOX®delta (CeramTec, TM) ceramic-on-ceramic bearing under adverse conditions [13] – compared to 1.84 mm^3/million cycles reported for third-generation ceramic BIOLOX®forte (CeramTec TM). Medium-term analysis of this new material shows promising results with no failure due to aseptic loosening. However, some reports of fractures of ceramic liners can be found in recent studies [36]. So far, no fracture of a BIOLOX®delta ceramic head has been published [16].

Metal-on-polyethylene combinations show osteolytic lesions in 11–26 % in medium- to long-term results, with osteolysis being the major risk for failure of the hip implant. According to the literature, a threshold value for osteolysis in polyethylene is 38 mm^3 per year. Under this value, osteolysis is unlikely to occur. The measured wear for ceramic articulations is much lower than this value; therefore osteolysis is not to be expected [37].

With the problem of wear and fracture rates sufficiently addressed by the new generation of ceramics, the new problem of acoustic emissions emerged. Reports on

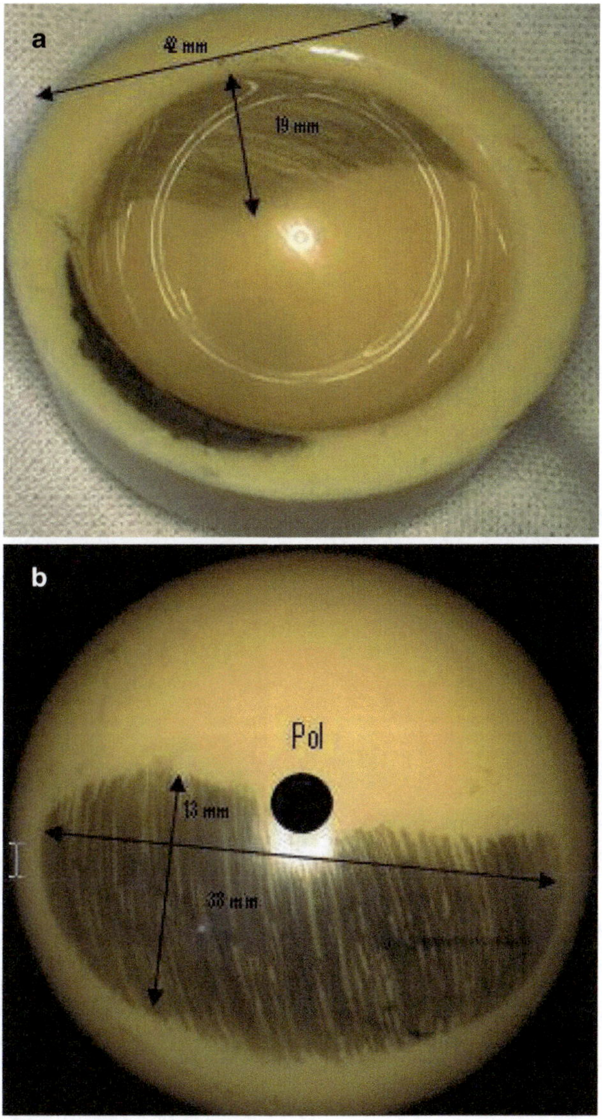

Fig. 8.7 (**a**, **b**) Retrievals after revision for noisy hip showing area of increased wear

noisy hips that can sometimes even feature a "squeaking" noise became widely known. Initial reports in 2006 showed varying incidences of 0.3–10.7 % for the squeaking and even up to 32.8 % for the generation of other noises like clicking, grating or grinding [34]. The reasons for the squeaking phenomenon are still under investigation. A multifactorial aetiology is suspected – including factors like stem design and material, fluid film disruption, stripe wear and microseparation. This was first described by Nevelos et al. and linked to joint laxity [7]. In an area of stripe wear, increased amounts of friction might be generated leading to vibration which is passed onto the components and generates an audible noise [30].

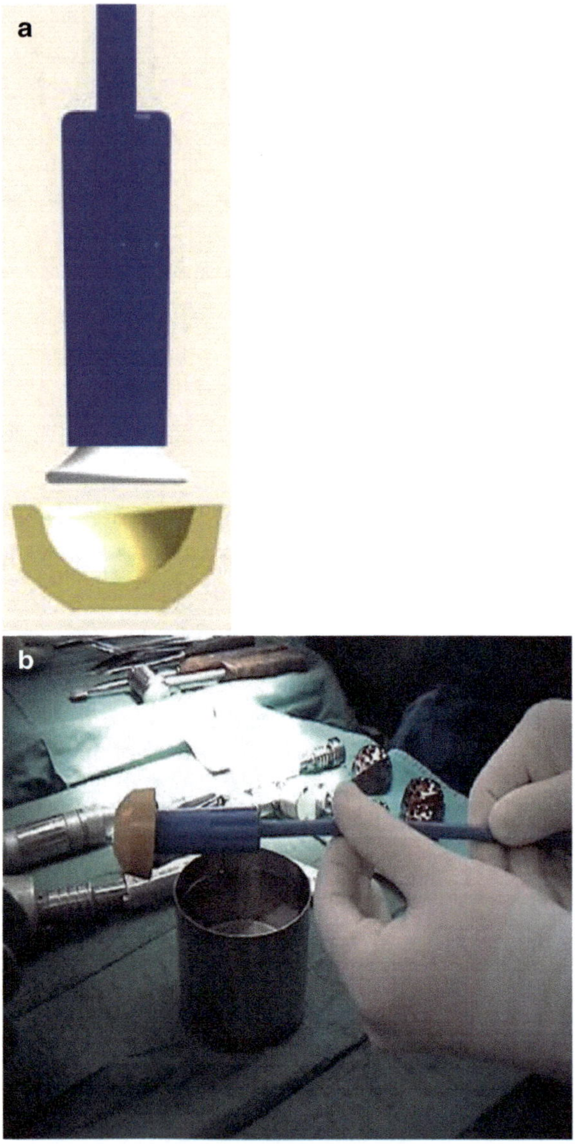

Fig. 8.8 (**a**, **b**) Suction device for safe handling of ceramic liner

Hard-on-hard bearings are more susceptible to mistakes in implantation technique than other bearings. Factors like component malposition, chipping during insertion and insufficient cleaning of the components can adversely affect the longevity of the material [14, 16].

To avoid damage of the material, we advocate a suction device for accurate and safe placement of the ceramic liner into the shell. It is crucial to ensure a clean and dry taper area. Debris on the interface between ceramic and metal has been associated with an increased risk of ceramic fracture due to point loads. The resulting failure is encountered between the first months or years after implantation [14] (Fig. 8.8).

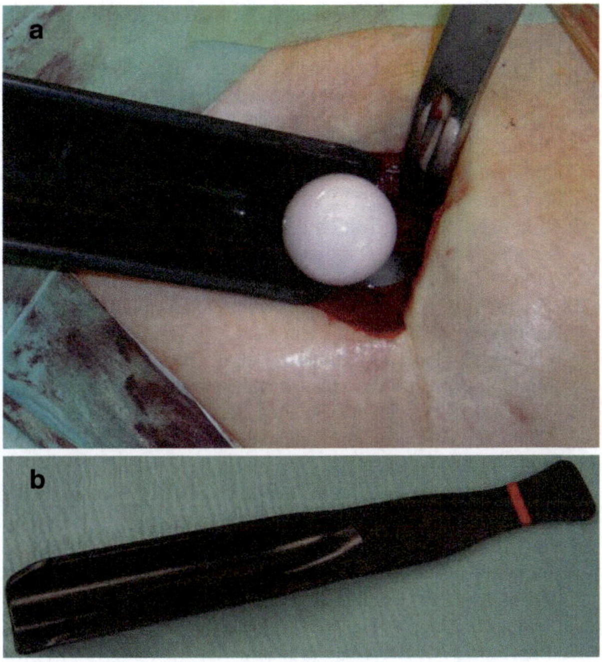

Fig. 8.9 (**a**, **b**) Shoehorn

Additionally we protect the head during repositioning with a "shoehorn" device, avoiding damage to the articulating surface of the head and the metallic shell, which could create stripe wear (Fig. 8.9).

We found an excellent midterm survival of 98.7 % for bearing-related causes in our series at a mean 10.6-year follow-up. This is in accordance with literature findings, which report 95–100 % survivorship for ceramic bearings around 10 years follow-up [18, 20, 22–29].

The low friction and high wear resistance paired with high biocompatibility make ceramic bearings the ideal option for long-term stability and therefore a reliable candidate for total hip arthroplasty in young and active patients.

References

1. Boutin P. Total arthroplasty of the hip by fritted aluminium prosthesis. Experimental study and 1st clinical applications. Rev Chir Orthop Reparatrice Appar Mot. 1972;58:29–46. French.
2. Mittelmeier H. Report on the first decennium of clinical experience with a cementless ceramic total hip replacement. Acta Orthop Belg. 1985;51:367–76.
3. Sedel L. Evolution of alumina-on-alumina implants: a review. Clin Orthop Relate Res. 2000;(379):48–54.
4. Boehler M, Knahr K, Plenk Jr H, Walter A, Salzer M, Schreiber V. Long-term results of uncemented alumina acetabular implants. J Bone Joint Surg Br. 1994;76-B:53–9.
5. Al-Hajar M, Jennings LM, Begand S, Oberbach T, Delfosse D, Fisher J. Wear of novel ceramic-on-ceramic bearings under adverse and clinically relevant hip simulator conditions. J Biomed Mater Res B Appl Biomater. 2013. doi:10.1002/jbm.b.32965. [Epub ahead of print].

6. Fisher J, Jin Z, Tipper J, Stone M, Ingham E. Tribology of alternative bearings. Clin Orthop Relat Res. 2006;453:25–34.
7. Nevelos J, Ingham E, Doyle C, Streicher R, Nevelos A, Walter W, Fisher J. Microseparation of the centers of alumina-alumina artificial hip joints during simulator testing produces clinically relevant wear rates and patterns. J Arthroplasty. 2000;15:793–5.
8. Nevelos J, Ingham E, Doyle C, Nevelo AB, Fisher J. The influence of acetabular cup angle on the wear of "BIOLOX Forte" alumina ceramic bearing couples in a hip joint simulator. J Mater Sci Mater Med. 2001;12:141–4.
9. Eskelinen A, et al. Total hip arthroplasty for primary osteoarthrosis in younger patients in the Finnish arthroplasty register. 4,661 primary replacements followed for 0-22 years. Acta Orthop. 2005;76:28–41.
10. Pospischill M, Knahr K. Cementless total hip arthroplasty using a threaded cup and rectangular tapered stem. J Bone Joint Surg Br. 2005;87-B(9):1210–5.
11. Clarke IC, Good V, Williams P, et al. Ultra-low wear rates for rigid on-rigid bearings in total hip replacements. Proc Inst Mech Eng H. 2000;214:331–47.
12. Tipper JL, Hatton A, Nevelos JE, et al. Alumina-alumina artificial hip joints. Part II: Characterisation of the wear debris from in vitro hip joint simulations. Biomaterials. 2002;23:3441–8.
13. Al-Hajjar M, Jennings LM, Leslie IJ, Fisher J. Ceramic-on-ceramic total hip replacement: the influence of cup inclination angle and head positioning. J Bone Joint Surg Br. 2011; 93-B(Suppl):67.
14. Parndorf T. The importance of clean taper conditions using ceramic hip implants. In: Cobb J, editor. Modern trends in THA bearings. Material and clinical performance. Berlin/Heidelberg: Springer; 2010. p. 97–102.
15. Hamilton WG, McAuley J, Dennis D, Blumenfeld T, Politi J. THA with delta ceramic. Clin Orthop Relat Res. 2010;468:358–66.
16. Hwang SK, et al. Fracture-dissociation of ceramic liner. Orthopedics. 2008;21(8):804.
17. Hannouche D, Nich C, Bizot P, Meunier A, Nizard R, Sedel L. Fractures of ceramic bearings: history and present status. Clin Orthop Relat Res. 2003;417:19–26.
18. Petsatodis GE, Papadopoulos PP, Papavasiliou KA, Hatzokos IG, Agathabgelidis FG, Christodoulou AG. Primary cementless total hip arthroplasty with an alumina ceramic-on-ceramic bearing: results after a minimum of twenty years of follow-up. J Bone Joint Surg Am. 2010;92(3):639–44.
19. Toni A. Osteolysis and ceramic-on-ceramic hip prosthesis :"fact or fairy tale?". In: Cobb J, editor. Modern trends in THA bearings. Material and clinical performance. Berlin/Heidelberg: Springer; 2010. p. 50–60.
20. Kim YH, Choi Y, Kim JS. Cementless total hip arthroplasty with ceramic-on-ceramic bearing in patients younger than 45 years with femoral head osteonecrosis. Int Orthop. 2010;34: 1123–7.
21. Capello WN, D'Antonio JA, Feinberg JR, et al. Ceramic-on-ceramic total hip arthroplasty: update. J Arthroplasty. 2008;23(7 Suppl):39–43.
22. Murphy SB. Two to 9 year clinical results of alumina ceramic-on-ceramic THA. Clin Orthop Relat Res. 2006;453:97–102.
23. Park YS, Park SJ, Lim SJ. Ten year results after cementless THA with sandwich-type alumina ceramic bearing. Orthopedics. 2010;33:796.
24. Chevilotte C, Pibarot V, Carret J-P, Bejui-Hugues J, Guyen O. Nine year follow-up of 100 ceramic-on-ceramic total hip arthroplasties. Int Orthop. doi:10.1007/s00264-010-1185-3. 2011;35(11):1599–1604.
25. Lewis PM, Al-Belooshi A, Olsen M, Schemitch EH, Waddell JP. Prospective randomized trial comparing alumina ceramic-on-ceramic bearings with ceramic-on-conventional polyethylene bearings in total hip arthroplasty. J Arthroplasty. 2010;25(3):392–7.
26. Lee YK, Ha YC, Yoo JJ, Koo KH, Toon KS, Kim HJ. Alumina-on-alumina total hip arthroplasty at minimum 10 year follow-up. J Bone Joint Surg Am. 2010;92:1715–8.

27. Kress AM, Schmidt R, Holzwart U, Forst R, Muller LA. Excellent results with cementless total hip arthroplasty and alumina-on-alumina pairing: minimum 10 year follow-up. Int Ortop. 2011;35:195–200.
28. Molloy D, Jack C, Esposito CA, Walter WL. Mid-term analysis suggests ceramic on ceramic hip arthroplasty is durable with minimal wear and low risk of squeak. HSS J. 2012; 8(3):291–4.
29. Sollarino G, Piazzolla A, Notarnicola A, Moretti L, Tafuri S, De Giogi S, Moretti B. Long-term results of 32-mm alumina-on-alumina THA for avascular necrosis of the femoral head. J Orthop Traumatol. 2012;13(1):21–7.
30. Chevilotte C, Trousdale RT, Chen Q, Guyen O, An K. The frank stitchfield award "Hip squeaking".a biomechanical study of ceramic-on-ceramic bearing surfaces. Clin Orthop Relat Res. 2009;468:345–50.
31. Swanson T, Peterson DJ, Seethala R, Bliss R, Spellmon Jr CA. Influence of prosthetic design on squeaking after ceramic-on-ceramic total hip arthroplasty. J Arthroplasty. 2010;25(6 Suppl):36–42.
32. Weiss C, Gdaniec P, Hoffmann N, Hothan A, Huber G, Morlock M. Squeak in hip endoprosthesis systems: an experimental study and a numerical technique to analyse design variants. Med Eng Phys. 2010;32(6):604–60.
33. Restrepo C, Parvizi J, Kurtz SM, Sharkey PF, Hozack WJ, Rothman RH. The noisy ceramic hip: is component malpositioning the cause? J Arthroplasty. 2008;23:643–9.
34. Jarret CA, Ranawat AS, Bruzzone M, Blum YC, Rodriguez JA, Ranawat CS. The squeaking hip: a phenomenon of ceramic-on-ceramic total hip arthroplasty. J Bone Joint Surg Am. 2009;91:1344–9.
35. Lusty PJ, Tai CC, Sew-Hoy RP, Walter WL, Walter WK, Zicat BA. Third generation alumina-on-alumina ceramic bearings in cementless total hip arthroplasty. J Bone Joint Surg Am. 2007;92:2676–83.
36. Oakley J. The early clinical results of alumina matrix composite ceramics in primary cementless hip arthroplasty. In: Cobb J, editor. Modern trends in THA bearings material and clinical performance. Berlin/Heidelberg: Springer; 2010. p. 179–84.
37. Dumbleton JH, Manley MT, Edidin AA. A literature review of the association between wear rate and osteolysis in total hip arthroplasty. J Arthroplasty. 2002;17:649–61.

Wear of Large Ceramic-on-Ceramic Bearings for Total Hip Arthroplasty and the Mechanical and Tribological Properties of Silicon Nitrides

9

Kim Lars Häußler, Roman Preuß, and Robert M. Streicher

9.1 Introduction

Dislocation is one of the major revision factors in total hip arthroplasty (THA) with a rate of 1–6 % for primary surgeries [1–4] and up to over 20 % for revision surgeries [5]. Using larger bearing couples has shown an increase of the range of motion and increased stability [6] and at the same time a reduction of the dislocation risk due to a less likelihood of component-on-component impingement [7, 8]. A large number of clinical retrospective studies have shown good early, midterm, and long-term outcomes of larger diameter THAs in terms of dislocation rates [8–11] compared to smaller diameter components.

Many studies have examined the wear behavior of these smaller diameter bearing couples using different material pairings up to 36 mm diameter [12–21]. Hard-on-soft articulations like metal or ceramic on ultrahigh-molecular-weight polyethylene have the highest wear rates followed by metal or ceramic on cross-linked polyethylene. Hard-on-hard bearings like metal-on-metal (MoM) and ceramic-on-ceramic (CoC) bearings showed the lowest wear rates. With the issues [22–28] and consequently decrease in usage of metal-on-metal articulations and the clinical benefit of using larger heads, CoC has gained a renaissance. Nevertheless, there exists a paucity of wear studies using larger diameter THAs (>36 mm), and therefore, the main purpose of the study reported was to compare the wear generated using large CoC bearings.

Recently, silicon nitride ceramics, which are normally used as high-performance bearings or in high-temperature industrial applications such as engine components, were investigated as a possible material for THAs due to its biocompatibility and

K.L. Häußler (✉) • R. Preuß • R.M. Streicher
Medical Products Division, CeramTec GmbH,
CeramTec-Platz 1-9, Plochingen, 73207, Germany
e-mail: k.haeussler@ceramtec.de, http://www.ceramtec.com

K. Knahr (ed.), *Tribology in Total Hip and Knee Arthroplasty*,
DOI 10.1007/978-3-642-45266-6_9, © EFORT 2014

promising mechanical and wear properties [29–33]. Therefore, a second aim of this study was to mechanically and tribologically characterize different silicon nitride ceramics and compare the results to the latest generation of ZPTA.

9.2 Materials and Methods

9.2.1 Hip Simulator Studies

Wear testing of three different CoC bearing couples (ball head and liner) made from zirconia-platelet-toughened alumina (ZPTA; BIOLOX®*delta*, CeramTec GmbH, Plochingen, Germany) was conducted in a servo-hydraulic hip simulator (Endolab GmbH, Rosenheim, Germany) up to five million cycles at a frequency of 1 Hz. The examined bearing diameters were 36, 40, and 44 mm. Standard gait conditions were applied to the bearing couples according to ISO14242-1 [34] and ISO14242-2 [35]. One cycle included a double peak load of 3 kN, flexion/extension of +25°/−18°, abduction/adduction of −4°/+7°, and internal/external rotation of −11°/+2°. All acetabular cups and thus liners were mounted at an inclination angle of 30° to the horizontal plane. The lubricant used consisted of newborn calf serum supplemented with ethylenediaminetetraacetic acid (1.8 g/l) to minimize precipitation of calcium phosphate onto the bearing surfaces and Patricine (10 ml/l) to retard bacterial growth. The protein content of the lubricant was 17 g/l. Every 500,000 cycles the lubricant was changed and replaced by fresh lubricant. Gravimetric wear measurements were performed after 500,000 cycles and afterwards every million cycles using a high precision balance (BP211D, Sartorius, Göttingen, Germany) with a resolution of 0.01 mg. Before the weighing process the ball heads and liners were disconnected from the tapers and metal backs, respectively, and thoroughly cleaned in an ultrasonic cleaner following a standard cleaning regime described in the ISO14242-2 [35]. To avoid metal transfer from the metal backs to the liners, a thin polyethylene film had been placed between the two components in the conical area. For each bearing diameter three different combinations regarding clearance and sphericity were chosen (Table 9.1). Combination 1 consisted of ball heads with a sphericity of less than 5 μm and liners with a sphericity of less than 7 μm. The diametrical clearance was 70 μm. Combination 2 and 3 consisted of ball heads with a sphericity of 15 μm and liners with a sphericity of less than 7 μm. The diametrical clearances were 240 and 20 μm, respectively.

Table 9.1 Geometrical parameters of the 36, 40, and 44 mm bearings

Bearing size	36 mm			40 mm			44 mm		
Combination number	1	2	3	1	2	3	1	2	3
Sphericity of the ball head in μm	<5	15	15	<5	15	15	<5	15	15
Sphericity of the liner in μm	<7	<7	<7	<7	<7	<7	<7	<7	<7
Clearance in μm	70	240	20	70	240	20	70	240	20

Data of weight measurements of liners and ball heads were accumulated and divided by the density of BIOLOX®*delta* ceramic (4.36 g/cm^3) to gain volumetric wear data. Linear regression analysis was performed over the first million cycles to gain the run-in volumetric wear rate and over five million cycles to gain the overall volumetric wear rate, i.e., mm^3/10^6 cycles. Statistical analysis was performed using a one-sided Wilcoxon rank-sum test with an α-level of 0.05.

9.2.2 Silicon Nitride Studies

Three different silicon nitride ceramics were tested. One of them was engineered in terms of an optimized strength (A), one in terms of an optimized hardness (B), and one in terms of an optimized toughness (C). Ring-on-disc wear tests were performed according to ISO 6474-2 [36] over a test period of 100 h. The rotation angle was ±25° and the frequency was 1 Hz. The test samples were axially loaded with a constant force of 1.5 kN to obtain a uniform contact pressure between the ring and the disc. The lubricant used was similar to that used for the hip simulator studies and consisted of 25 % calf serum diluted with distilled water, ethylenediaminetetraacetic acid (1.86 g/l) to bind the calcium phosphate, and Patricine (10 ml/l) to retard bacteria-induced degradation. The resulting protein content was 15.75 g/l. All test samples had a special design to enhance the fixation in the testing machines (Fig. 9.1) and were polished to achieve a roughness (Ra)

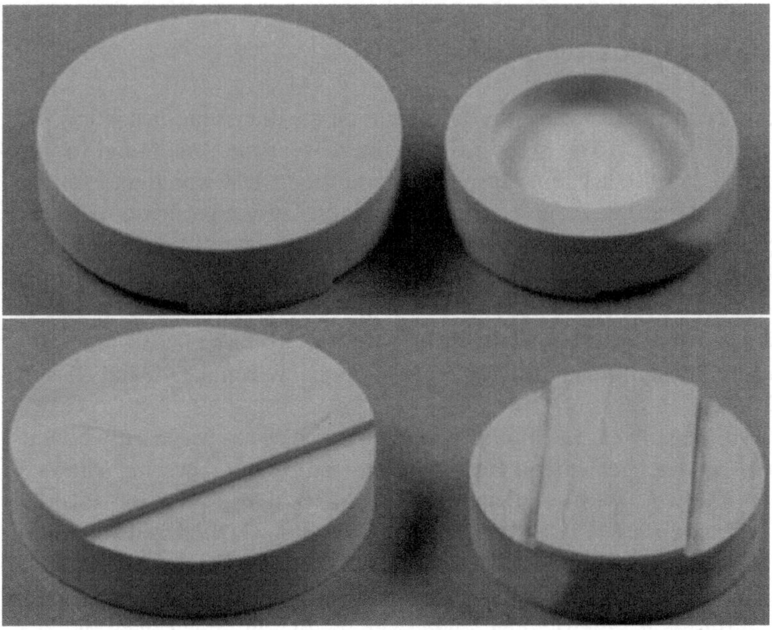

Fig. 9.1 Specially designed ring-on-disc test samples to enhance fixation in the testing machine

between 0.03 and 0.06 μm. Torque measurements were performed at the beginning and end of the tests. Volumetric wear determination was conducted by first scanning the wear profile of the discs at six positions at intervals of 60° using a surface scanning device (Surftest SJ-401, Mitutoyo, Neuss, Germany) and then multiplying the mean value of the wear profile area by the mean diameter of the wear profile.

Flexural strength was measured in 4-point bending according to DIN EN 843-1 [37] using 30 ground specimens for each group with cross-section dimensions of 3×4 mm. The outer span was 40 or 30 mm, and the inner span was 20 or 10 mm depending on the specimen length. The load was applied using a material testing machine (Zwick 1445, Zwick GmbH & Co. KG, Ulm, Germany) at a crosshead speed of 2.75 or 3.75 mm/min, respectively. Fracture toughness was also measured in four point bending according to ISO 23146 [38] using the single-edge v-notch beam method on five specimens for each group (dimension, 3×4×45 mm). The notch was prepared using a razor blade. The outer span was 40 mm, the inner span 20 mm, and the crosshead speed was 1 mm/min. Vickers hardness HV1 was determined according to DIN EN 843-4 [39] using a Semi Makrovickers 5112 (ITW Test & Measurement GmbH, Düsseldorf, Germany) at ten indentation points in a distance of 0.5 mm from indentation point to indentation point with a load of 9.807 N. Statistical analysis was performed using a two-sided Wilcoxon rank-sum test with an α-level of 0.05.

9.3 Results

9.3.1 Hip Simulator Studies

The run-in linear wear rate was dependent on the diameter, increasing with bigger diameter (Fig. 9.2). The highest run-in linear wear rate was found for the 44 mm bearing (0.263 ± 0.021 $mm^3/10^6$ cycles) and the lowest was found for the 36 mm bearing (0.045 ± 0.017 $mm^3/10^6$ cycles). Statistically significant differences were found between all groups ($p < 0.05$). Contrary, the overall linear wear rate did not show a diameter dependency (Fig. 9.2). The 40 mm bearing exhibited the highest overall linear wear rate (0.051 ± 0.001 $mm^3/10^6$ cycles), whereas the 44 mm bearing showed the lowest overall linear wear rate (0.032 ± 0.008 $mm^3/10^6$ cycles). A statistically significant difference was found between the 40 and 44 mm bearing ($p < 0.05$).

Run-in linear wear rate of the 40 and 44 mm bearing was hardly affected by the different geometrical parameters whereas the 36 mm bearing shows twice as much run-in wear with small and large clearance than with a mid-tolerance clearance and sphericity (Fig. 9.3). The 36 mm bearing showed a distinct influence of the three clearances with the 70 μm clearance resulting in the lowest overall linear wear rate (0.018 $mm^3/10^6$ cycles) (Fig. 9.3). For the 40 mm bearings, no influence of the different geometrical parameters on the overall linear wear rate was found. The 44 mm bearing showed a similar trend compared to the 36 mm bearing with the mid-tolerance clearance resulting in the lowest wear rate (0.024 $mm^3/10^6$ cycles).

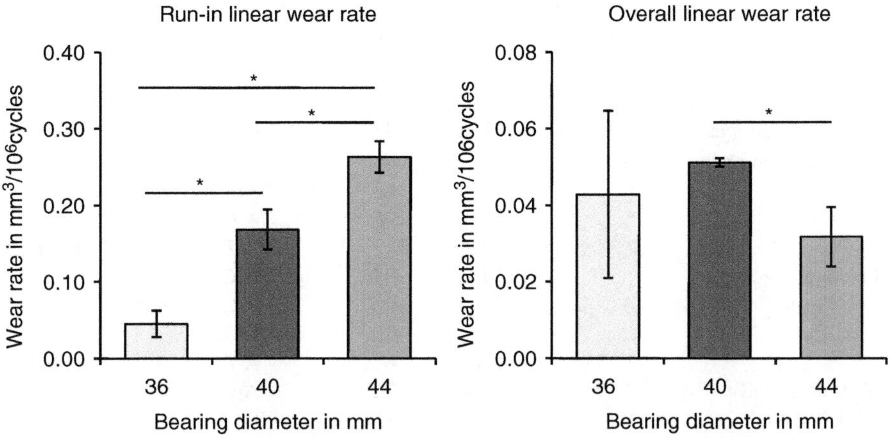

Fig. 9.2 Mean values and standard deviations of the cumulative (ball head and liner) run-in and overall linear wear rate plotted over the different bearing diameters. The *asterisk* denotes a statistically significant difference ($p<0.05$)

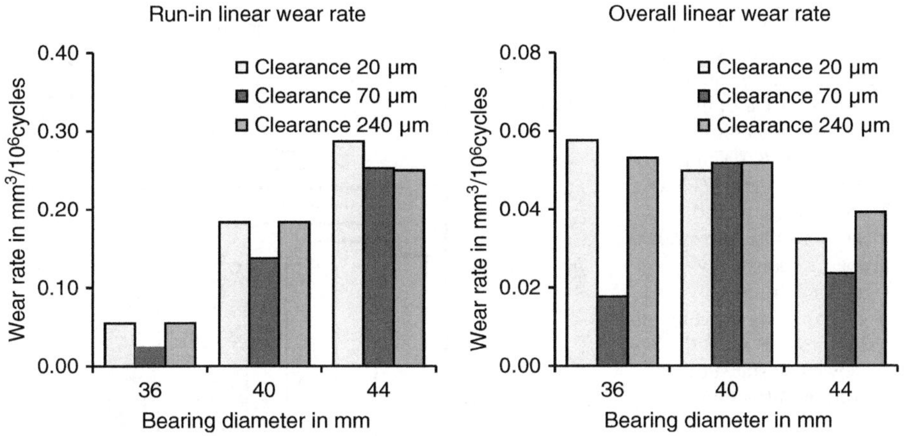

Fig. 9.3 Single values of the cumulative run-in and total linear wear rate dependent on the different diametrical clearances plotted over the different bearing diameters

9.3.2 Silicon Nitride Studies

The different silicon nitrides all achieved good results in terms of mechanical properties, but the values for all examined properties were inferior to BIOLOX®*delta* except for the hardness, where silicon nitride B showed comparable results to the ZPTA (Table 9.2).

The volumetric wear measured using the ring-on-disc setup showed that ZPTA vs. ZPTA couplings were superior to all other couplings tested (0.05 ± 0.01 mm^3) (Fig. 9.4). The highest volumetric wear was found for silicon nitride A (135.72 ± 7.17 mm^3). Except for the comparison between group B vs. B and C vs. C, all other comparisons between groups resulted in statistically significant differences ($p<0.05$).

Table 9.2 Mean values and standard deviations of the mechanical properties of the three different silicon nitride ceramics (A, B, C) compared to reference values obtained with BIOLOX®*delta* (ZPTA)

Mechanical property	Material	Mean	Standard deviation	$p<0.05$
Bending strength in Mpa	A	1,104	95	A-B, A-C, A-ZPTA
	B	965	60	AB, B-ZPTA
	C	943	74	A-C, C-ZPTA
	ZPTA	1,390	–	A-ZPTA, B-ZPTA, C-ZPTA
Fracture toughness in MPa·m$^{0.5}$	A	5.6	0.0	A-C, A-ZPTA
	B	5.5	0.1	B-C, B-ZPTA
	C	5.7	0.1	B-C, C-ZPTA
	ZPTA	6.4	–	A-ZPTA, B-ZPTA, C-ZPTA
Vickers hardness HV1 in Gpa	A	15.6	0.2	A-C, A-ZPTA
	B	18.9	1.0	B-C
	C	15.3	0.5	B-C, C-ZPTA
	ZPTA	19.1	–	A-ZPTA, C-ZPTA

The last column depicts statistically significant differences between the mechanical properties of the different materials

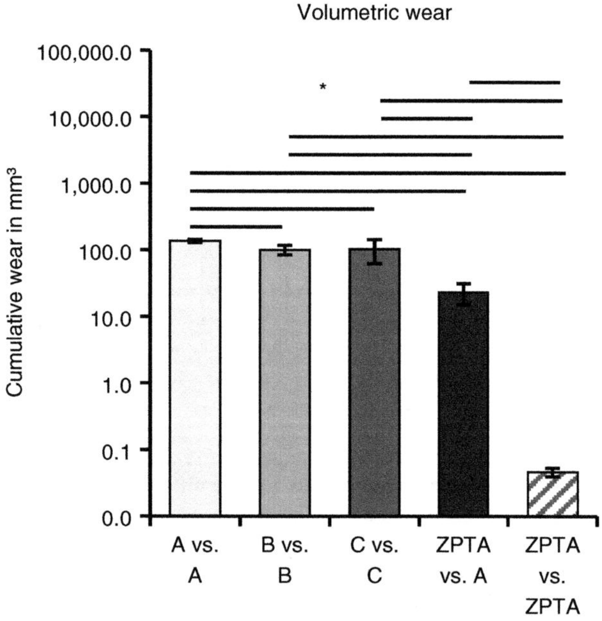

Fig. 9.4 Mean values and standard deviations of the cumulative (ring and disc) volumetric wear of the different silicon nitride ceramics (*A*, *B*, *C*) compared to BIOLOX®*delta* (ZPTA). The ordinate is scaled logarithmically. The *asterisk* denotes a statistically significant difference ($p<0.05$). Only the comparison of group B vs. B to C vs. C showed no statistically significant difference

Except for material C, chip-offs at the edges of the ring samples after the wear testing were found for all other combinations using silicon nitride ceramics (Fig. 9.5). BIOLOX®*delta* vs. BIOLOX®*delta* specimens also did not show any rim chipping.

The torques measured at the end of the ring-on-disc tests were highest and almost equal for the silicon nitrides A, B, and C (9.0±0.7 Nm, 9.2±0.5 Nm, 9.5±0.5 Nm),

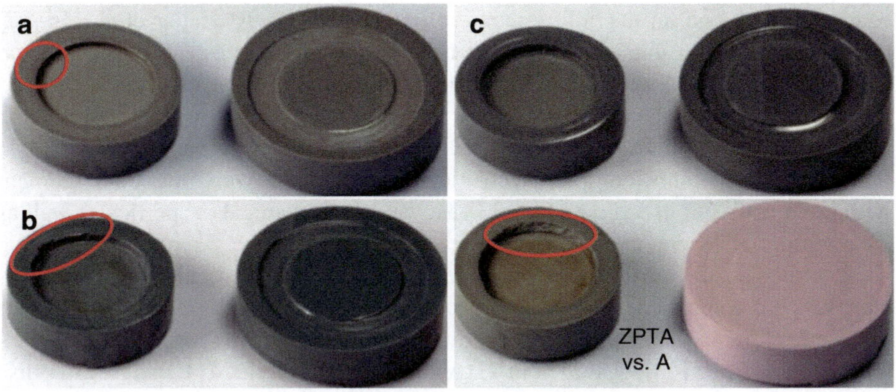

Fig. 9.5 Ring and disc samples of the different silicon nitride ceramics (*A*, *B*, *C*) and silicon nitride A against ZPTA after the ring-on-disc tests. The *red circles* highlight the chip-offs at the edges of the ring samples

followed by the ZPTA vs. A coupling (7.7 ± 1.6 Nm). The BIOLOX®*delta* vs. BIOLOX®*delta* coupling showed lowest torque values (5.2 ± 1.1 Nm).

9.4 Discussion

The goals of the current study were first to gain wear data using larger CoC bearings under standard gait conditions and gain insight into the effects of different geometrical parameters like the clearance and sphericity of ball head and liner on the wear behavior of these larger bearings. Secondly, this study examined mechanical and tribological properties of different silicon nitride ceramics which possibly could be used as an alternative bearing.

Interestingly, this study detected a diameter dependency of the wear rates during the run-in phase up to one million cycles, which could not be found for the overall wear rates. This is probably due to a larger contact area for the larger bearings in combination with a bedding-in process where possibly small surface irregularities resulting from the hard machining process were removed, thus showing higher run-in wear rates for larger bearings.

Effects of different geometrical parameters of the components were most distinct for the 36 mm bearings where the wear rates were higher using ball heads with a sphericity deviation of 15 μm in combination with 20 and 240 μm clearances. These results could be caused by a combination of sphericity deviations of the ball head and contact area which could be larger for the small clearance resulting in lower contact stresses and lower for the large clearance resulting in higher contact stresses. Both possibilities could possibly cause an increase of the wear rate. The effect of a clearance at the lower and upper tolerance limit is part of a currently running study taking into account the main limitation of the small sample size of this study.

The result of the current study that there is no diameter dependency of the wear rates under standard gait conditions was affirmed by comparing the wear rates to recent literature using BIOLOX®*delta* bearings. Kaddick and Pfaff [21] used 22.2 mm bearings and found an overall wear rate of 0.02 $mm^3/10^6$. Al-Hajjar et al. [16, 17] performed studies using 28 and 36 mm bearings and found wear rates of 0.05 and 0.01 $mm^3/10^6$, respectively. They also could show that the wear rate under standard gait conditions is not dependent on different bearing diameters. But when introducing microseparation conditions, a larger bearing size did result in higher wear rates.

Silicon nitrides showed good mechanical properties and were in good agreement with previously published data [32, 33]. However, mechanical properties as well as wear properties were inferior compared to BIOLOX®*delta*. Wear determination using a ring-on-disc setup could be indeed regarded as a screening test, and it is clear that the contact conditions differ from clinical applications. Peak stresses of a THA move due to varying loading conditions and thus varying angles of the resultant hip joint force [40], also seen in THA slide track analysis [41]. In a ring-on-disc setup, these peak stresses do not move and are localized at the edges of the contact zone between the two components. Nevertheless the ring-on-disc setup represents a worst-case scenario. If chipping at the edges during these wear tests occurs, there also could be a risk of damage or fracture to THA components under in vivo conditions and especially during edge loading due to microseparation [42]. Therefore, the silicon nitrides examined in this study could bear a risk of fracture and seem unsuitable as hard-hard bearing for THA. However, Bal et al. [32, 33] conducted hip simulator wear tests under standard gait conditions using silicon nitride bearings (28 mm) and found volumetric wear of 0.2 mm^3 after one million cycles and extrapolated the data to ten million cycles resulting in a volumetric wear of 0.65 mm^3. These results are encouraging but were still inferior to the results of the current study using BIOLOX®*delta* couplings considering that a higher load of 3 kN were used in our study compared to 2 kN of the study by Bal et al..

This study has shown extremely low wear rates of BIOLOX®*delta*, superior to earlier generations of ceramic materials [18, 19] and MoM bearings [20, 21, 43]. Under standard gait conditions, equal wear rates were found when using larger diameter bearings. Silicon nitride ceramics examined in this study seemed to be unsuitable for use as bearing material in THA due to their inferior wear properties.

Acknowledgments The authors would like to acknowledge Endolab GmbH for conducting the wear studies.

References

1. Berry DJ, von Knoch M, Schleck CD, Harmsen WS. Effect of femoral head diameter and operative approach on risk of dislocation after primary total hip arthroplasty. J Bone Joint Surg Am. 2005;87:2456–63.
2. Byström S, Espehaug B, Furnes O, Havelin LI, Norwegian Arthroplasty Register. Femoral head size is a risk factor for total hip luxation: a study of 42,987 primary hip arthroplasties from the Norwegian Arthroplasty Register. Acta Orthop Scand. 2003;74:514–24.
3. Khatod M, Barber T, Paxton E, Namba R, Fithian D. An analysis of the risk of hip dislocation with a contemporary total joint registry. Clin Orthop Relat Res. 2006;447:19–23.
4. Phillips CB, Barrett JA, Losina E, Mahomed NN, Lingard EA, Guadagnoli E, Baron JA, Harris WH, Poss R, Katz JN. Incidence rates of dislocation, pulmonary embolism, and deep infection

during the first six months after elective total hip replacement. J Bone Joint Surg Am. 2003;85-A:20–6.
5. AOA. Australian Orthopaedic Association National Joint Replacement Registry, Hip and Knee Arthroplasty-Annual report. 2012. https://aoanjrr.dmac.adelaide.edu.au/documents/10180/60142/Annual%20Report%202012?version=1.3&t=1361226543157
6. Jr Lombardi AV, Skeels MD, Berend KR, Adams JB, Franchi OJ. Do large heads enhance stability and restore native anatomy in primary total hip arthroplasty? Clin Orthop Relat Res. 2011;469:1547–53.
7. Stroh DA, Issa K, Johnson AJ, Delanois RE, Mont MA. Reduced dislocation rates and excellent functional outcomes with large-diameter femoral heads. J Arthroplasty. 2013;28(8):1415–20.
8. Berton C, Girard J, Krantz N, Migaud H. The Durom large diameter head acetabular component: early results with a large-diameter metal-on-metal bearing. J Bone Joint Surg Br. 2010;92:202–8.
9. Beaulé PE, Schmalzried TP, Udomkiat P, Amstutz HC. Jumbo femoral head for the treatment of recurrent dislocation following total hip replacement. J Bone Joint Surg Am. 2002;84-A:256–63.
10. Sikes CV, Lai LP, Schreiber M, Mont MA, Jinnah RH, Seyler TM. Instability after total hip arthroplasty: treatment with large femoral heads vs constrained liners. J Arthroplasty. 2008;23:59–63.
11. Smith TM, Berend KR, Jr Lombardi AV, Jr Emerson RH, Mallory TH. Metal-on-metal total hip arthroplasty with large heads may prevent early dislocation. Clin Orthop Relat Res. 2005;441:137–42.
12. Clarke IC, Green DD, Williams PA, Kubo K, Pezzotti G, Lombardi A, Turnbull A, Donaldson TK. Hip-simulator wear studies of an alumina-matrix composite (AMC) ceramic compared to retrieval studies of AMC balls with 1-7 years follow-up. Wear. 2009;267:702–9.
13. Clarke IC, Good V, Williams P, Schroeder D, Anissian L, Stark A, Oonishi H, Schuldies J, Gustafson G. Ultra-low wear rates for rigid-on-rigid bearings in total hip replacements. Proc Inst Mech Eng H. 2000;214:331–47.
14. Oonishi H, Clarke IC, Good V, Amino H, Ueno M. Alumina hip joints characterized by run-in wear and steady-state wear to 14 million cycles in hip-simulator model. J Biomed Mater Res A. 2004;70:523–32.
15. Stewart TD, Tipper JL, Insley G, Streicher RM, Ingham E, Fisher J. Long-term wear of ceramic matrix composite materials for hip prostheses under severe swing phase microseparation. J Biomed Mater Res B Appl Biomater. 2003;66:567–73.
16. Al-Hajjar M, Fisher J, Tipper JL, Williams S, Jennings LM. Wear of 36-mm BIOLOX® delta ceramic-on-ceramic bearing in total hip replacements under edge loading conditions. Proc Inst Mech Eng H. 2013;227:535–42.
17. Al-Hajjar M, Leslie IJ, Tipper J, Williams S, Fisher J, Jennings LM. Effect of cup inclination angle during microseparation and rim loading on the wear of BIOLOX® delta ceramic-on-ceramic total hip replacement. J Biomed Mater Res B Appl Biomater. 2010;95:263–8.
18. Nevelos JE, Ingham E, Doyle C, Nevelos AB, Fisher J. Wear of HIPed and non-HIPed alumina-alumina hip joints under standard and severe simulator testing conditions. Biomaterials. 2001;22:2191–7.
19. Stewart T, Tipper J, Streicher R, Ingham E, Fisher J. Long-term wear of HIPed alumina on alumina bearings for THR under microseparation conditions. J Mater Sci Mater Med. 2001;12:1053–6.
20. Essner A, Sutton K, Wang A. Hip simulator wear comparison of metal-on-metal, ceramic-on-ceramic and crosslinked UHMWPE bearings. Wear. 2005;259:992–5.
21. Kaddick C, Pfaff HG. Results of hip simulator testing with various wear couples. In: Proceedings 7th international BIOLOX symposium. Stuttgart: Georg Thieme Verlag; 2002. p. 16–20.
22. Bernthal NM, Celestre PC, Stavrakis AI, Ludington JC, Oakes DA. Disappointing short-term results with the DePuy ASR XL metal-on-metal total hip arthroplasty. J Arthroplasty. 2012;27:539–44.

23. Campbell P, Ebramzadeh E, Nelson S, Takamura K, De Smet K, Amstutz HC. Histological features of pseudotumor-like tissues from metal-on-metal hips. Clin Orthop Relat Res. 2010;468:2321–7.
24. Dahlstrand H, Stark A, Anissian L, Hailer NP. Elevated serum concentrations of cobalt, chromium, nickel, and manganese after metal-on-metal alloarthroplasty of the hip: a prospective randomized study. J Arthroplasty. 2009;24:837–45.
25. Langton DJ, Jameson SS, Joyce TJ, Hallab NJ, Natu S, Nargol AVF. Early failure of metal-on-metal bearings in hip resurfacing and large-diameter total hip replacement: a consequence of excess wear. J Bone Joint Surg Br. 2010;92:38–46.
26. Long WT, Dastane M, Harris MJ, Wan Z, Dorr LD. Failure of the Durom Metasul acetabular component. Clin Orthop Relat Res. 2010;468:400–5.
27. Ollivere B, Darrah C, Barker T, Nolan J, Porteous MJ. Early clinical failure of the Birmingham metal-on-metal hip resurfacing is associated with metallosis and soft-tissue necrosis. J Bone Joint Surg Br. 2009;91:1025–30.
28. Pandit H, Glyn-Jones S, McLardy-Smith P, Gundle R, Whitwell D, Gibbons CLM, Ostlere S, Athanasou N, Gill HS, Murray DW. Pseudotumours associated with metal-on-metal hip resurfacings. J Bone Joint Surg Br. 2008;90:847–51.
29. Bal BS, Rahaman MN. Orthopedic applications of silicon nitride ceramics. Acta Biomater. 2012;8:2889–98.
30. Guedes e Silva CC, König Jr B, Carbonari MJ, Yoshimoto M, Allegrini Jr S, Bressiani JC. Tissue response around silicon nitride implants in rabbits. J Biomed Mater Res A. 2008;84:337–43.
31. Mazzocchi M, Gardini D, Traverso PL, Faga MG, Bellosi A. On the possibility of silicon nitride as a ceramic for structural orthopaedic implants. Part II: chemical stability and wear resistance in body environment. J Mater Sci Mater Med. 2008;19:2889–901.
32. Bal BS, Khandkar A, Lakshminarayanan R, Clarke I, Hoffman AA, Rahaman MN. Fabrication and testing of silicon nitride bearings in total hip arthroplasty: winner of the 2007 'HAP' PAUL Award. J Arthroplasty. 2009;24:110–6.
33. Bal BS, Khandkar A, Lakshminarayanan R, Clarke I, Hoffman AA, Rahaman MN. Testing of silicon nitride ceramic bearings for total hip arthroplasty. J Biomed Mater Res B Appl Biomater. 2008;87:447–54.
34. ISO14242-1. Implants for surgery – wear of total hip-joint prostheses – part 1: loading and displacement parameters for wear-testing machines and corresponding environmental conditions for test. 2012.
35. ISO14242-2. Implants for surgery – wear of total hip-joint prostheses – part 2: methods of measurement. 2000.
36. ISO6474-2. Implants for surgery – ceramic materials – part 2: composite materials based on a high-purity alumina matrix with zirconia reinforcement. 2012.
37. DIN_EN843-1. Hochleistungskeramik – Mechanische Eigenschaften monolithischer Keramik bei Raumtemperatur – Teil 1: Bestimmung der Biegefestigkeit; Deutsche Fassung. 2006.
38. ISO23146. Fine ceramics (advanced ceramics, advanced technical ceramics) — test methods for fracture toughness of monolithic ceramics—single-edge V-notch beam (SEVNB) method. 2008.
39. DIN_EN843-4. Hochleistungskeramik – Mechanische Eigenschaften monolithischer Keramik bei Raumtemperatur – Teil 4: Härteprüfung nach Vickers, Knoop und Rockwell; Deutsche Fassung. 2005.
40. Bergmann G, Graichen F, Rohlmann A, Bender A, Heinlein B, Duda GN, Heller MO, Morlock MM. Realistic loads for testing hip implants. Biomed Mater Eng. 2010;20:65–75.
41. Saikko V, Calonius O. Slide track analysis of the relative motion between femoral head and acetabular cup in walking and in hip simulators. J Biomech. 2002;35:455–64.
42. Stewart TD, Tipper JL, Insley G, Streicher RM, Ingham E, Fisher J. Severe wear and fracture of zirconia heads against alumina inserts in hip simulator studies with microseparation. J Arthroplasty. 2003;18:726–34.
43. Firkins PJ, Tipper JL, Ingham E, Stone MH, Farrar R, Fisher J. Influence of simulator kinematics on the wear of metal-on-metal hip prostheses. Proc Inst Mech Eng H. 2001;215:119–21.

Ceramic-on-Ceramic Total Hip Replacement: Five Cases of Early *Delta* Ceramic Liner Fracture

10

Ellen McCourt, M. Mawdsley, and J.M. Loughead

Over other bearing surfaces, ceramic-on-ceramic (CoC) articulations in total hip replacements (THR) have the advantages of reduced wear, reduced osteolysis, improved maintenance of lubrication and improved biocompatibility [1–3]; however, they are more brittle and have a higher tendency to fracture [4].

BIOLOX®*delta* (CeramTec AG, Plochingen, Germany) is a fourth-generation ceramic. It is thought to prevent cracking by restraining the phase transformation due to the insertion of yttria-stabilised tetragonal zirconia into the alumina matrix [5]. This offers several advantages over older ceramics including increased mechanical strength allowing the use of thinner-walled liners and larger-diameter heads. With increased use of *delta* ceramic, there has been a reduction in the fracture rate associated with CoC articulations. The composition of *delta* ceramic is designed to maximise mechanical strength. It is an aluminium oxide matrix composed of 80 % alumina, 17 % zirconia and 3 % strontium oxide. Zirconia provides increased strength and acts to reduce the initiation and propagation of cracks [6]. Strontium augments this by diffusing crack energy through formation of platelet type crystals. These improved mechanical properties have enabled the manufacture of thinner liners, which have in turn allowed the use of larger femoral heads, the advantage being to reduce dislocation rate, reduce rate of impingement and improve stability [7].

There are very few reported cases of early *delta* ceramic liner fractures. Many more reports exist for alumina ceramic liner and head fractures, the majority of

E. McCourt (✉) • M. Mawdsley • J.M. Loughead
Trauma and Orthopaedics, Queen Elizabeth Hospital, Gateshead, UK
e-mail: ellenmccourt1@gmail.com

K. Knahr (ed.), *Tribology in Total Hip and Knee Arthroplasty*,
DOI 10.1007/978-3-642-45266-6_10, © EFORT 2014

Table 10.1 Summary of five cases presented

	Age (M/F)	Anything noted on post operative x-ray? (any symptoms noted at follow up?)	Time from surgery to fracture (weeks)
Case 1	66 F	Malseating noted on check x-ray. (Early subjective clunking which resolved)	6
Case 2	68 F	No abnormality noted on check x-ray. (No abnormal symptoms)	12
Case 3	55 F	No abnormality noted on check x-ray. (Trendelenburg gait and squeaking hip)	28
Case 4	76 M	Subtle malseating changes on lateral x-ray. (Some clicking of hip)	32
Case 5	72 M	Malseating noted on check x-ray. (Minor discomfort, medically poor candidate for revision)	6

which have failed between 14 and 48 months postoperatively [1–4, 7–12]. Literature review exposed one Korean case of early *delta* ceramic liner fracture at 4 months [5] and one later case from Iran occurring 18 months postoperation [8]. We present five cases of *delta* ceramic liner fracture in total hip replacements occurring less than 12 months after index surgery.

We examined five cases of early *delta* ceramic liner fracture occurring in the Queen Elizabeth Hospital (QEH), Gateshead, an NHS Foundation Trust in the north-east of England, between 2011 and 2012 (Table 10.1). We used the term 'early' to refer to a fracture occurring less than 12 months after the index procedure. Subsequently we have discussed the optimal recognition of patients at risk of liner fracture and how to best manage these individuals.

The National Joint Registry in the United Kingdom (UK) reported over 71,000 total hip replacements (THR) in 2011, of which 17,000 used ceramic-on-ceramic (CoC) articulations [13]. For the same time period, the QEH performed 899 total hip replacements of which 100 were CoC.

The QEH managed five cases of early *delta* CoC liner fractures over 12 months. Two different THR systems were used. Two cases involved Corail©/Pinnacle© (DePuy, Warsaw, IN), and three cases involved Taperloc©/Exceed© (Biomet, Warsaw, IN). Procedures were not all carried out by the same surgeon and all occurred within 9 months of the index procedure.

Revision surgery included retention of the original acetabular component, removal of debris and careful seating of a new *delta* ceramic liner and head. In two cases a sleeved option head was used. All cases have been followed up beyond 1 year with satisfactory outcomes and no further complications.

Case 1 (Figs. 10.1, 10.2 and 10.3)

A 66-year-old female with an unremarkable past medical history underwent primary THR for osteoarthritis. Review of her postoperative images demonstrates gross malseating of the ceramic liner. She experienced some early subjective clunking of the hip that resolved spontaneously without treatment.

Six weeks postoperatively she experienced sudden groin pain radiating down the thigh when transferring from standing to sitting and a crunching sensation on all movements. Radiograph at this stage demonstrated catastrophic liner fracture. She underwent urgent revision surgery; the hip was washed out and the head and liner replaced with ceramic components. Although some debris remained in the soft tissues, she has experienced no further complications.

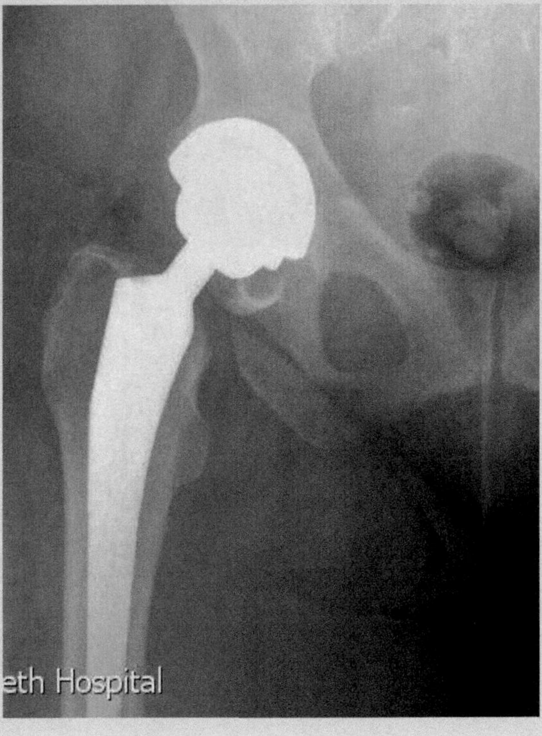

Fig. 10.1 Case 1: Immediate post-op radiograph; gross malseating of liner

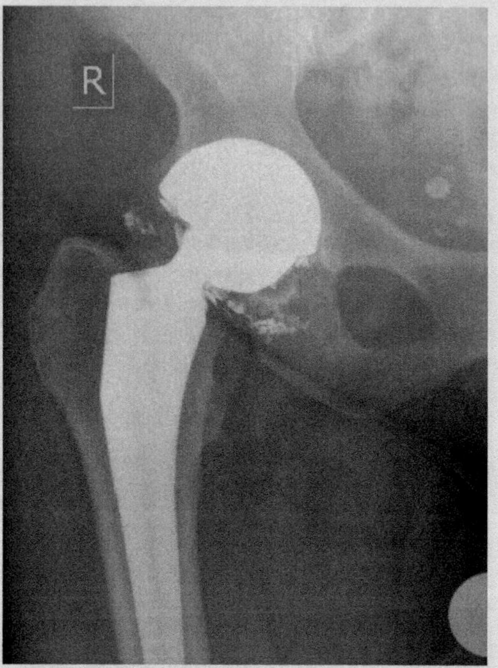

Fig. 10.2 Case 1: Radiograph at presentation at 6 weeks

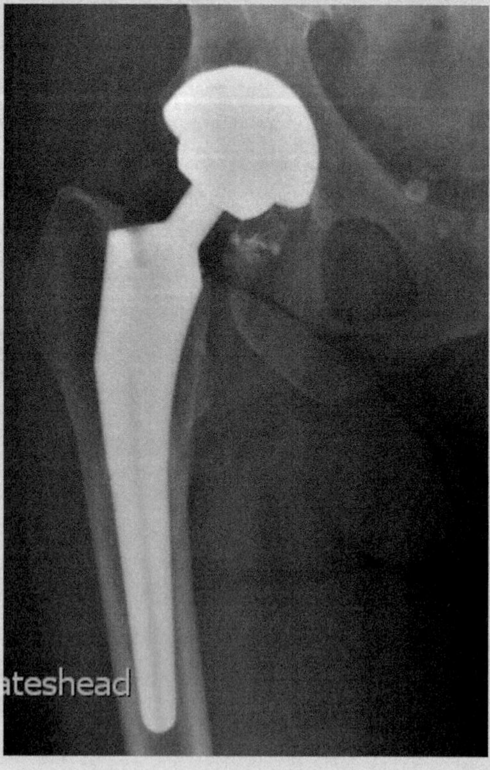

Fig. 10.3 Case 1: Radiograph after revision procedure

Case 2
A 68-year-old female with a past medical history of diabetes mellitus underwent a right total hip replacement for osteoarthritis. At follow-up 4 weeks later, she was mobilising with the aid of one stick, pain-free with no gait abnormalities. Three months after surgery she presented to clinic with sudden onset of grating sensation in right hip with associated creaking. She experienced no pain and had no recent trauma. Retrospective review of initial postoperative radiographs showed subtle liner malseating, and repeat x-rays demonstrated liner fracture. She underwent revision surgery and has had no further complications on follow-up.

Case 3
A fit and well 55-year-old female underwent a left total hip replacement. At follow-up 6 weeks later, she was noted to have a Trendelenburg gait and was referred for physiotherapy. She had no concerns. Seven months after surgery she developed a squeak in her left hip associated with increasing pain and decreasing mobility. Radiographs showed a fractured ceramic liner. Retrospectively there was evidence of subtle liner malseating. She returned to theatre 2 weeks later for revision surgery. Both head and liner were replaced with *delta* ceramic components. At follow-up 6 weeks and 6 months, she has a persisting Trendelenburg gait but otherwise is experiencing no adverse symptoms.

Case 4 (Figs. 10.4, 10.5, 10.6 and 10.7)
A 76-year-old male with no significant medical co-morbidities underwent primary THR for osteoarthritis. Postoperative review of AP radiograph revealed an acceptable position of the articulations. However, retrospectively, the lateral x-ray demonstrates subtle malseating of the ceramic liner.

Thirty-two weeks post-op, this patient presented with acute hip symptoms. Liner fracture was clearly visible on the x-ray. There was also evidence of stem subsidence. He underwent urgent revision, washout and replacement of the ceramic articulations with *delta* ceramic components. The stem was found to be stable intraoperatively. He has experienced no further complications on follow-up.

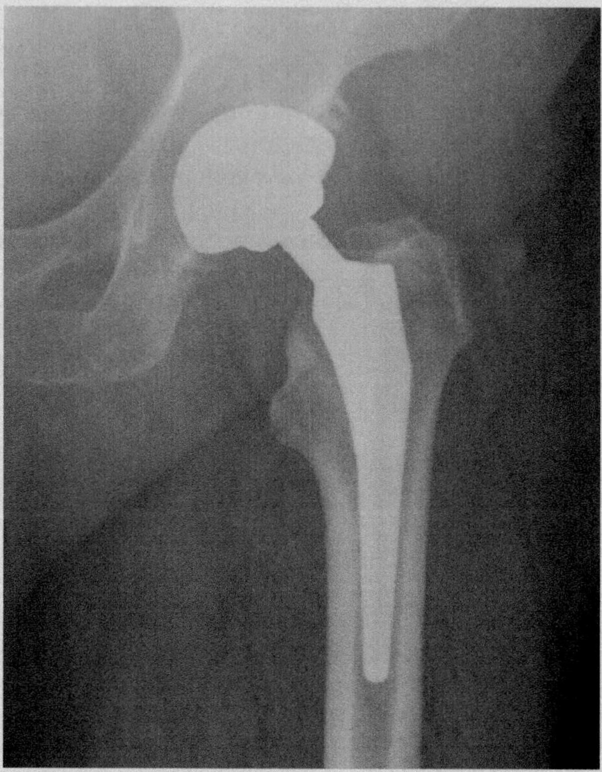

Fig. 10.4 Case 4: Immediate post-op AP radiograph; subtle malseating of liner

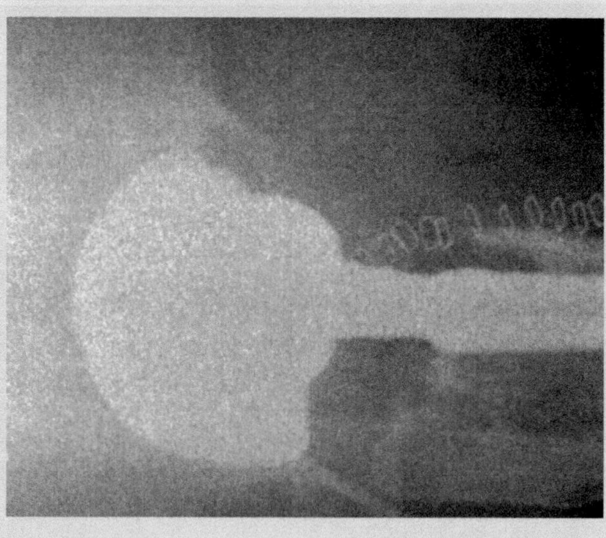

Fig. 10.5 Case 4: Immediate post-op lateral radiograph; subtle malseating of liner

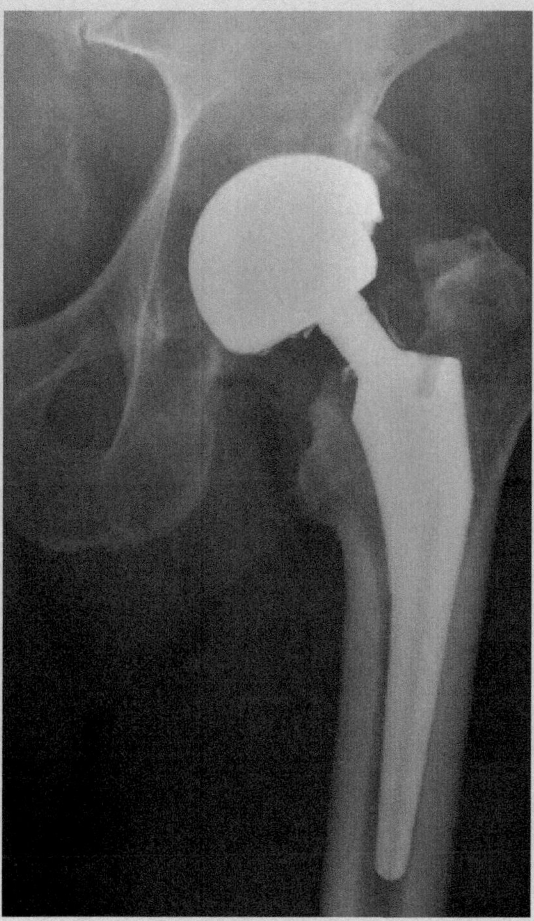

Fig. 10.6 Case 4: Radiograph at presentation at 32 weeks

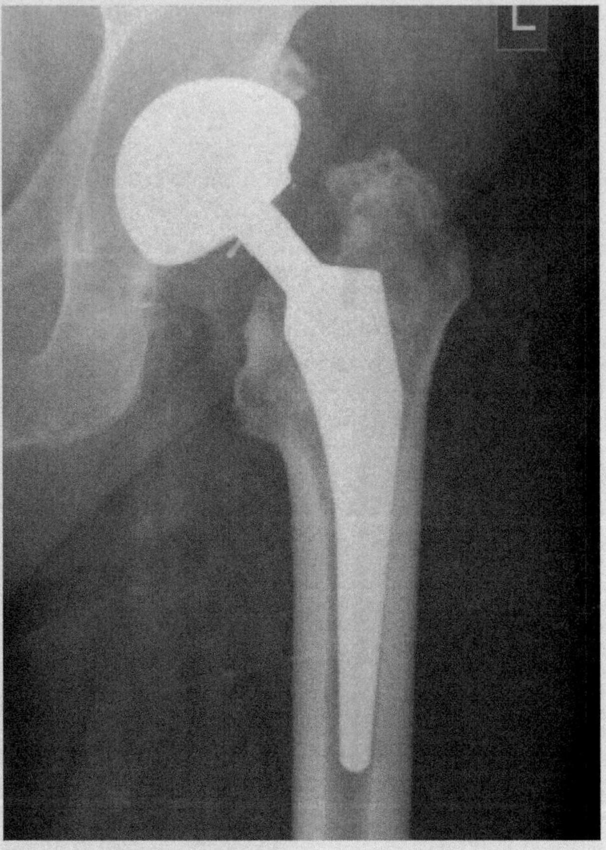

Fig. 10.7 Case 4: Radiograph after revision procedure

Case 5 (Figs. 10.8, 10.9 and 10.10)
A 72-year-old male with significant medical co-morbidities underwent a CoC THR. Six weeks postoperatively malseating of the ceramic liner was noted. He was experiencing minor discomfort at this time. However, in view of his past medical history a decision was made to manage him conservatively rather than subject him to the risks of a further anaesthetic. Unfortunately he subsequently progressed to catastrophic failure with his hip symptoms increasing over time. He then required urgent revision surgery without the luxury of elective pre-op planning.

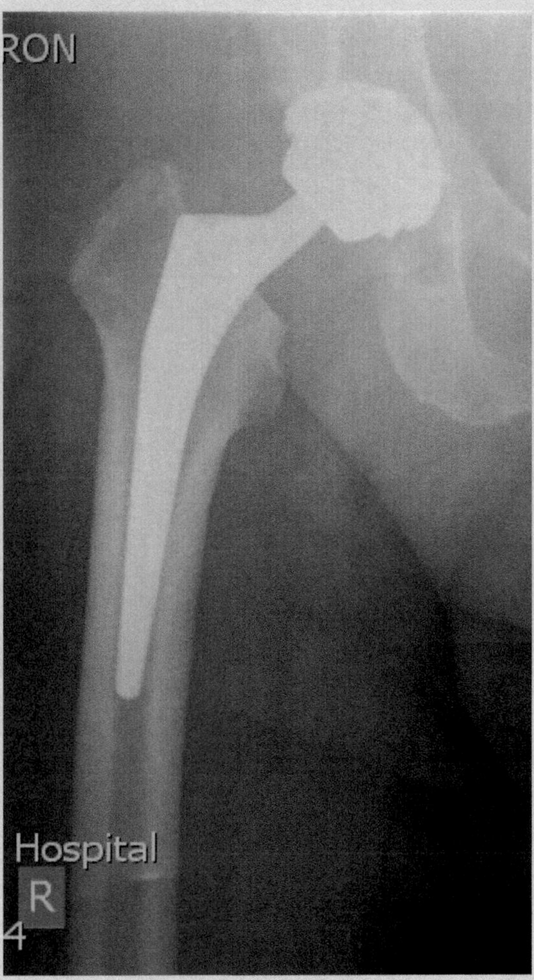

Fig. 10.8 Case 5: Radiograph at 6 week follow-up

Fig. 10.9 Case 5: Radiograph at 12 months

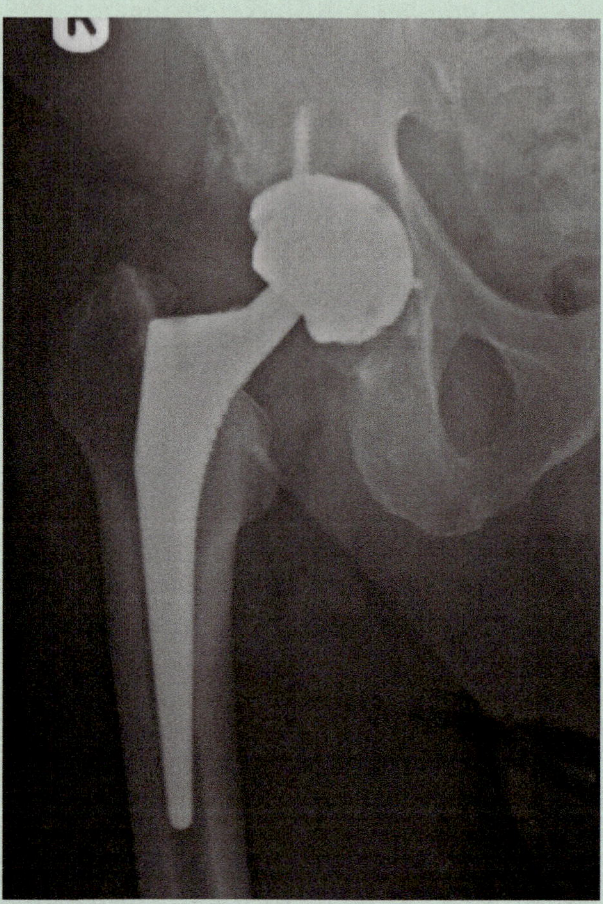

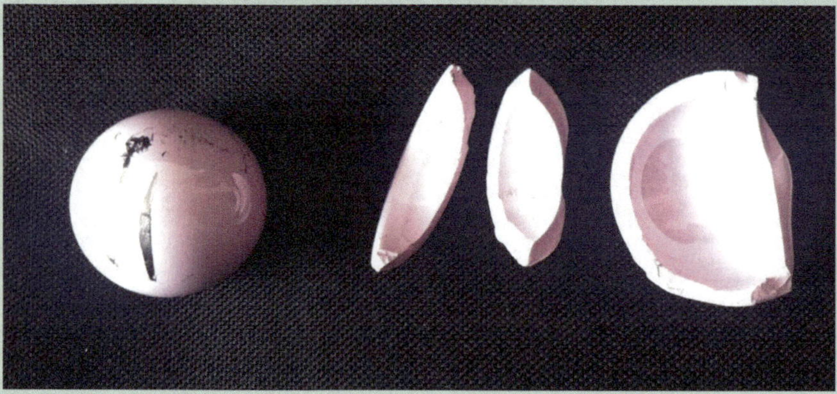

Fig. 10.10 Fractured delta ceramic liner

10.1 Discussion

The first and second generation of ceramics were associated with high fracture rates across all components of 13 and 5%, respectively [3]. Early ceramics are now thought to have been inadequately designed for their role. Third-generation ceramics which were more pure with smaller grain size and improved technical knowledge were associated with a much improved fracture rate of 0–0.004 % [3, 8]. Initially, ceramic-on-ceramic total hip replacements were associated with high rates of loosening [2]; polyethylene ceramic sandwich cups were introduced to counteract the rigid nature of ceramic.

Previous published case studies reporting ceramic liner fracture have predominantly discussed ceramic-polyethylene-titanium sandwich liners. Collectively they have associated liner fracture with stress concentrated on the rim of the liner, flaws in the ceramic and impingement between rim and femoral head [1–4, 7–12]. Several cases from Asian populations have associated peripheral liner stress with loaded hip flexion such when rising from sitting [7]. Liner fracture is also associated with malpositioning of the liner at initial surgery generating stress in the liner.

However fracturing of ceramic liners has been associated with several factors other than the composition of the ceramic. Trauma, level of activity and a high BMI are thought to increase risk of liner fracture [1–4, 7–12]. We found no common precipitating patient factors, and no cases followed trauma or excessive physical activity. There were also no consistent prodromal symptoms.

Intra-operative events have also been linked to fracture in previous generations of ceramic. Accurate alignment of all components is imperative. Actions resulting in peripheral chipping, such as incomplete sitting of the liner, have been associated with fracture [1–4, 7–12] alongside inaccurate acetabular cup positions, which increase the edge loading, or result in impingement [3]. Several previously published case studies report placement error as the prodrome to ceramic liner fracture [4]. This correlates with our findings. All cases presented demonstrated some degree of malseating visible when retrospectively viewing the initial postoperative radiographs.

We noted two distinct types of malseating:

- *Gross malseating*, readily evident on anteroposterior radiograph, often associated with dissociation of the liner and catastrophic failure.
- *Subtle malseating*, more evident on lateral radiograph usually resulting in rim fractures.

Conclusion

Between 2008 and 2011 there was an increase in 10 % of the use of CoC THR in the UK. Rates of revision of CoC and metal-on-polyethylene (MoP) components are comparable at 1.90 % CoC and 1.91 % MoP [13]. However our cases have highlighted a notable risk of ceramic liner fracture regardless of prosthesis used, occurring less than 12 months from initial surgery.

We advocate the need for meticulous technique in seating ceramic liners, a careful review of postoperative radiographs for component malposition and, when required, a low threshold for early revision surgery.

We would advise against nonoperative treatment of malseated ceramic liners which have been noted on x-ray, particularly in symptomatic patients, even if these symptoms are mild, in order to avoid catastrophic failure and the introduction of large volumes of ceramic debris in the joint.

With the use of larger femoral heads and thinner *delta* ceramic liners, there are reduced rates of dislocation, reduced rates of impingement and improved joint stability. The age of the ceramic head fracture may well be over, but are we facing a new dawn, the age of the ceramic liner fracture?

References

1. Min B, Kwang-Soon S, Chul-Hyung K, et al. Delayed fracture of a ceramic insert with modern ceramic total hip replacement. J Arthroplasty. 2007;22(1):136–9.
2. Hasegawa M, Akhiro S, Hitoshi H, Uchida A. Ceramic acetabular liner fracture in total hip arthroplasty with ceramic sandwich cup. J Arthroplasty. 2003;18(5):658–61.
3. Diwanji SR, Seon JK, Song EK, Yoon TR. Fracture of the ABC ceramic liner: a report of 3 cases. Clin Orthop Relat Res. 2007;464:242–6.
4. McCarthy MJH, Halawa M. Lining up the liner: 2 case reports of early ceramic liner fragmentation. J Arthroplasty. 2007;22:8.
5. Hwang SK, Oh JR, Her MS, et al. Fracture dissociation of a ceramic liner. Orthopedics. 2008;31(8):804.
6. www.exac.com/products/hip/acetabular-systems/biolox-delta. CeramTec: BIOLOX®delta. Accessed 2013.
7. Hamilton WG, McAuley JP, Dennis DA, et al. THA with delta ceramic on ceramic: results of a multicenter investigational device exemption trial. Clin Orthop Relat Res. 2010;468(2):358.
8. Taheriazam A, Mohajer MA, Aboulghasemian M, Hajipour B. Fracture of the alumina bearing couple delta ceramic liner. Orthopedics. 2012;35(1):e91.
9. Szymanski C, Gueriot S, Boniface O, et al. Sandwich type ceramic liner fracture rate with Atlas III socket: a study of 144 primary total hip replacements at a mean 74 month follow up. Orthop Traumatol Surg Res. 2011;97:494–500.
10. Ha YC, Kim SY, Kim HJ, et al. Ceramic liner fracture after cementless alumina on alumina total hip replacement. Clin Orthop Relat Res. 2006;458:106–10.
11. Toni A, Traina F, Sudanese A, et al. Early diagnosis of ceramic liner fracture; guidelines based o 12 year clinical experience. J Bone Joint Surg Am. 2006;88(Supl 4):55–63.
12. Chotai PN, Su EP. Fracture of the titanium sleeve encased third generation ceramic liner in a modern total hip arthroplasty. Orthopedics. 2011;34(10):e682.
13. UK National Joint Registry. http://www.njrcentre.org.uk/njrcentre/default.aspx.

Part IV

Metal-on-Metal: Still an Option?

Current Concepts in Metal-on-Metal Articulations

11

K.-P. Günther, J. Schmitt, F. Hannemann, J. Lützner, A. Seidler, C. Kopkow, E. Haase, S. Kirschner, and A. Hartmann

Total hip replacement (THR) for patients with osteoarthritis is one of the most successful surgical interventions in general inducing substantial improvement of health-related quality of life of affected patients [1]. Implant survival can be limited, however, by mechanical wear of bearing materials, which often leads to aseptic loosening. Increasing demands in young and physically active patient groups

K.-P. Günther (✉)
University Hospital Carl Gustav Carus Dresden, University Centre of Orthopaedics and Traumatology, Fetscherstr. 74, 01307 Dresden, Germany
e-mail: klaus-peter.guenther@uniklinikum-dresden.de

J. Schmitt • C. Kopkow
Centre for Evidence-Based Health Care, Fetscherstr. 74, 01307 Dresden, Germany

University of Dresden, Occupational and Social Medicine, Fetscherstr. 74, 01307 Dresden, Germany

F. Hannemann • S. Kirschner
University Hospital Carl Gustav Carus Dresden, University Centre of Orthopaedics and Traumatology, Fetscherstr. 74, 01307 Dresden, Germany

Centre for Evidence-Based Health Care, Fetscherstr. 74, 01307 Dresden, Germany

J. Lützner • A. Hartmann
University Hospital Carl Gustav Carus Dresden, University Centre of Orthopaedics and Traumatology, Fetscherstr. 74, 01307 Dresden, Germany

A. Seidler
University of Dresden, Occupational and Social Medicine, Fetscherstr. 74, 01307 Dresden, Germany

E. Haase
Centre for Evidence-Based Health Care, Fetscherstr. 74, 01307 Dresden, Germany

K. Knahr (ed.), *Tribology in Total Hip and Knee Arthroplasty*,
DOI 10.1007/978-3-642-45266-6_11, © EFORT 2014

resulted in the development of bearing materials with improved wear characteristics. These "hard-on-hard"-bearings are characterized by potential combinations of highly cross-linked polyethylene, ceramic, or metal cup inserts with ceramic or metal heads.

Metal-on-metal (MoM) bearings have been applied in conventional THR for several decades with promising results from early applications [2–5]. Low wear potential of mechanically well-investigated prostheses, no relevant risk of material fracture, and a high design variability seemed to justify the application of MoM bearings even in hip resurfacing arthroplasty (HRA) and large-head total hip replacement (LH-THR) [6, 7]. However, wear and corrosion of these implants may lead to a release of metal products into the surrounding tissue and body fluids as well as the internal organs. Metal accumulation may result in local as well as systemic adverse effects (i.e., toxicity, teratogenicity, and carcinogenicity). Recent reports on pseudotumor formation after resurfacing [8, 9] and high failure rates of specific THR and LH-THR implants [10, 11] induced a very controversial discussion on the indication as well as necessity of clinical follow-up investigations after implantation of MoM implants [12–14]. The aim of this chapter is to summarize the current knowledge on the potential risks of MoM and to provide recommendations about appropriate handling of patients with implanted MoM THR.

11.1 Types of MoM Implants

Survival rates as well as the release of metal ions from the prosthesis show relevant differences according to the type of MoM implants. By convention, the following design categories of MoM bearing articulations, which can be used for hip arthroplasty, are differentiated (Fig. 11.1a–c):

1. Small-head MoM THR: Modular metal head on a hip stem with a modular metal insert in a metal socket and a head diameter of 32 mm or less
2. Large-head MoM THR: Modular metal head on a hip stem with a metal cup and a head diameter of 36 mm or more (the metal cup can be either a modular insert or a monobloc cup)
3. Resurfacing (HRA): Metal resurfacing head with a monobloc metal cup

11.2 Survival Rates of Contemporary MoM Implants

11.2.1 Small-Head THR

In clinical studies, survival rates depend on the type of metal bearing: For Metasul®, good 10-year results of 94–98 % survival [15–17] are reported. The results of other implants with lower carbide concentrations, however, are significantly worse [18–20]. There are also some reports indicating the development of local adverse reactions to metal debris in small-head MoM THR [21, 22].

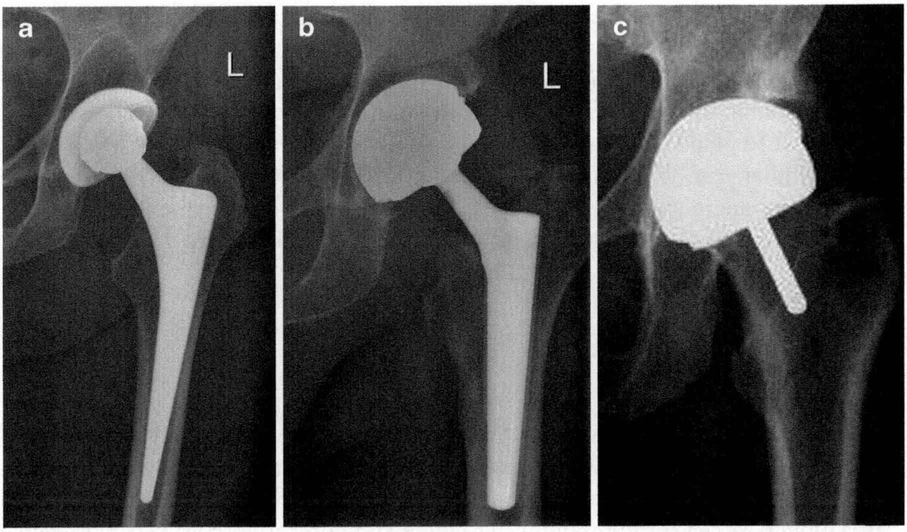

Fig. 11.1 Examples of small-head MoM THR (**a**), large-head MoM THR (**b**), and hip resurfacing arthroplasty (**c**)

In the Australian Arthroplasty Registry [23], the 11-year revision rate for MoM THR with a head diameter of ≤32 mm is 6.0 %. It is similar to the revision rate for ceramic-on-ceramic (5.8 %) as well as for ceramic on highly cross-linked PE (5.7 %) and significantly better than the revision rates for conventional polyethylene with ceramic heads (9.3 %) and metal heads (8.9 %).

From currently available data, it can be concluded that high-quality MoM bearings with head diameters of ≤32 mm seem to show sufficient 10-year survival rates which meet current international benchmarks for the performance of modern primary joint replacement. Metal products are probably released, however, from small-head MoM implants as well as from all other MoM implants. As systematic investigations of large patient cohorts are currently not available, it is not possible to determine the potential risk of local adverse reactions in those patients.

11.2.2 Large-Head MoM THR

Recently, high revision rates have been reported for large-head MoM implants after relatively short follow-up: 3.5 years postoperatively, Bosker et al. [10] report 39 % CT-diagnosed pseudotumors in patients with a revision rate of 12 %, of a Magnum/ReCap® configuration even in short- and medium-term reports that document the poor performance of these implants due to a high incidence of pseudotumor formation. Meyer et al. [24] described the results of a histological investigation in 114 revised implants out of a series of 650 operated patients (805 hips). They conclude that the high failure rate may be due to a combination of elevated metal ion release and fretting corrosion at the taper due to the large head diameter. In the Australian Registry [23], the 10-year cumulative percent revision of MoM implants with a head diameter of 36 mm and more is four times higher (20.3 %) than the revision rate of ceramic-on-ceramic bearings with similar diameter. In the National Joint Registry of England and Wales, a cumulative revision rate of 7.6 % for MoM heads with a diameter of 36 mm in women aged 60–70 is calculated after 7 years, while the revision rate in the same cohort is 2.8 % for ceramic-on-ceramic [25].

Due to the unsatisfactory results, several organizations have recently recommended a "time-out" for large-head MoM THR.

11.2.3 Resurfacing

In a recent meta-analysis, Van der Weegen et al. [26] reported a HRA survival of 84–100 % in 29 articles (10,621 resurfaced hips) with a mean follow-up of 0.6–10.5 years. The number of available investigations with long-term follow-up is still very limited [27–30], representing all single-surgeon series. Survival rates range from 87.0 to 95.5 %, and only two series reported a revision rate of less than 10 % after 10 years, which can be considered as a benchmark of satisfactory performance of a primary THA according to the National Institute of Clinical Excellence (NICE). We have recently published the results of a long-term follow-up study [31], where the overall survival rate of 88 % did also not meet this full 10-year benchmark. We could, however, observe a superior survival rate of 93 % in a cohort of male patients. In the meantime, it is well known that better results can be obtained with HRA in male patients. Additional factors which seem to support improved survival rates are sufficient implant size (>50 mm head size), patient age, and surgeon's experience. Design characteristics have also to be taken into account.

A major limitation of all published long-term studies is the lack of systematic investigation regarding the prevalence of local ARMD (adverse reaction to metal debris) even in clinically and radiographically well-performing implants. Neither in our own investigation nor in other long-term studies has it been tried to visualize local soft tissue reactions to metallic debris. Even when no osteolytic changes can be seen on plain radiographs, the potential presence of ARMD cannot be excluded.

Hip registry data can also not provide this information, as they do only report the rate of revision procedures. Nevertheless, the results of these registries are very important. The first registry which provides long-term survival rates is published in Australia [23]. HRA revision rates 11 years postoperatively are 9.5 % for HRA and 7.2 % for conventional THA. Obviously, there is a substantial difference between male and female gender, as the revision rate in female patients (16.9 %) is three times higher than the revision rate in male patients (6.1 %). The 10-year revision rate for HRA with femoral head size ≥50 mm is below 5 %, while implants with a head size ≤49 mm show a 12 % revision rate. In the Australian database, the 7-year revision rate is 5.1 % for BHR® resurfacing and 23.4 % for ASR® resurfacing. As extremely bad results for the latter implant have also been documented in clinical studies [11], this prosthesis has been withdrawn from the market.

Five years postoperatively, the prosthesis survival in British Registries [32] is 94 % for HRA and 96–99 % for conventional THA. In summary, the survival rates of HRA in registries are generally lower than in conventional implants, but comparable results can be achieved in subgroups of male patients with well-performing implants and sufficient head size as well as adequate positioning. However, it is also not possible to gain information on the incidence of metal-related problems from registry data in general.

11.3 Release of Metal Products from Implants

MoM hip replacements may release metallic products (i.e., particles, ions, metallo-organic compounds) due to wear and corrosion [33, 34]. Metal ions from the corresponding alloying element (i.e., cobalt, Co; chromium, Cr; titanium, Ti; nickel, Ni; molybdenum, Mo) can be measured in the joint itself as well as in surrounding tissue and body fluids. As the risk of local adverse reactions of MoM THR has been reported to correlate with the level of systemic metal ion concentrations [8, 9, 35–39], metal ion determination is used as a surrogate measure for metal exposure.

We have recently performed a systematic review to summarize the clinical and epidemiological evidence concerning the impact of MoM implants on metal ion levels in body fluids [40]. Overall, 104 studies (11 RCTs, 14 cohort studies, 1 case–control study, 55 cross-sectional studies, 23 case series) totaling 9,957 patients with measurement of metal ions in body fluids could be analyzed regarding study as well as patient characteristics, type and position of implants, details of metal ion assessment (i.e., type of metal ions, medium of assessment, method of analysis), and clinical outcome.

An important result of this systematic review is that the median as well as the maximum serum Co and Cr levels were consistently higher at all postoperative assessments in patients who received large-head MoM THR and HRA when compared to patients after small-head MoM THR. Maximum Co concentrations after implantation of small-head MoM implants ranged between 0.72 and 26.0 μg/L, while the highest Co concentrations were observed after large-head MoM THR (range of maximum values, 1.8–79.3 μg/L) and after HRA (range of maximum values, 1.4–124.9). In some studies, median Co concentrations peaked at 12 months' follow-up and declined after the run-in period. Other investigations showed stable and/or increased median serum Co concentrations until 4 years postoperatively.

Conclusions on the association of patient characteristics (i.e., age and gender) on metal ion concentration could not be drawn due to a lack of standardization in the design and reporting of the epidemiological studies included.

Metal ion concentration is most often measured in whole blood and serum, preferred technique is inductively coupled plasma mass spectrometry (ICP-MS).

From this review, it can be concluded that after hip replacement with contemporary MoM bearings, the release of metal ions is highest in stemmed implants with large heads followed by resurfacing devices and also – but on a lower level – small heads.

11.4 Metal-Related Adverse Events

As the implantation of MoM hip arthroplasty leads to a release of metal products (i.e., particles, ions, metallo-organic compounds), a deposition of these substances in body fluids, lymph nodes, bone marrow, and internal organs is possible. This can lead to local as well as systemic adverse events.

11.4.1 Local Adverse Events

Local tissue responses to metal particles are often described as "metallosis." Willert et al. [41] have introduced a more specific concept of "aseptic lymphocytic vasculitis-associated lesion" (ALVAL) based on a lymphocyte-dominated immunological response within the periprosthetic tissues from MoM implants. Pandit et al. [42] described the occurrence of "pseudotumors," which are cystic/solid masses developing in relation to failed metal prostheses. Finally, Natu et al. [43] developed the term "adverse reactions to metal debris" (ARMD), which summarizes the histopathology seen in association with MoM hip arthroplasties including ALVAL, lymphoid neogenesis, granulomatous inflammation, and metallosis. The clinical spectrum of adverse local events is large and can range from small asymptomatic cysts to large cystic or solid soft tissue masses (pseudotumors, Fig. 11.2a–d) as well as large osteolyses with bone destruction around the prosthesis (Fig. 11.3). The most appropriate diagnostic tools to assess the severity of bone and soft tissue destruction are conventional radiographs/CT and MRI with metal artifact reduction sequence (MARS-MRI).

Currently, it is difficult to determine the prevalence of ARMD in MoM THR, as the number of systematic studies with appropriate screening techniques and follow-up is very small. The published incidence of pseudotumors in large-head MoM THA and HRA ranges from 0 to 61 % in different series [9, 36, 44, 45]. In small-head MoM bearings, no systematic studies exist.

In several recent investigations, an association between elevated metal ion levels and the occurrence of ARMD has been assessed. Some authors have even tried to define cutoff levels for well-functioning versus bad functioning prostheses [8, 9, 11, 35–37, 39]. While initially in the Medicines and Healthcare Products Regulatory Agency Medical Device Alert [46], a threshold level of 7 μg/L cobalt and/or chromium has been reported, those studies tend to recommend lower levels of 3.5–4.5 μg/L [35, 39].

11.4.2 Systemic Adverse Events

Potential systemic risks of an exposition to cobalt and/or chromium after MoM hip arthroplasty are toxicity, carcinogenicity, and teratogenicity. As the currently available database of systemic risks is very small, it is very difficult to give valid recommendations.

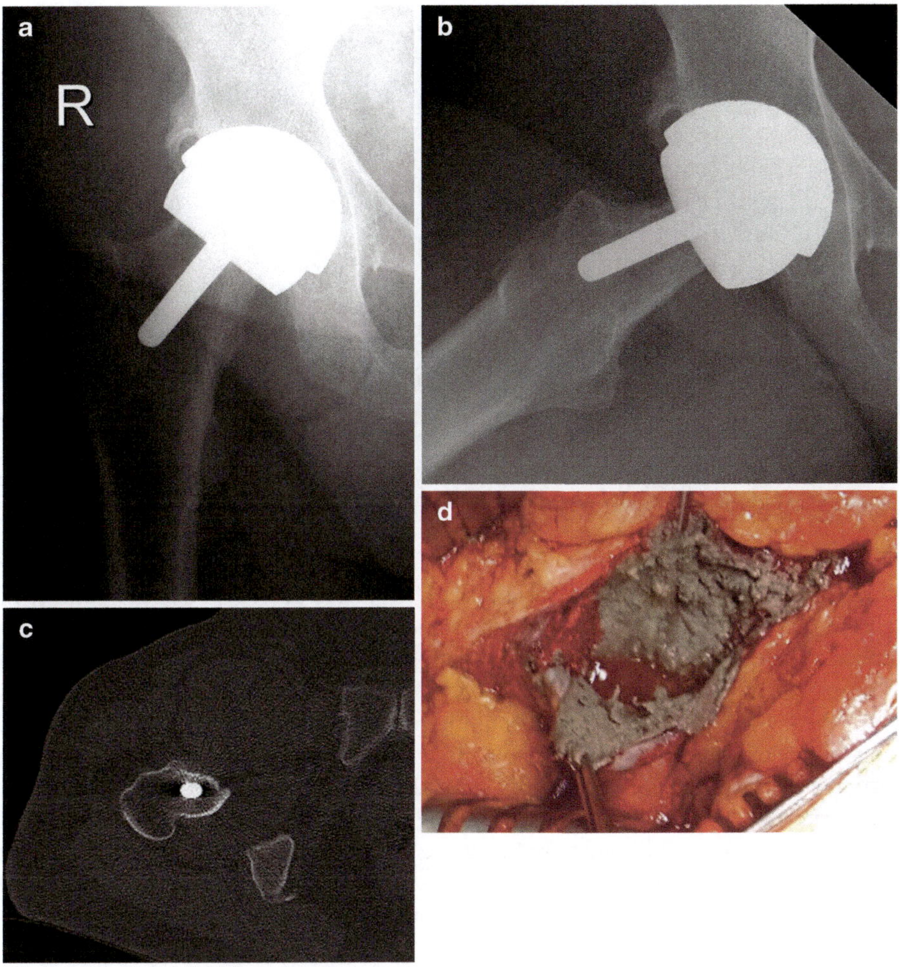

Fig. 11.2 ARMD after hip resurfacing 2005: ap-radiograph of right hip (**a**) and lateral view (**b**) 7 years postoperatively show no relevant osteolysis. A large pseudotumor is diagnosed in the CT, however, anteriorly to the hip joint (**c**), and the intraoperative exposure (**d**) confirms the diagnosis

In several cross-sectional surveys, no clinically relevant impairment of kidney function has been reported even after long follow-up times [16, 47–49]. In a recent case–control study, Prentice et al. [50] described an elevated total body bone mineral density with decreased bone turnover, lower cardiac ejection fraction, and larger left ventricular end-diastolic diameter in HRA patients versus patients with conventional THR. The differences in bone and cardiac function were very small, and no evidence of difference in neuropsychological, renal tubular, hepatic, or endocrine function between patients with and without MoM implants could be identified. These findings, however, indicate that exposure to metal products in patients with well-functioning MoM THR may have a systemic effect.

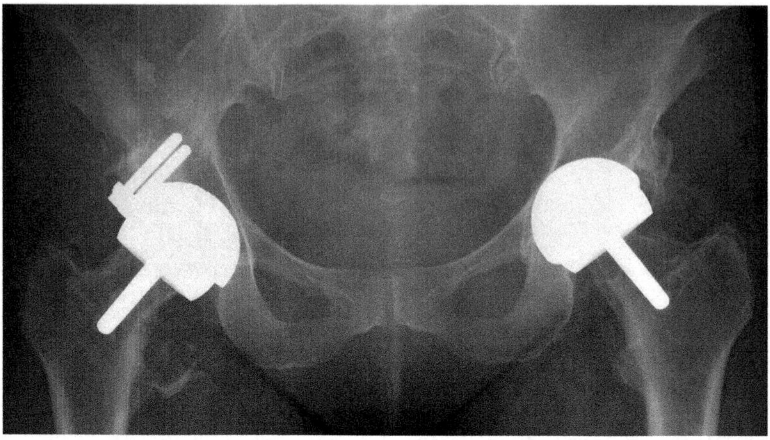

Fig. 11.3 Large acetabular as well as femoral osteolyses on both sides 10 years after hip resurfacing in a 42-year-old female patient

Regarding carcinogenicity, Dunstan et al. [51] have described a larger number of chromosomal aberrations (structural aberrations aneuploidy gain) in a MoM patient cohort when compared to individuals without metal implants. In epidemiological studies and analyses from large arthroplasty registries, conflicting results have been published: Some authors describe slightly elevated incidence of prostate, bladder, and kidney cancer as well as melanoma [52, 53] and higher cancer mortality [54] in patients with MoM THR when compared with other patient groups. It is emphasized, however, that long-term results have been achieved with historic types of MoM implants and cannot be transferred to those with modern design. In a large cohort from the Finnish Arthroplasty Registry, Mäkela et al. [55] could not find an elevated overall risk of cancer in patients with MoM hip implants when compared to the general population. An interesting observation has been reported from a long-term study after total knee replacement [56]: An analysis of the Swedish Knee Arthroplasty Registry showed that cancer risks after knee replacement were elevated, when compared to the overall national cancer incidence in Sweden. The greatest increases in risk were observed for leukemia subtypes and myelodysplastic syndromes, but increases in risk were also observed for breast cancer, prostate cancer, and melanoma. These findings suggest that a potential release of metal products and an association with systemic adverse effects is not only limited to patients with MoM implants but can probably occur also in other patients with all types of metal implants.

One major concern is the potential transplacental transfer of metal products during pregnancy. Two studies have found a transplacental passage of metal ions in women with HRA [57, 58]. They could not identify any teratologic effects, however, and the ion levels in newborns were significantly lower than the levels in their mother's blood. One other study [59] did not find elevated metal ion levels in newborns after small-head MoM THA in their mothers at all. A clear limitation of all investigations to date is that no measurement of core blood was performed up to now in female patients with extremely high metal ion levels. In summary, a teratogenic potential of chromium and cobalt is well known, but there are no documented clinical cases at the moment. Due to the potential of transplacental metal ion transfer, however, MoM THR is not anymore recommended in female patients during childbearing age.

In summary, the database regarding local as well as systemic adverse effects of MoM THR and HRA is not substantial enough to provide detailed conclusions. The potential risk for the development of adverse reactions seems to be associated with the type of implants, as small-head MoM THR have a relatively low incidence of local complications, while adverse tissue reactions to HRA and mainly large-head THR can be very destructive. Although it is unclear yet, whether a carcinogenic potential of MoM implants is substantially different from that of other metallic implants, patients should be informed about this potential risk, and MoM is definitely not indicated in females during childbearing age.

11.5 Recommendations for the Follow-Up of Patients with MoM Implants

Following an international and interdisciplinary expert conference, which was endorsed by several organizations including European Federation of National Associations of Orthopaedics and Traumatology (EFORT), clinically relevant advice on how to treat and monitor current and future patients with MoM THR can be given [60].

11.5.1 Routine Follow-Up Investigations After MoM Implantation

Due to the special risks of MoM bearings, systematic follow-up is recommended for all patients and all implants. For small-head MoM THR, a systematic follow-up comparable to conventional THR is sufficient. A closer follow-up is recommended, however, for large-head MoM (annual follow-up for the life of the joint) as well as HRA. In the latter, annual follow-up for the first 5 years is recommended, then according to local protocols for patients with conventional THR. If metal ion levels are normal at year one and two postoperatively, the frequency of further annual follow-up investigations may be changed to local protocols for conventional THR. In patients with risk factors such as small-size HRA (<50 mm femoral component), female gender, and low coverage arc, annual follow-up for the life of the joint is recommended.

All patients should undergo radiographic examination during follow-up. In case of clinical/radiographic abnormality, additional imaging (ultrasound, CT scan, and/or MARS-MRI) is recommended. Ordinary MRI without MARS technique is ineffective. In case of Co values above a certain threshold (within the range of 2–7 μg/L), additional imaging (e.g., ultrasound, CT scan, and/or MARS-MRI) is recommended.

Monitoring of metal ions should be performed at the time of regular follow-up in asymptomatic patients. In all symptomatic patients, additional monitoring is recommended between regular follow-up investigations. Metal ion determination of body fluids can be performed in blood, serum, and urine (at present measurement of whole blood is most practicable); cobalt should be monitored as reference substance. Ion measurement must be performed under the rules of internal/external quality control (GF-AAS and ICP-MS are considered as valid). The preferred reporting units should be micrograms/l (= ppb). The threshold value for clinical concern is expected to be within the range of 2–7 μg/L (exact levels have still to be determined within this range). In increased values above the threshold, additional imaging even in asymptomatic patients is recommended. Recommendations are based on local effects; critical values for systemic effects have not yet been established for patients after MoM implantation.

11.5.2 Indications for Revision of MoM Implants for Safety Reason

The appropriate management for local ARMD is based on the differentiation, whether a patient has symptoms: In asymptomatic patients, small fluid collection indicative of ARMD needs close monitoring (repeated imaging is recommended). In symptomatic patients and/or patients with progressive osteolysis, large or expanding pseudotumor, and/or progressive neck thinning, and/or cobalt ions above threshold level, revision may be considered.

If the metal ions levels are elevated at first detection, but the patient is asymptomatic, the levels should be confirmed through repeated measurement in asymptomatic patients. Above a threshold of 2–7 μg/L (exact level still to be determined), additional imaging and closer follow-up is recommended. In case of pathological results of additional imaging and/or further significant increase of cobalt level, revision surgery should be discussed with the patient, as significant metal accumulation with local ARMD is to be expected (especially in cobalt values >20 μg/L). In case of excessive elevation (cobalt approximately 20 μg/L or above), because of potential osteolysis, tissue necrosis, and long-term health effects, revision surgery should also be discussed with the patient. The individual risk-to-benefit ratio should always be considered before intervention.

Routine monitoring of metal ions after removal of MoM bearings is not recommended, as no effective interventions can currently be recommended in case of increased metal ions.

11.5.3 Further Topics to Consider

The recommendations also include detailed aspects of appropriate communication with patients as well as surgeons and other medical disciplines. One important issue is detailed information about the benefits, risks, uncertainties, and recommended monitoring concerning MoM bearings in order to support informed decision making (i.e., concerning the implantation of MoM bearings as well as indication for revision in problem cases with implanted MoM bearings).

Finally, a list of future research needs has been provided by the expert group, which contains important aspects of preclinical as well as clinical research. Primary issues of experimental work should address, for example, the determination of production mechanisms and internal distribution of metal products in different implants, impact of additional metal ions (i.e., titanium), as well as interaction between wear/corrosion of MoM interfaces and taper connections. Future clinical research should include aspects of metal ion determination (i.e., reproducibility of metal ion measurements among different labs, investigation of urine as screening tool, ion levels after implantation of other artificial implant). As it is not possible at the moment to define generally accepted cutoff levels for metal ions indicating malfunction, it is important to investigate effects of long-term exposure to metal ion concentrations between 2 and 7 μg/L. Furthermore, it is necessary to determine distribution paths of particles/ions/metallo-organic compounds and the clinical relevance of their potential systemic effects. Also the true incidence of ARMD in all different types of MoM implants (including assessment of correlations between the presence of wear/corrosion at taper connections and the presence/extent of adverse local tissue reactions) has to be analyzed.

References

1. Learmonth ID, Young C, Rorabeck C. The operation of the century: total hip replacement. Lancet. 2007;370:1508–19.
2. Dorr LD, Wan Z, Longjohn DB, Dubois B, Murken R. Total hip arthroplasty with use of Metasul metal-on-metal articulation. Four to seven-year results. J Bone Joint Surg Am. 2000;82-A(6):789–98.
3. Rieker CB, Köttig P. In vivo tribological performance of 231 metal-on-metal hip articulations. Hip Int. 2002;12(2):73–6.
4. Wagner M, Wagner H. Medium-term results of a modern metal-on-metal system in total hip replacement. Clin Orthop Relat Res. 2000;379:123–33.
5. Weber BG. Experience with the Metasul total hip bearing system. Clin Orthop Relat Res. 1996;329(Suppl):S69–77.
6. Amstutz HC, Beaule PE, Dorey FJ, Le Duff MJ, Campbell PA, Gruen TA. Metal-on-metal hybrid surface arthroplasty: two to six-year follow-up study. J Bone Joint Surg Am. 2004;86-A(1):28–39.
7. McMinn DJW, Daniel J, Ziaee H, Pradhan C. Indications and results of hip resurfacing. Int Orthop. 2011;35(2):231–7.
8. Kwon YM, Ostlere SJ, McLardy-Smith P, Athanasou NA, Gill HS, Murray DW. "Asymptomatic" pseudotumors after metal-on-metal hip resurfacing arthroplasty. Prevalence and metal ion study. J Arthroplasty. 2011;26(4):511–8.
9. Matthies AK, Skinner JA, Osmani H, Henckel J, Hart AJ. Pseudotumors are common in well-positioned low-wearing metal-on-metal hips. Clin Orthop Relat Res. 2012;470(7):1895–906.
10. Bosker BH, Ettema HB, Boomsma MF, Kollen BJ, Maas M, Verheyen CC. High incidence of pseudotumour formation after large-diameter metal-on-metal total hip replacement: a prospective cohort study. J Bone Joint Surg Br. 2012;94(6):755–61.
11. Langton DJ, Jameson SS, Joyce TJ, Gandhi JN, Sidaginamale R, Mereddy P, Lord J, Nargol AVF. Accelerating failure rate of the ASR total hip replacement. J Bone Joint Surg Br. 2011;93 B(8):1011–6.

12. Cohen D. How safe are metal-on-metal implants?. BMJ. 2012;344.
13. Godlee F. Serious risks from metal-on-metal hip implants. BMJ. 2012;344.
14. Heneghan C, Langton D, Thompson M. Ongoing problems with metal-on-metal hip implants. BMJ. 2012;344:e1349.
15. Eswaramoorthy V, Moonot P, Kalairajah Y, Biant LC, Field RE. The Metasul metal-on-metal articulation in primary total hip replacement. Clinical and radiological results at ten years. J Bone Joint Surg Br. 2008;90-B:1278–83.
16. Grübl A, Marker M, Brodner W, Giurea A, Heinze G, Meisinger V, Zehetgruber H, Kotz R. Long-term follow-up of metal-on-metal total hip replacement. J Orthop Res. 2007;25(7): 841–8.
17. Zenz P, Stiehl JB, Knechtel H, Titzer-Hochmaier G, Schwagerl W. Ten year follow-up of the non-porous Allofit cementless acetabular component. J Bone Joint Surg Br. 2009; 91-B:1443–7.
18. Korovessis P, Petsinis G, Repanti M, Repantis T. Metallosis after contemporary metal-on-metal total hip arthroplasty. Five to nine-year follow-up. J Bone Joint Surg Am. 2006;88(6): 1183–91.
19. Milosev I, Trebse R, Kovac S, Cor A, Pisot V. Survivorship and retrieval analysis of Sikomet metal-on-metal total hip replacements at a mean of seven years. J Bone Joint Surg Am. 2006; 88(6):1173–82.
20. Park YS, Moon YW, Lim SJ, Yang JM, Ahn G, Choi YL. Early osteolysis following second-generation metal-on-metal hip replacement. J Bone Joint Surg Am. 2005;87(7):1515–21.
21. Baur W, Honle W, Willert HG, Schuh A. Pathological findings in tissue surrounding revised metal/metal articulations. Orthopade. 2005;34(3):225–6. 8–33.
22. Gruber FW, Bock A, Trattnig S, Lintner F, Ritschl P. Cystic lesion of the groin due to metallosis: a rare long-term complication of metal-on-metal total hip arthroplasty. J Arthroplasty. 2007;22(6):923–7.
23. Australian Orthopaedic Association, National Joint Replacement Registry. Hip and knee arthroplasty – annual report 2012. University of Adelaide. 2012. https://aoanjrr.dmac.adelaide.edu.au/documents/10180/60142/Annual%20Report%202012?version=1.2&t=1355186837517.
24. Meyer H, Mueller T, Goldau G, Chamaon K, Ruetschi M, Lohmann CH. Corrosion at the cone/taper interface leads to failure of large-diameter metal-on-metal total hip arthroplasties. Clin Orthop Relat Res. 2012;470(11):3101–8.
25. National Joint Registry. National Joint Registry for England and Wales. 9th annual report. Surgical data to 31st December 2011. http://www.njrcentre.org.uk/njrcentre/Portals/0/Documents/England/Reports/9th_annual_report/NJR%209th%20Annual%20Report%202012.pdf
26. van der Weegen W, Hoekstra HJ, Sijbesma T, Bos E, Schemitsch EH, Poolman RW. Survival of metal-on-metal hip resurfacing arthroplasty: a systematic review of the literature. J Bone Joint Surg Br. 2011;93(3):298–306.
27. Amstutz HC, Le Duff MJ, Campbell PA, Gruen TA, Wisk LE. Clinical and radiographic results of metal-on-metal hip resurfacing with a minimum ten-year follow-up. J Bone Joint Surg Am. 2010;92(16):2663–71.
28. Baker RP, Pollard TC, Eastaugh-Waring SJ, Bannister GC. A medium-term comparison of hybrid hip replacement and Birmingham hip resurfacing in active young patients. J Bone Joint Surg Br. 2011;93(2):158–63.
29. Daniel J, Ziaee H, Kamali A, Pradhan C, Band T, McMinn DJ. Ten-year results of a double-heat-treated metal-on-metal hip resurfacing. J Bone Joint Surg Br. 2010;92(1):20–7.
30. Treacy RB, McBryde CW, Shears E, Pynsent PB. Birmingham hip resurfacing: a minimum follow-up of ten years. J Bone Joint Surg Br. 2011;93(1):27–33.
31. Hartmann A, Lützner J, Kirschner S, Witzleb WC, Gunther KP. Do survival rate and serum ion concentrations 10 years after metal-on-metal hip resurfacing provide evidence for continued use? Clin Orthop Relat Res. 2012;470(11):3118–26.

32. National Joint Registry. National Joint Registry for England and Wales. 8th annual report. Surgical data to 31st December 2010. 2011.
33. Ishida T, Clarke IC, Donaldson TK, Shirasu H, Shishido T, Yamamoto K. Comparing ceramic-metal to metal-metal total hip replacements–a simulator study of metal wear and ion release in 32- and 38-mm bearings. J Biomed Mater Res B Appl Biomater. 2009;91(2):887–96.
34. Yan Y, Neville A, Dowson D, Williams S, Fisher J. Effect of metallic nanoparticles on the biotribocorrosion behaviour of Metal-on-Metal hip prostheses. Wear. 2009;267:683–8.
35. Hart AJ, Sabah SA, Bandi AS, Maggiore P, Tarassoli P, Sampson B, Skinner JA. Sensitivity and specificity of blood cobalt and chromium metal ions for predicting failure of MoM hip replacement. J Bone Joint Surg Br. 2011;93-B:1308–13.
36. Kwon YM, Thomas P, Summer B, Pandit H, Taylor A, Beard D, Murray DW, Gill HS. Lymphocyte proliferation responses in patients with pseudotumors following metal-on-metal hip resurfacing arthroplasty. J Orthop Res. 2010;28(4):444–50.
37. Langton DJ, Jameson SS, Joyce TJ, Hallab NJ, Natu S, Nargol AVF. Early failure of metal-on-metal bearings in hip resurfacing and large-diameter total hip replacement: a consequence of excess wear. J Bone Joint Surg Br. 2010;92-B(1):38–46.
38. Langton DJ, Joyce TJ, Jameson SS, Lord J, van Orsouw M, Holland JP, Nargol AVF, De Smet KA. Adverse reaction to metal debris following hip resurfacing: the influence of component type, orientation and volumetric wear. J Bone Joint Surg Br. 2011;93-B(2):164–71.
39. van der Straeten C, Grammatopoulos G, Gill HS, Calistri A, Campbell P, De Smet KA. The 2012 Otto Aufranc Award: the interpretation of metal ion levels in unilateral and bilateral hip resurfacing. Clin Orthop Relat Res. 2012;471(2):377–85.
40. Hartmann A, Hannemann F, Lutzner J, Seidler A, Drexler H, Gunther KP, Schmitt J. Metal ion concentrations in body fluids after implantation of hip replacements with metal-on-metal bearing – systematic review of clinical and epidemiological studies. PLoS One. 2013;8(8):e70359.
41. Willert HG, Buchhorn GH, Fayyazi A, Flury R, Windler M, Koster G, Lohmann CH. Metal-on-metal bearings and hypersensitivity in patients with artificial hip joints. A clinical and histomorphological study. J Bone Joint Surg Am. 2005;87(1):28–36.
42. Pandit H, Glyn-Jones S, McLardy-Smith P, Gundle R, Whitwell D, Gibbons CL, Ostlere S, Athanasou N, Gill HS, Murray DW. Pseudotumours associated with metal-on-metal hip resurfacings. J Bone Joint Surg Br. 2008;90(7):847–51.
43. Natu S, Sidaginamale RP, Gandhi J, Langton DJ, Nargol AV. Adverse reactions to metal debris: histopathological features of periprosthetic soft tissue reactions seen in association with failed metal on metal hip arthroplasties. J Clin Pathol. 2012;65(5):409–18.
44. Daniel J, Holland J, Quigley L, Sprague S, Bhandari M. Pseudotumors associated with total hip arthroplasty. J Bone Joint Surg Am. 2012;94(1):86–93.
45. Williams DH, Greidanus NV, Masri BA, Duncan CP, Garbuz DS. Prevalence of pseudotumor in asymptomatic patients after metal-on-metal hip arthroplasty. J Bone Joint Surg Am. 2011;93(23):2164–71.
46. Medicines and Healthcare Products Regulatory Agency (MHRA). Medical Device Alert. All metal-on-metal (MoM) hip replacements. MDA/2012/008. MHRA, London. 2012. http://www.mhra.gov.uk/home/groups/dts-bs/documents/medicaldevicealert/con155767.pdf.
47. Daniel J, Ziaee H, Pradhan C, Pynsent PB, McMinn DJW. Renal clearance of cobalt in relation to the use of metal-on-metal bearings in hip arthroplasty. J Bone Joint Surg Am. 2010; 92-A(4):840–5.
48. Marker M, Gruebl A, Riedl O, Heinze G, Pohanka E, Kotz R. Metal-on-metal hip implants: do they impair renal function in the long-term? A 10-year follow-up study. Arch Orthop Trauma Surg. 2008;128(9):915–9.
49. Yang J, Shen B, Zhou Z, Pei F, Kang P. Changes in cobalt and chromium levels after metal-on-metal hip resurfacing in young, active Chinese patients. J Arthroplasty. 2011;26(1):65–70.
50. Prentice JR, Clark MJ, Hoggard N, Morton AC, Tooth C, Paley MN, Stockley I, Hadjivassiliou M, Wilkinson JM. Metal-on-metal hip prostheses and systemic health: a cross-sectional association study 8 years after implantation. PLoS One. 2013;8(6):e66186.

51. Dunstan E, Ladon D, Whittingham-Jones P, Carrington R, Briggs TW. Chromosomal aberrations in the peripheral blood of patients with metal-on-metal hip bearings. J Bone Joint Surg Am. 2008;90(3):517–22.
52. Onega T, Baron J, MacKenzie T. Cancer after total joint arthroplasty: a meta-analysis. Cancer Epidemiol Biomarkers Prev. 2006;15(8):1532–7.
53. Visuri T, Pukkala E, Pulkkinen P, Paavolainen P. Decreased cancer risk in patients who have been operated on with total hip and knee arthroplasty for primary osteoarthrosis. A meta-analysis of 6 Nordic cohorts with 73,000 patients. Acta Orthop Scand. 2003;74(3):351–60.
54. Visuri T, Borg H, Pulkkinen P, Paavolainen P, Pukkala E. A retrospective comparative study of mortality and causes of death among patients with metal-on-metal and metal-on-polyethylene total hip prostheses in primary osteoarthritis after a long-term follow-up. BMC Musculoskelet Disord. 2010;11(78):78.
55. Mäkelä KT, Visuri T, Pulkkinen P, Eskelinen A, Remes V, Virolainen P, Junnila M, Pukkala E. Risk of cancer with metal-on-metal hip replacements: population based study. BMJ. 2012; 345:e4646.
56. Wagner P, Olsson H, Lidgren L, Robertsson O, Ranstam J. Increased cancer risks among arthroplasty patients: 30 year follow-up of the Swedish Knee Arthroplasty Register. Eur J Cancer. 2011;47(7):1061–71.
57. de Souza RM, Wallace D, Costa ML, Krikler SJ. Transplacental passage of metal ions in women with hip resurfacing: no teratogenic effects observed. Hip Int. 2012;22(1):96–9.
58. Ziaee H, Daniel J, Datta AK, Blunt S, McMinn DJ. Transplacental transfer of cobalt and chromium in patients with metal-on-metal hip arthroplasty: a controlled study. J Bone Joint Surg Br. 2007;89(3):301–5.
59. Brodner W, Grohs JG, Bancher-Todesca D, Dorotka R, Meisinger V, Gottsauner-Wolf F, Kotz R. Does the placenta inhibit the passage of chromium and cobalt after metal-on-metal total hip arthroplasty? J Arthroplasty. 2004;19(8 Suppl 3):102–6.
60. Hannemann F, Hartmann A, Schmitt J, Lutzner J, Seidler A, Campbell P, Delaunay CP, Drexler H, Ettema HB, Garcia-Cimbrelo E, Huberti H, Knahr K, Kunze J, Langton DJ, Lauer W, Learmonth I, Lohmann CH, Morlock M, Wimmer MA, Zagra L, Gunther KP. European multidisciplinary consensus statement on the use and monitoring of metal-on-metal bearings for total hip replacement and hip resurfacing. Orthop Traumatol Surg Res. 2013;99(3):263–71.

Why Is There a Continuing Role for Metal-on-Metal in Hip Replacement?

12

Julien Girard and Henri Migaud

12.1 Introduction

In 2013, total hip arthroplasty (THA) with metal-on-metal (MoM) bearing is still a debated controversy. In fact, the introduction of hard-on-hard bearing (MoM or ceramic on ceramic (CoC)) with excellent tribological properties tries to solve the problem of polyethylene wear. Indeed, THA (especially in young and active patients) showed a very high complication rate with short durability of both components. This is strongly correlated with high polyethylene wear resulting from the active lifestyle population of this "millennium" patient [8, 11]. On the other hand, hard-on-hard bearing shows some disadvantages. CoC bearing has the advantage of having chemical inertness properties. But the acetabular fixation and the head or insert fracture risk remains an ongoing problematic concern [1, 15]. MoM bearing has been problematic since its appearance in the 1960s with the McKee-Farrar THA [4]. The acetabular loosening frequencies were one of the reasons why they were not implanted in the 1970s [7]. At the end of the 1980s, excellent tribological improvements led Weber [24] to reintroduce the MoM bearing. A metallic insert was set in a polyethylene cup, and bone fixation was obtained by acrylic cement. At the beginning of the 1990s, this bearing was reintroduced in a cementless version,

J. Girard, PhD, MD (✉)
Department of Orthopedic Surgery, Roger Salengro Hospital, University of Lille, Lille, France

Department of Sport and Medicine, University of Lille 2, Lille, France

Orthopaedic Department, Lille University Hospital,
2 avenue Oscar Lambret, Lille Cedex 59037, France
e-mail: j_girard_lille@yahoo.fr

H. Migaud, MD
Department of Orthopedic Surgery, Roger Salengro Hospital, University of Lille, Lille, France

K. Knahr (ed.), *Tribology in Total Hip and Knee Arthroplasty*,
DOI 10.1007/978-3-642-45266-6_12, © EFORT 2014

the sandwich being fixed to the acetabulum by press-fit cup [5]. Despite favourable results reported since its reintroduction, there are in 2013 some authors who claim for a relative ending of MoM bearing use. For them, some concerns still exist after a MoM implantation. One of them is the soft tissue reactions or adverse reactions to metal debris (aseptic lymphocyte-dominated vasculitis-associated lesion, pseudotumor, etc.) [25]. Another concern is the release of blood metallic ion and its potential side effects [2, 3]. Through the authors' experience, this article shows that there is a continuing role for MoM hip replacement.

12.2 Author's Experience with the MoM Bearing

12.2.1 MoM THA for Very Young Patients Under 30 Years Old

To date, it is still unclear whether THA provides excellent long-term results in young and active patients. We reported the results of 48 MoM THAs (28-mm head diameter) inserted as a primary hip arthroplasty in patients under the age of 30 years. We evaluated the survival rate with a mean follow-up of 8.1 years [10]. There were 24 males and 12 females, with a mean age of 25 years at the time of surgery (range 15–30). The results were compared with a matched control group of THA using hard-on-soft bearing. The hard-on-soft control group (42 cases (38 patients)) was selected by matching follow-up, sex ratio, BMI and mean age at the procedure. From the hard-on-soft group, the annual linear wear was 0.14 mm/year. From the MoM group, two revisions occurred, one for impingement secondary to cup malposition and one for acetabular loosening with osteolysis. The revision rate was significantly lower than with the hard-on-soft group (45.4 % vs 4.1 %) despite a higher activity level (Devane 4 or 5; 87 % vs 41 %) in the MoM group. The 10-year survivorship was 90 % with a MoM bearing (95 % confidence interval; range 82.4–95.1 %) and still 90 % at 15 years of follow-up, 80.1 % with a ceramic-on-polyethylene bearing (95 % confidence interval; range 72.2–90.3 %) and 60.3 % with a metal-on-polyethylene bearing (95 % confidence interval; range 52.2–69.5 %). We concluded that these encouraging medium-term results in our patients suggest that THA with MoM bearing may be a good solution for very young patients suffering from hip osteoarthritis. Moreover, the lack of or a low osteolysis rate is important for young and active patients because it could lead to easier revision with excellent bone stock preservation.

12.2.2 Hip Resurfacing in Patients Under 30 Years Old

The concept of hip resurfacing seems very attractive for this specific population by associating a hard-on-hard bearing component limiting the wear, a large femoral head dramatically reducing the risk of dislocation, and the femoral bone stock preservation. We studied 22 patients with 24 hips [11]. The mean age at operation was 24.9 years (17.1–29.9). At an average follow-up of 24.6 months (18–34), there was no revision. The mean UCLA activity score improved from a mean of 5.5 (1–9) preoperatively to 7.6 (1–10) postoperatively. The mean Harris hip score increased from 43.9 (19–67) to 89.3 (55–100), and no dislocation was observed in this group. Despite the challenge in performing hip resurfacing in very young and active population with dysplastic cases, the clinical and radiological short-term results in this series are encouraging and demonstrate comparable outcomes to standard THA at this early stage.

This study supports the use of MoM hip resurfacing as a suitable alternative to conventional THA for this complex group of patients. Moreover, the specific advantages of hip resurfacing (bone stock preservation, excellent stability, low risk of dislocation, large diameter of the articulation, biomechanical restoration, etc.) made this procedure a very attractive option for younger patients.

12.2.3 MoM THA for Young and Active Patients Under 50 Years Old

The current authors reported 39 MoM cementless 28-mm THAs (30 patients with a mean age of 39 (23–49)) and compared it to a control group including 39 ceramic-on-polyethylene cementless hip replacement in 28 mm (32 patients with a mean age of 40 (15–49)) [19]. The mean follow-up was 151 months (144–166). At the revision, the mean Oxford score was 15.3 points (12–35). The median concentration of cobalt was 1 μg/L (0.4–4.8), and the median concentration of chromium was 1.2 μg/L (0.1–5.6). The 12-year survivorship with revision for any reason as end point was 70 % (confidence interval at 95 %, 63–77 %) for the ceramic-on-polyethylene cohort versus 100 % in the MoM cohort. MoM bearings improved arthroplasty survivorship and reduced the rate of osteolysis compared to hard-on-soft bearing in young and active patients after a minimum 12-year follow-up. Moreover, current wrought metal-on-metal implants with a 28-mm-diameter head and high carbide concentration did not produce the high rates of osteolysis and allergic reactions that may be observed with cast low-carbide metal-on-metal bearings after a shorter duration of follow-up.

12.2.4 MoM Bearing Use for Difficult Primary Cases and/or Revision

Considering its excellent tribological properties, hard-on-hard bearing is preferred for young and active patients. In this specific population, acetabular reconstructions can be justified (correlated with dysplastic hip, previous acetabular surgery, etc.). In such cases, the use of a cementless cup with hard-on-hard bearing could not be possible. Such reconstructions can indeed impose reinforcement ring use only compatible with metal-on-metal bearing. We reported 23 THAs using a MoM cup cemented directly into a Muller™ reinforcement ring. The mean follow-up was 6.1 years (5–10) [12]. At the final follow-up, Harris hip score increased from 62.2 (39–85) to

95.2 (84–100). We did not observe revision for aseptic loosening or fixation failure. Acetabular bone grafts (6 autologous and 16 allografts) systematically showed osteointegration. Only one revision was performed on the femoral side because of femoral shaft fracture. Considering a reoperation and bearing revision as end points, survival rates were, respectively, 95.8 and 100 %. The mean blood concentration of chromium, cobalt and titanium were, respectively, 1.85, 1.24 and 9.62 μg/L. Ion levels were not correlated with stem size, activity level, gender or clinical scores. The possibility of the use of a hard-on-hard bearing couple in a reinforcement ring opens attractive perspectives for the MoM bearing. Indeed, this system allows us to propose a hard-on-hard bearing couple for young and active subjects when acetabular bone stock does not allow a metal-back cementless cup (acetabular deformity or, especially, in revision cases) but requires the use of a reinforcement ring and bone grafts.

12.2.5 MoM as a Bearing Component That Prevents THA Revision in Patients Younger than 30 Years

We reported a multicenter study that was made in 23 French centres specializing in THA for young patients with a case control study to assess the risk factors for revision THAs inserted in patients under the age of 30 [12, 13]. Fifty-five patients (77 cases) that had revision of a THA inserted less than 30 years old were compared to a nonrevised group, including 819 THAs inserted in patients younger than 30 years. For these 77 revisions, the primary THA was made in very young patients (mean 19.7 years (12–29)). These 77 revisions were performed because of aseptic loosening in 40 cases (51 %), wear in 19 (24 %), recurrent dislocation in 4 (6 %), implant breakage in 3 (4 %), infection in 6 (8 %) and osteolysis in 5 (7 %). A multivariable analysis identified three factors related to a higher risk of revision: younger age at primary THA (OR 1.14 [1.07–1.19]), higher number of previous surgeries (OR 5.41 [2.67–10.98]) and use of hard-on-soft bearings instead of hard bearings (mainly MoM) (OR 3.42 [1.91–6.1]). According to these results, cementless or cemented primary THA design has no correlation with revision probability. This study on the basis of a large population identified the low survivorship of THA (10-year survival rate was 36 % (95 % confidence interval, 21–51 %) and confirmed the interest of MoM articulation to reduce the risk of revision. The use of a hard-on-soft bearing appeared to be an important and independent risk factor for mechanical failure.

12.2.6 Running Activity After Hip Resurfacing Arthroplasty: A Prospective Study

The ability to return to sports activities after hip arthroplasty seems to be more and more important for the "millennium" young and active patient. However, as the component wear of prosthetic metal-polyethylene bearings is directly related to the level of patient activity, it seems logical to advise THA patients against long-term participation in activities with repeated movements.

A prospective, consecutive series of 202 patients (215 MoM hip resurfacings) were assessed to evaluate the possible resumption of running activity (time spent, weekly mileage and return to competition) [9]. Of this initial cohort, 40 patients (43 resurfacings, 21 %) practised running preoperatively. At last follow-up, 33/40 patients (36/43 hips) still practised running ($p=0.74$), in that 91.6 % (who ran preoperatively) had returned to running at last follow-up. Mean average recovery time before running at a level assessed as good by patients was 16.4 weeks (5–36).

The excellent hip function found in resurfacing patients may be due to the conservative nature of the resurfacing procedure on the femoral head that conserves bone stock as well as mechanoreceptors and allows closer approximation to the normal proximal femoral anatomy. Running is possible after MoM hip resurfacing, and runners can even recover some degree of competition, but the short follow-up of this series of hip resurfacing in athletes should be interpreted with caution regarding implant survival.

Conclusion

According to our experience, in active and young patients, MoM bearing implantation reduces significantly the rates of wear/osteolysis and reoperation especially versus hard-on-soft bearing. On the other hand, a MoM insertion is not an easy and straightforward surgical procedure. This bearing is very sensitive to malposition on the acetabular side (i.e. edge loading or cam effect). But the very low dislocation rate and the ability to return to high-impact sports activity observed with large diameter head are strongly encouraging for the use of these components. The main concern is the occurrence of adverse tissue reaction mainly secondary to cup malposition with too vertical cups [14]. But it seems necessary to clarify some points. The use of MoM bearing in women of childbearing age is still controversial [26]. However, the use of metallic device in spine surgery in the adolescent (or knee arthroplasty [18] for a long time without any adverse effect seems reassuring [6]. To date, there is a scientific evidence that carcinogenicity is increased in subjects receiving MoM hip prostheses compared to those receiving metal-on-polyethylene or ceramic-on-polyethylene hip prostheses [22, 23]. The metal allergy is still controversial, and a preoperative diagnosis seems impossible. A positive metallic test is not correlated with in vitro side effects and seems to be not recommended. Despite these few controversies, MoM articulations still retain strong advantages. With an adequate design and appropriate tribological properties, MoM bearing constitutes a very high resistant articulation. It is the only bearing to securely perform hip resurfacing. Moreover it is the only hard-on-hard bearing that could be used in difficult primary cases (as protusio, hip dysplasia, etc.) as well as in revision surgery [12, 13]. Unlike the ceramic-on-ceramic bearing, the rate of squeaking is very low (close to zero for most authors) and compares favourably with the 2.7–21 % rate observed after a ceramic-on-ceramic bearing [16, 20]. In the same way, the rupture rate observed after MoM bearing is zero when it reaches from 0.1 to 7.4 %

with a ceramic-on-ceramic couple [17, 21]. The new generation of correctly designed MoM in small diameter has overcome 10 years and almost reached 15 years of follow-up [19] without serious adverse effect despite these components being mainly used in young and active patients. This uneventful follow-up is in the author's opinion the major reason to keep on using MoM articulations as long as these are well designed and manufactured and correctly inserted.

Conflict of Interest Julien Girard is a consultant for Zimmer, Wright Medical Technology and Smith and Nephew. Henri Migaud is a consultant for Zimmer and Tornier.

References

1. Allain J, Roudot-Thoraval F, Delecrin J, Anract P, Migaud H, Goutallier D. Revision total hip arthroplasty performed after fracture of a ceramic femoral head. A multicenter survivorship study. J Bone Joint Surg Am. 2003;85:825–30.
2. Brodner W, Bitzan P, Meisinger V, Kaider A, Gottsauner-Wolf F, Kotz R. Elevated serum cobalt with metal-on-metal articulating surfaces. J Bone Joint Surg Br. 1997;79:316–22.
3. Brodner W, Bitzan P, Meisinger V, Kaider A, Gottsauner-Wolf F, Kotz R. Serum cobalt levels after metal-on-metal total hip arthroplasty. J Bone Joint Surg Am. 2003;85:2168–73.
4. Dandy DJ, Theodorou BC. The management of local complications of total hip replacement by the McKee-Farrar technique. J Bone Joint Surg Br. 1975;57:30–5.
5. Delaunay CP. Metal-on-metal bearings in cementless primary total hip arthroplasty. J Arthroplasty. 2004;19:35–40.
6. del Rio J, Beguiristain J, Duart J. Metal levels in corrosion of spinal implants. Eur Spine J. 2007;16:1055–61.
7. Dobbs HS. Survivorship of total hip replacements. J Bone Joint Surg Br. 1980;62:168–72.
8. Eskelinen A, Remes V, Helenius I, Pulkkinen P, Nevalainen J, Paavolainen P. Total hip arthroplasty for primary osteoarthritis in younger patients in the Finnish arthroplasty register. 4,661 primary replacements followed for 0–22 years. Acta Orthop. 2005;76:28–41.
9. Fouilleron N, Wavreille G, Endjah N, Girard J. Running activity after hip resurfacing arthroplasty: a prospective study. Am J Sports Med. 2012;40:889–94.
10. Girard J, Bocquet D, Autissier G, Fouilleron N, Migaud H. Metal-on-metal hip arthroplasty in patients thirty years of age or younger. J Bone Joint Surg Am. 2010;92:2419–26.
11. Girard J, Miletic B, Migaud H, Krantz N. Hip resurfacing in patients under 30 years-old: an attractive option for young and active patients. Int Orthop. 2012;36:1789–94.
12. Girard J, Combes A, Herent S, Migaud H. Metal-on-metal cups cemented into reinforcement rings: a possible new acetabular reconstruction procedure for young and active patients. J Arthroplasty. 2011;26:282–8.
13. Girard J, Glorion C, Bonnomet F, Fron D, Migaud H. Risk factors for revision of hip arthroplasties in patients younger than 30 years. Clin Orthop Relat Res. 2011;469:1141–7.
14. Glyn-Jones S, Pandit H, Kwon YM, Doll H, Gill HS, Murray DW. Risk factors for inflammatory pseudotumour formation following hip resurfacing. J Bone Joint Surg Br. 2009;91:1566–74.
15. Hamadouche M, Boutin P, Daussange J, et al. Alumina-on-alumina total hip arthroplasty: a minimum 18.5-year follow-up study. J Bone Joint Surg Am. 2002;84:69–77.
16. Jarrett CA, Ranawat AS, Bruzzone M, Blum YC, Rodriguez JA, Ranawat CS. The squeaking hip: a phenomenon of ceramic-on-ceramic total hip arthroplasty. J Bone Joint Surg Am. 2009;91:1344–9.

17. Koo KH, Ha YC, Jung WH, Kim SR, Yoo JJ, Kim HJ. Isolated fracture of the ceramic head after third-generation alumina-on-alumina total hip arthroplasty. J Bone Joint Surg Am. 2008;90:329–36.
18. Luetzner J, Krummenauer F, Lengel AM, Ziegler J, Witzleb WC. Serum metal ion exposure after total knee arthroplasty. Clin Orthop Relat Res. 2007;461:136–42.
19. Migaud H, Putman S, Krantz N, Vasseur L, Girard J. Cementless metal-on-metal versus ceramic-on-polyethylene hip arthroplasty in patients less than 50 years of age: a comparative study at 12- to 14-year follow-up. J Bone Joint Surg Am. 2011;93:137–42.
20. Restrepo C, Parvizi J, Kurtz SM, Sharkey PF, Hozack WJ, Rothman RH. The noisy ceramic hip: is component malpositioning the cause? J Arthroplasty. 2008;23:643–9.
21. Szymanski C, Guériot S, Boniface O, Deladerrière JY, Luneau S, Maynou C. Sandwich type ceramic liner fracture rate with the Atlas III™ socket: a study of 144 primary total hip replacements at a mean 74 months' follow-up. Orthop Traumatol Surg Res. 2011;97:494–500.
22. Tharani R, Dorey FJ, Schmalzried TP. The risk of cancer following total hip or knee arthroplasty. J Bone Joint Surg Am. 2001;83:774–9.
23. Visuri T, Pukkala E, Paavolainen P, Pulkkinen P, Riska EB. Cancer risk after metal on metal and polyethylene on metal total hip arthroplasty. Clin Orthop Relat Res. 1996;329:280–9.
24. Weber BG. Experience with the Metasul total hip bearing system. Clin Orthop Relat Res. 1996;329(Suppl):S69–77.
25. Willert HG, Buchhorn GH, Fayyazi A, et al. Metal-on-metal bearings and hypersensitivity in patients with artificial hip joints. A clinical and histomorphological study. J Bone Joint Surg Am. 2005;87:28–36.
26. Ziaee H, Daniel J, Datta AK, Blunt S, McMinn DJ. Transplacental transfer of cobalt and chromium in patients with metal-on-metal hip arthroplasty: a controlled study. J Bone Joint Surg Br. 2007;89:301–5.

Long-Term Results of Metal-on-Metal Total Hip Replacement After a Minimum of Seventeen Years' Follow-Up

13

Richard Lass, Alexander Grübl, Alexander Kolb, Stephan Domayer, Claudia Csuk, Bernd Kubista, Alexander Giurea, and Reinhard Windhager

13.1 Introduction

The indication for total hip arthroplasty, especially in young patients, has increased over the past 20 years. Accelerated risk of polyethylene wear and subsequent prosthetic loosening due to osteolysis has led to a renaissance of metal-on-metal bearings. Failures of the first-generation metal-on-metal total hip replacements were attributed to suboptimal surgical technique, excessive or negative clearance, poor fixation, and neck-socket impingement. Second-generation metal-on-metal bearings for total hip arthroplasty were successfully reintroduced in 1988 by Weber [1], following improvements in manufacturing, better clearance, and a better understanding of the factors influencing their wear [2–4]. However, there may be different survival rates based on bearing materials, manufacturing technologies, and femoral component designs. In vitro wear of low-carbon alloy has been shown to be higher than that of high-carbon alloy, resulting in decreased in vivo survival [5]. For high-carbon alloy with 28-mm metal-on-metal articulation (Metasul®, Zimmer, Winterthur, Switzerland), the survival with revision for any reason has ranged between 94.4 % at 12.3 years [6], 98.7 % at 12.4 years [7], 94.0 % at 13 years [8], and 92.2 % at 16.4 years [9].

These hard bearing surfaces seem advantageous, especially for young and active patients [10, 11], but concerns remain regarding the effects of prolonged exposure to increased level of metal ions, such as hypersensitivity [12, 13], carcinogenicity [14, 15], and fetal exposure to ions in pregnant women [16, 17].

At the 10-year follow-up, 73 of the original 98 patients were available for clinical and radiographic examination [18]. The probability of survival was 98.6 % at

R. Lass, MD (✉) • A. Kolb • S. Domayer • C. Csuk • B. Kubista • A. Giurea • R. Windhager
Department of Orthopedics, Medical University of Vienna,
Währinger Gürtel 18-20, Vienna A-1090, Austria
e-mail: richard.lass@meduniwien.ac.at

A. Grübl
Department of Orthopedics, Sanatorium Hera, Löblichgasse 14, Vienna A-1090, Austria

K. Knahr (ed.), *Tribology in Total Hip and Knee Arthroplasty*,
DOI 10.1007/978-3-642-45266-6_13, © EFORT 2014

10 years. The Harris hip score was 92.1 points, and the University of California, Los Angeles (UCLA), activity score was 6.4 points after 10 years. Small osteolytic lesions and radiolucent lines were found in Gruen zones 1, 7, 8, and 14. The median serum cobalt concentration of the 22 patients with their hip replacement as the only source of cobalt was 0.75 μg/L (range, 0.3–50.1 μg/L) and did not differ from short- and intermediate-term follow-up values [19]. There was no evidence of an increased rate of primary malignancy or renal failure in the study group.

This study was undertaken as a concise follow-up of this previous report of the 10-year follow-up with a second-generation metal-on-metal hip prosthesis [18] to provide information about long-term survival, clinical outcome, radiographic appearance, and serum metal concentration at a mean follow-up of 17.9 years.

13.2 Materials and Methods

13.2.1 Patients

Between November 1992 and May 1994, 105 cementless primary total hip prostheses with metal-on-metal articulating surfaces were implanted in 98 patients [18]. There were 54 female and 44 male patients with an average age of 56 years (range, 22–79 years) and a mean body mass index of 27.2 kg/m^2. The most common diagnoses were primary osteoarthritis (56.1 %), secondary osteoarthritis due to dysplasia of the hip (18.1 %), and avascular necrosis of the femoral head (15.2 %). Surgery was performed through a transgluteal, lateral approach in supine position under general or spinal anesthesia. Routine prophylaxis against heterotopic bone formation (indomethacin 50 mg, three times per day) was administered for 7 days.

13.2.2 Implant

The implant used in this study is a tapered rectangular stem made of titanium-aluminum-niobium alloy (Zweymüller® Alloclassic®, Zimmer GmbH, Winterthur, Switzerland) and a conical screw cup made of pure titanium (CSF®, Zimmer GmbH, Winterthur, Switzerland). It holds the articulating surface embedded in an ultrahigh molecular weight polyethylene liner. The ball head with a diameter of 28 mm is made of a wrought cobalt-based Co-28Cr-6Mo alloy with a carbon content of 0.2 % (Metasul®, Zimmer, Winterthur, Switzerland). Primary stability of the femoral component is achieved by press-fit implantation into a precisely prepared osseous bed.

13.2.3 Clinical and Radiographic Follow-Up

We retrospectively evaluated the clinical and radiographic results at a minimum of 17 years after implantation between May 2011 and March 2012 according to the methods used at the time of the 10-year follow-up visits [18]. Institutional review board approval was obtained for the ongoing follow-up evaluation at our institution.

The clinical examination was performed using the Harris hip score and the UCLA score. Additionally, all patients were asked to fill in a questionnaire requesting information on possible cardiovascular or renal diseases or malignancies and other metal implants, including orthopedic implants, plates and screws, cerclage wires, and dental prostheses or pacemakers. All patients were asked about intake of cobalt- or vitamin B^{12}-containing nutritional supplements, smoking and drinking habits, and sports activities, including the 72 h prior to the follow-up visit, as this may alter the serum levels.

Anteroposterior and lateral radiographs of the hip were taken at the follow-up visit and investigated for radiolucent lines and osteolytic areas using Gruen zones and the DeLee classification [20, 21]. Additionally, the inclination of the acetabular component was measured, and para-articular ossifications were graded using the classification of Brooker [22].

13.2.4 Serum Analysis

This procedure was performed according to our previous study protocol at 10-year follow-up [18]. Blood samples were taken using Vacutainer® glass tubes (Becton, Dickinson and Company, Franklin Lakes, NJ) without additives. In order to avoid bias of the serum metal concentrations, all patients with a contralateral hip replacement and cobalt- or chromium-containing devices of any kind or those who were taking cobalt-containing nutritional supplements were excluded from the serum metal analysis. Furthermore, patients with known renal insufficiency were excluded as cobalt and chromium might have accumulated in these patients. As in our previous study, an atomic absorption spectrometer (5100-ZL, Perkin Elmer, Shelton, CT) at wavelengths of 242.5 and 357.9 nm was used to determine the cobalt and chromium levels. Additionally, we analyzed creatinine values in order to detect renal insufficiency. The detection limit of cobalt and chromium in serum was 0.3 μg/L, and the creatinine reference value was 0.5–1.1 mg/dL in our laboratory.

13.2.5 Statistical Analysis

The Kaplan-Meier method [23] was used to estimate the implant survival probabilities, counting revision of both components for aseptic failure and for any reason as the terminating event and censoring patients at the time of their death or at the end of the follow-up period.

The correlation between postoperative serum ion values and the mean values of age, gender, BMI, Harris hip score, UCLA activity score, and acetabular component inclination was calculated by using the Spearman's rank correlation coefficient.

Statistical analysis was performed using the Statistical Package for the Social Sciences (SPSS), version 20.0 (SPSS®, Chicago, Illinois). Statistical significance was set at $p < 0.05$.

13.2.6 Source of Funding

The authors did not receive grants or outside funding in support of their research for preparation of this manuscript. No authors received payments or other benefits from a commercial entity (Zimmer GmbH, Winterthur, Switzerland). No commercial entity paid or directed, or agreed to pay or direct, any benefits to any research fund, foundation, educational institution, or other charitable or nonprofit organization with which the authors are affiliated.

13.3 Results

13.3.1 Patients

At a minimum of 17 years of follow-up, 49 (52 hips) of the original 98 patients (105 hips) were available for clinical examination, 34 (34.7 %) died, 14 (14.2 %) were lost to follow-up, and 1 patient was bedridden and could only be contacted by telephone. All of the 34 deceased patients had retained their implant, and the cause of death was not associated with the implant in any case. All of these patients had been followed postoperatively, and all had well-functioning hips at the time of death. Most of the patients lost to follow-up are living abroad, leaving no contact information to get in touch with them. All of them had no signs of implant failure at the latest available follow-up.

The patients' average age at the time of the latest follow-up was 70.9 years (range, 45.9–90.6 years).

13.3.2 Implant

Eight hips in eight patients underwent revision between the time of implantation of the prosthesis and the 17 years' follow-up. Aseptic loosening of the implant combined with focal osteolysis was the reason for three cup revisions (2.8 %) and one stem revision (0.9 %).

The other hips were reoperated for late infection (0.9 %), for posttraumatic recurrent dislocation (0.9 %), for para-articular ossifications (0.9 %), and for metallosis from impingement between the head and liner (0.9 %).

13.3.3 Clinical and Radiographic Follow-Up

After excluding the revision cases, 41 patients (44 hips) were available for clinical and radiographic evaluation after a minimum of 17 years of follow-up. The average Harris hip score decreased from 92.1 (range, 43.8–100 points) at 10 years to 88.8 (range, 44.0–100 points), and the average UCLA score increased from 6.4 (range,

Table 13.1 Distribution of radiolucent lines (rl) and osteolytic lesions (o) of the stem (Gruen zones) and the cup (DeLee classification) at a minimum of 10 years and 17 years of follow-up

Zone	rl[a] (10 a) (%)	rl[a] (17 a) (%)	o[b] (10 a) (%)	o[b] (17 a) (%)
Stem (Gruen) 1	17.1	25	3.9	2.2
2	–	–	–	–
3	–	–	–	–
4	–	–	–	–
5	–	–	–	–
6	–	–	1.3	–
7	6.6	22.7	1.3	4.5
8	7.9	20.4	1.3	2.2
9	–	–	–	–
10	–	–	–	–
11	–	–	–	–
12	–	–	–	–
13	–	–	–	–
14	6.6	27.3	1.3	4.5
Cup (DeLee) I	–	6.8	2.6	2.2
II	1.3	4.5	2.6	–
III	7.9	2.2	–	2.2
IV	–	9.1	1.3	–
V	–	9.1	–	–
VI	2.6	4.5	–	–

[a]Radiolucent lines
[b]Osteolytic lesions in percent (%)

1–10 points) at 10 years to 6.7 (range, 2–10 points). The patient with the HHS of 44 is a 73-year-old man, who has still retained his implant. He has only little pain and an excellent range of motion in his “study hip” but also achieved a contralateral hip some years ago, which prevents him from walking properly for longer distances, and he still needs crutches. Therefore, the HHS score is quite low.

At mean 17.9 years, the radiographs showed radiolucent lines predominantly in Gruen zones 1, 7, 8, and 14 with 25, 22.7, 20.4, and 27.3 %, whereas at 10 years, we could find only 17.1, 6.6, 7.9, and 6.6 %, respectively. Osteolysis was identified in zones 7 and 14 in 4.5 % and in zones 1 and 8 in 2.2 %, compared to 3.9 % in zone 1 and 1.3 % in zones 6, 7, 8, and 14 in our previous study. Radiolucent lines around the acetabular component were seen in 9.1 % in zones IV and V, in 6.8 % in zone I, in 4.5 % in zones II and VI, and in 2.2 % in zone III of DeLee. At 10 years’ follow-up, radiolucent lines were seen in 7.9 % in zone III, in 2.6 % in zone VI, and in 1.3 % in zone II. Osteolytic lesions were identified in 2.2 % in zones I and III, compared to 2.6 % in zones I and II and 1.3 % in zone IV in the previous study (see Table 13.1 and Figs. 13.1 and 13.2). Para-articular ossifications grades I and II according to Brooker were seen in 9.1 % and grade III in 4.5 %, and no ossifications grade IV were found at all. The mean inclination of the acetabular component was 48° (range, 36°–59°).

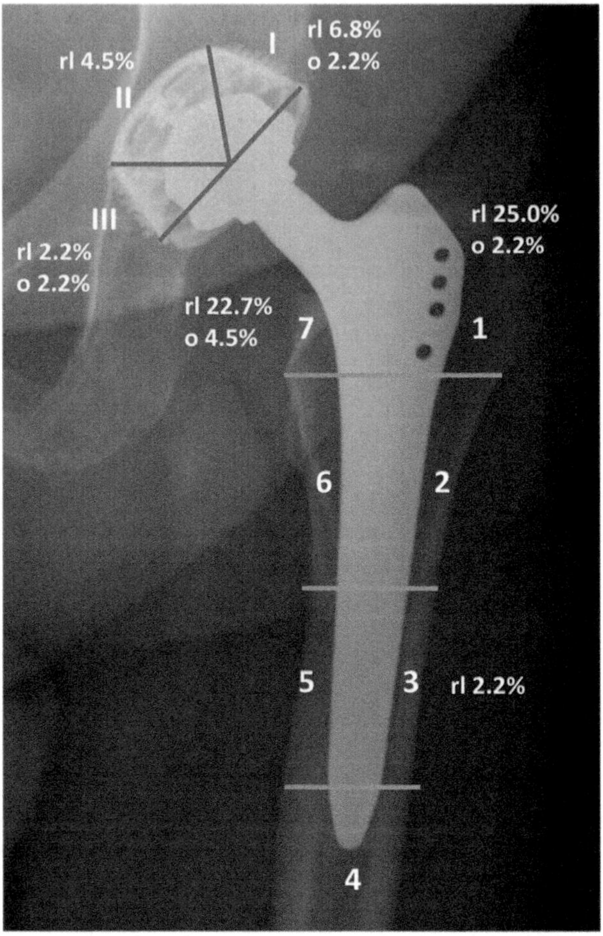

Fig. 13.1 Distribution of radiolucent lines (*rl*) and osteolytic lesions (*o*) on anteroposterior radiographs of the stem (Gruen zones) and the cup (DeLee classification) at a minimum of 17 years

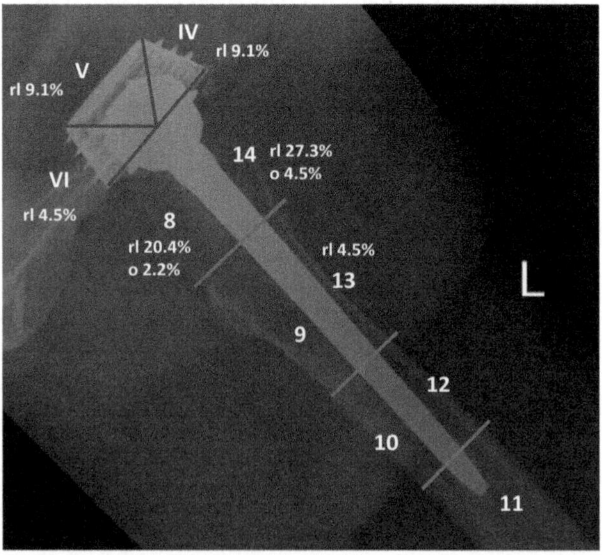

Fig. 13.2 Distribution of radiolucent lines (*rl*) and osteolytic lesions (*o*) on lateral radiographs of the stem (Gruen zones) and the cup (DeLee classification) at a minimum of 17 years

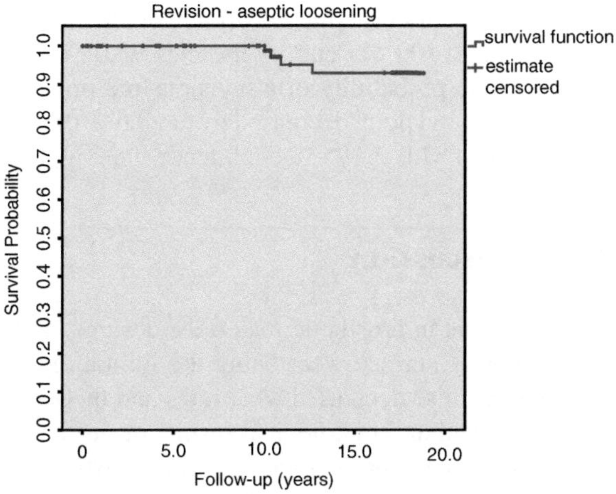

Fig. 13.3 The cumulative rate of survival of the prostheses, counting revision of both components with aseptic failure as the end point at 18.8 years, was 93.0 % (95 % confidence interval, 89.5–96.5 %)

13.3.4 Serum Analysis

Of the 22 patients evaluated at the 10 years' follow-up, only eight patients were left, who qualified for serum metal analysis, as their hip replacement was the only known source of cobalt and chromium and they had no chronic renal failure at the time of surgery.

After a minimum of 17 years, the median serum cobalt concentration decreased from 0.75 μg/L (range, 0.3–50.1 μg/L) at 10 years to 0.70 μg/L (range 0.4–5.1 μg/L). The median serum chromium level decreased from 0.95 μg/L (range, 0.3–58.6 μg/L) at 10 years to 0.70 μg/L (range 0.4–2.1 μg/L).

There were three patients with an established diagnosis of chronic renal failure at the time of surgery. All of them underwent kidney transplantation and were excluded from the analysis of the creatinine level. The median serum creatinine level of the analyzed 38 patients at the latest follow-up visit was 0.95 mg/dL compared to 0.86 mg/dL at 10 years' follow-up. In the 17-year period since the arthroplasty, no diagnosis of acute or chronic failure was established in any of the remaining patients.

Seven patients were diagnosed with a primary malignant tumor between the time of implantation of the prosthesis and the 17 years' follow-up. Since our previous study [18], two additional cases (one breast cancer, one lymphatic leukemia) were diagnosed. In total, there were two cases of rectum carcinoma, two cases of breast cancer, two cases of chronic lymphatic leukemia, and one patient with cancer of unknown primary in the follow-up. This is still consistent with the expected incidence rate of malignancies for the given period of time and number of patients [24].

13.3.5 Survival Analysis

The cumulative rate of survival of the prostheses, counting revision of both components with aseptic failure as the end point at 18.8 years, was 93.0 % (95 % confidence interval, 89.5–96.5 %; see Fig. 13.3). The cumulative rate of survival with aseptic failure as the end point of the stem was 97.9 % (95 % confidence interval, 95.8–100 %) and of the cup 95.0 % (95 % confidence interval, 92.1–97.9 %). The probability of a revision-free implant survival with revision for any reason as the end point decreased from 98.6 % (95 % confidence interval, 96–100 %) at 10 years to 87.0 % (95 % confidence interval, 82.6–91.4 %) at 18.8 years.

13.4 Discussion

Improvements in prosthetic materials, designs, and implant fixation for THA have led to bearing surface wear being the limitation of this technology. Hard-on-hard bearings promise decreased wear rates and increased survival.

The clinical and radiological results of our present study, the longest follow-up of a series of cementless total hip arthroplasties with a 28-mm high-carbon metal-on-metal bearing (Metasul®), show a cumulative rate of survival of the prostheses with aseptic failure as the end point of 93.0 % and with revision for any reason of 87.0 % at 18.8 years. These results continue to be comparable to other hard-on-hard bearings at a minimum of 17 years postoperatively.

Kolb et al. [25] reported the probability of survival of the identical stem and cup (Zweymüller® Alloclassic®/CSF®, Zimmer GmbH, Winterthur, Switzerland) with an ultrahigh molecular weight polyethylene-on-alumina bearing of 65 % (95 % confidence interval, 0.55–0.73) at a minimum of 20 years postoperatively. Excessive polyethylene wear was the most frequent cause (67 %), and aseptic loosening of the cup (20 %) was the second most common cause for revision surgery in this study. Petsatodis et al. [26] evaluated the clinical and radiographic results of 109 primary total hip arthroplasties with a cementless alumina ceramic-on-ceramic prosthesis. The cumulative rate of survival of the prostheses was 84.4 % at 20.8 years.

Recent comparative studies of alternative bearings show contradictive results. Milosev et al. [27] could show higher survival with ceramic-on-ceramic bearings (95.6 %) than with the metal-on-metal components (87.9 %) when revision for any reason was the end point. However, the difference was not significant at the 10-year follow-up. Opposite results were obtained in a meta-analysis by Shetty et al. [28], who could identify MoM to be the optimal bearing for young active patients. In his study, these bearings resulted in a significantly higher rate of survival than that of metal-on-polyethylene and ceramic-on-ceramic bearings.

Despite low wear, aseptic loosening remains the main reason for revision of MoM bearings. The deposition of cobalt-chrome wear particles in periprosthetic tissues induces spectrum of necrotic and inflammatory changes. This periprosthetic soft-tissue lesions have been described generally as adverse reaction to metal debris (ARMD) [29], including metallosis [30], aseptic lymphocytic vasculitis-associated lesions (ALVAL) [12], and pseudotumors [31]. It has been presumed that these abnormal soft-tissue reactions may be attributed to two etiologies: wear-related cellular cytotoxicity and hypersensitivity [32]. Hart et al. showed that the prevalence of pseudotumors was similar in patients with well-functioning hip prosthesis and well-positioned acetabular component, as well as in patients with a painful hip.

The presence of a cystic pseudotumor may not necessarily indicate the need for revision arthroplasty [33]. In our recent study, there were no patients with similar symptoms, but we did not perform magnetic resonance imaging to evaluate the prevalence of pseudotumors in well-functioning hip prosthesis. Willert et al. [12] described the histological features of ALVAL also in non-MoM bearing surfaces. However, the ceramic wear particles are more biocompatible than metal debris [34].

In our study, we could find no significant or consistent correlation between the mean postoperative serum ion levels and the mean values of age, gender, BMI, Harris hip score, and UCLA activity score. This is in agreement with results of several studies showing that metal ion levels are not acutely affected by patient activity [11, 35, 36].

In terms of acetabular component inclination, we found no significant correlation between cobalt and chromium serum concentrations in our study patients. This is supported by Imanishi et al. [36]. In contrast, Hart et al. [37] found that acetabular inclination angle was strongly positively correlated with the rate of wear, but acetabular version and combined version of the acetabular and femoral components showed a poor correlation with the rate of wear. This is also supported by hip simulator analysis [38].

In our radiological follow-up, we could find an increase in the number of the radiolucent lines predominantly in the proximal part of the stem (Gruen zones 1, 7, 8, 14). We did not find significant changes for the distal parts of the stem, for the cup, or for the osteolytic lesions. We could not find a correlation between the radiological changes and clinical symptoms. This is supported by several long-term studies, relating to the Zweymüller® Alloclassic® stem, which have failed to confirm that these radiological changes have clinical relevance for aseptic loosening [25, 39].

Despite concerns regarding chromosome aberrations and translocations, the International Agency for Research on Cancer concluded that there is inadequate evidence in humans regarding the carcinogenicity of orthopedic implants [40]. A meta-analysis by Onega, Baron, and MacKenzie [41] comprising 1,435,356 person-years of follow-up and a recent analysis by Visuri et al. [42] of 310,341 person-years have shown no overall increase in cancer after joint replacement [43]. Visuri noted, however, that the mean follow-up at 11 years was too short, compared to the latency for some tumors (20–40 years). Therefore, it seems to be important to continue surveillance at long-term follow-ups of more than 20 years. In our study group, we could not show an increase in cancer incidence at a mean follow-up of 17.9 years.

Our study confirmed that no renal function impairment was related to elevated serum metal levels. The median serum creatinine level at the latest follow-up visit was 0.95 mg/dL. This is supported by Corradi et al. [44], who found a median serum creatinine level in the MoM group of 1.1 mg/dL, and no difference to the control group without any metal exposure.

There is overall consensus that the blood cobalt or chromium level of a well-functioning MoM hip is approximately 2 μg/L. It may thus be presumed that raised metal ion levels up to a certain level is a feature of MoM bearings and does not necessarily represent underlying pathogenesis. However, higher levels may be the reason for adverse changes [43]. Hart et al. [45] showed that blood levels of cobalt were doubled in painful hips compared with well-functioning hips and defined a cutoff level of 7 μg/L (7 parts per billion, ppb), for either cobalt or chromium to predict failure of MoM hips. This cutoff level is also used by the Medicines and Healthcare Products Regulatory Agency (MRHA).

After a minimum of 17 years, the median serum cobalt concentration decreased in our patient population from 0.75 μg/L (range, 0.3–50.1 μg/L) at 10 years to 0.70 μg/L (range 0.4–5.1 μg/L), and the median serum chromium level decreased from 0.95 μg/L (range, 0.3–58.6 μg/L) at 10 years to 0.70 μg/L (range 0.4–2.1 μg/L). Brodner et al. [46] reported a median serum cobalt concentration of 1 μg/L at 1 year and 0.7 μg/L at 5 years after surgery in a prospective randomized study using the same type of implant. This is in accordance with Savarino et al. [47], showing that the conspicuous ion release with metal-on-metal bearings tended to decrease over time. In fact, the median value for Co at a follow-up of 5 years was 0.89 μg/L, whereas in the long-term population, they observed a median value of 0.58 μg/L.

There are many complex issues associated with the analysis of metal ions, including collecting technique, analysis, and reporting of the results. Daniel et al. [48] highlighted differences between whole blood and plasma concentration, meaning that they should not be used interchangeably, and their interconversion is unreliable. We measured ion levels in the serum, exactly as in our previous study [18], following the recommendation of MacDonald et al. [49], regarding the use of serum analysis for comparing purposes. De Smet et al. [50] concluded that there is a correlation between the metal ion concentrations of serum and joint aspirate and component wear.

This study has some limitations. One limitation is that we did not consider the regional dissemination or the local determination, such as in the synovial fluid, which could offer better information about wear and local reactions at the components level. In patients with increased serum metal ion level, we additionally performed a joint aspiration to evaluate the local metal ion concentrations and performed a correlation analysis. Spearman correlations evaluated that there was no significant relationship between the serum cobalt or chromium level and the local metal level.

Furthermore, we did not perform an ultrasound or magnetic resonance imaging for local tissue reaction evaluation. Further investigations to compare the local and systematic parameters in the same patient group, a Metal Artifact Reduction Sequence Magnetic Resonance Imaging (MARS MRI) evaluation series and a concise follow-up of more than 20 years will be necessary to evaluate chronic adverse reactions to the metal debris.

Another limitation is the quite high number of 14 patients (14.3 %) lost to follow-up. Most of the patients lost to follow-up are living abroad, leaving no contact information to get in touch with them. Some of them were in our hospital just for the operation. All of them had no signs of implant failure at the latest available follow-up.

All of the 34 deceased patients had retained their implant, and the cause of death was not associated with the implant in any case. All of these patients had been followed postoperatively, and all had well-functioning hips at the time of death.

Of the 22 patients evaluated at the 10 years' follow-up, only eight patients were left, who qualified for serum metal analysis, as their hip replacement was the only known source of cobalt and chromium and they had no chronic renal failure at the time of surgery. Most of the 22 patients achieved a contralateral hip or a total knee arthroplasty in the meantime, 2 patients were deceased, and 2 patients were lost to follow-up.

This is to our knowledge the first minimum 17 years' follow-up publication of clinical and radiological results, as well as the serum metal concentrations of cementless total hip arthroplasties with a 28-mm high-carbon metal-on-metal bearing (Metasul®). We were investigating the systemic dissemination of metal bearing wear, which in turn did not show an increased number of severe general effects, such as carcinogenicity or renal failure caused by the prolonged exposure to increased level of metal ions in our study population. Serum cobalt and chromium levels did not differ from those reported at 10-year follow-up. Our recent study showed superior results to certain bearings, like polyethylene on ceramic, implanted in the same time period as our study population, but even comparable results to other hard-on-hard bearings at a minimum of 17 years' follow-up.

References

1. Weber BG. Experience with the Metasul total hip bearing system. Clin Orthop Relat Res. 1996;(329 Suppl):S69–77.
2. Goldsmith AA, Dowson D, Isaac GH, Lancaster JG. A comparative joint simulator study of the wear of metal-on-metal and alternative material combinations in hip replacements. Proc Inst Mech Eng H. 2000;214(1):39–47.
3. Schmalzried TP, Peters PC, Maurer BT, Bragdon CR, Harris WH. Long-duration metal-on-metal total hip arthroplasties with low wear of the articulating surfaces. J Arthroplasty. 1996;11(3):322–31.
4. Sieber HP, Rieker CB, Kottig P. Analysis of 118 second-generation metal-on-metal retrieved hip implants. J Bone Joint Surg Br. 1999;81(1):46–50.
5. Rieker CB, Schon R, Kottig P. Development and validation of a second-generation metal-on-metal bearing: laboratory studies and analysis of retrievals. J Arthroplasty. 2004;19(8 Suppl 3):5–11.
6. Saito S, Ishii T, Mori S, Hosaka K, Ootaki M, Tokuhashi Y. Long-term results of metasul metal-on-metal total hip arthroplasty. Orthopedics. 2010;33(8).
7. Hwang KT, Kim YH, Kim YS, Choi IY. Cementless total hip arthroplasty with a metal-on-metal bearing in patients younger than 50 years. J Arthroplasty. 2011;26(8):1481–7.
8. Randelli F, Banci L, D'Anna A, Visentin O, Randelli G. Cementless Metasul metal-on-metal total hip arthroplasties at 13 years. J Arthroplasty. 2012;27(2):186–92.
9. Dastane M, Wan Z, Deshmane P, Long WT, Dorr LD. Primary hip arthroplasty with 28-mm Metasul articulation. J Arthroplasty. 2011;26(4):662–4.
10. Migaud H, Jobin A, Chantelot C, Giraud F, Laffargue P, Duquennoy A. Cementless metal-on-metal hip arthroplasty in patients less than 50 years of age: comparison with a matched control group using ceramic-on-polyethylene after a minimum 5-year follow-up. J Arthroplasty. 2004;19(8 Suppl 3):23–8.
11. Heisel C, Silva M, Skipor AK, Jacobs JJ, Schmalzried TP. The relationship between activity and ions in patients with metal-on-metal bearing hip prostheses. J Bone Joint Surg Am. 2005;87(4):781–7.
12. Willert HG, Buchhorn GH, Fayyazi A, Flury R, Windler M, Koster G, Lohmann CH. Metal-on-metal bearings and hypersensitivity in patients with artificial hip joints. A clinical and histomorphological study. J Bone Joint Surg Am. 2005;87(1):28–36.
13. Davies AP, Willert HG, Campbell PA, Learmonth ID, Case CP. An unusual lymphocytic perivascular infiltration in tissues around contemporary metal-on-metal joint replacements. J Bone Joint Surg Am. 2005;87(1):18–27.

14. Ladon D, Doherty A, Newson R, Turner J, Bhamra M, Case CP. Changes in metal levels and chromosome aberrations in the peripheral blood of patients after metal-on-metal hip arthroplasty. J Arthroplasty. 2004;19(8 Suppl 3):78–83.
15. Keegan GM, Learmonth ID, Case CP. Orthopaedic metals and their potential toxicity in the arthroplasty patient: a review of current knowledge and future strategies. J Bone Joint Surg Br. 2007;89(5):567–73.
16. Ziaee H, Daniel J, Datta AK, Blunt S, McMinn DJ. Transplacental transfer of cobalt and chromium in patients with metal-on-metal hip arthroplasty: a controlled study. J Bone Joint Surg Br. 2007;89(3):301–5.
17. MacDonald SJ. Metal-on-metal total hip arthroplasty: the concerns. Clin Orthop Relat Res. 2004;(429):86–93.
18. Grubl A, Marker M, Brodner W, Giurea A, Heinze G, Meisinger V, Zehetgruber H, Kotz R. Long-term follow-up of metal-on-metal total hip replacement. J Orthop Res. 2007;25(7): 841–8.
19. Berendes E, Schmidt C, Van Aken H, Hartlage MG, Rothenburger M, Wirtz S, Scheld HH, Brodner G, Walter M. A-type and B-type natriuretic peptides in cardiac surgical procedures. Anesth Analg. 2004;98(1):11–9. table of contents.
20. Gruen TA, McNeice GM, Amstutz HC. "Modes of failure" of cemented stem-type femoral components: a radiographic analysis of loosening. Clin Orthop Relat Res. 1979;(141):17–27.
21. DeLee JG, Charnley J. Radiological demarcation of cemented sockets in total hip replacement. Clin Orthop Relat Res. 1976;(121):20–32.
22. Brooker AF, Bowerman JW, Robinson RA, Riley Jr LH. Ectopic ossification following total hip replacement. Incidence and a method of classification. J Bone Joint Surg Am. 1973; 55(8):1629–32.
23. Kaplan E, Meier P. Nonparametric estimation from incomplete observations. J Am Stat Assoc. 1958;53:457–81.
24. Statistik Austria. Jahrbuch der Gesundheitsstatistik 2002. Wien: Statistik Austria; 2004.
25. Kolb A, Grubl A, Schneckener CD, Chiari C, Kaider A, Lass R, Windhager R. Cementless total hip arthroplasty with the rectangular titanium Zweymuller stem: a concise follow-up, at a minimum of twenty years, of previous reports. J Bone Joint Surg Am. 2012;94(18):1681–4.
26. Petsatodis GE, Papadopoulos PP, Papavasiliou KA, Hatzokos IG, Agathangelidis FG, Christodoulou AG. Primary cementless total hip arthroplasty with an alumina ceramic-on-ceramic bearing: results after a minimum of twenty years of follow-up. J Bone Joint Surg Am. 2010;92(3):639–44.
27. Milosev I, Kovac S, Trebse R, Levasic V, Pisot V. Comparison of ten-year survivorship of hip prostheses with use of conventional polyethylene, metal-on-metal, or ceramic-on-ceramic bearings. J Bone Joint Surg Am. 2012;94(19):1756–63.
28. Shetty V, Shitole B, Shetty G, Thakur H, Bhandari M. Optimal bearing surfaces for total hip replacement in the young patient: a meta-analysis. Int Orthop. 2011;35(9):1281–7.
29. Langton DJ, Jameson SS, Joyce TJ, Hallab NJ, Natu S, Nargol AV. Early failure of metal-on-metal bearings in hip resurfacing and large-diameter total hip replacement: a consequence of excess wear. J Bone Joint Surg Br. 2010;92(1):38–46.
30. Korovessis P, Petsinis G, Repanti M, Repantis T. Metallosis after contemporary metal-on-metal total hip arthroplasty. Five to nine-year follow-up. J Bone Joint Surg Am. 2006; 88(6):1183–91.
31. Pandit H, Glyn-Jones S, McLardy-Smith P, Gundle R, Whitwell D, Gibbons CL, Ostlere S, Athanasou N, Gill HS, Murray DW. Pseudotumours associated with metal-on-metal hip resurfacings. J Bone Joint Surg Br. 2008;90(7):847–51.
32. Campbell P, Ebramzadeh E, Nelson S, Takamura K, De Smet K, Amstutz HC. Histological features of pseudotumor-like tissues from metal-on-metal hips. Clin Orthop Relat Res. 2010;468(9):2321–7.
33. Hart AJ, Satchithananda K, Liddle AD, Sabah SA, McRobbie D, Henckel J, Cobb JP, Skinner JA, Mitchell AW. Pseudotumors in association with well-functioning metal-on-metal hip

prostheses: a case–control study using three-dimensional computed tomography and magnetic resonance imaging. J Bone Joint Surg Am. 2012;94(4):317–25.
34. Germain MA, Hatton A, Williams S, Matthews JB, Stone MH, Fisher J, Ingham E. Comparison of the cytotoxicity of clinically relevant cobalt-chromium and alumina ceramic wear particles in vitro. Biomaterials. 2003;24(3):469–79.
35. Vendittoli PA, Mottard S, Roy AG, Dupont C, Lavigne M. Chromium and cobalt ion release following the Durom high carbon content, forged metal-on-metal surface replacement of the hip. J Bone Joint Surg Br. 2007;89(4):441–8.
36. Imanishi T, Hasegawa M, Sudo A. Serum metal ion levels after second-generation metal-on-metal total hip arthroplasty. Arch Orthop Trauma Surg. 2010;130(12):1447–50.
37. Hart AJ, Ilo K, Underwood R, Cann P, Henckel J, Lewis A, Cobb J, Skinner J. The relationship between the angle of version and rate of wear of retrieved metal-on-metal resurfacings: a prospective, CT-based study. J Bone Joint Surg Br. 2011;93(3):315–20.
38. Angadji A, Royle M, Collins SN, Shelton JC. Influence of cup orientation on the wear performance of metal-on-metal hip replacements. Proc Inst Mech Eng H. 2009;223(4):449–57.
39. Grubl A, Chiari C, Giurea A, Gruber M, Kaider A, Marker M, Zehetgruber H, Gottsauner-Wolf F. Cementless total hip arthroplasty with the rectangular titanium Zweymuller stem. A concise follow-up, at a minimum of fifteen years, of a previous report. J Bone Joint Surg Am. 2006;88(10):2210–5.
40. Antoniou J, Zukor DJ, Mwale F, Minarik W, Petit A, Huk OL. Metal ion levels in the blood of patients after hip resurfacing: a comparison between twenty-eight and thirty-six-millimeter-head metal-on-metal prostheses. J Bone Joint Surg Am. 2008;90 Suppl 3:142–8.
41. Onega T, Baron J, MacKenzie T. Cancer after total joint arthroplasty: a meta-analysis. Cancer Epidemiol Biomarkers Prev. 2006;15(8):1532–7.
42. Visuri T, Pulkkinen P, Paavolainen P, Pukkala E. Cancer risk is not increased after conventional hip arthroplasty. Acta Orthop. 2010;81(1):77–81.
43. Haddad FS, Thakrar RR, Hart AJ, Skinner JA, Nargol AV, Nolan JF, Gill HS, Murray DW, Blom AW, Case CP. Metal-on-metal bearings: the evidence so far. J Bone Joint Surg Br. 2011;93(5):572–9.
44. Corradi M, Daniel J, Ziaee H, Alinovi R, Mutti A, McMinn DJ. Early markers of nephrotoxicity in patients with metal-on-metal hip arthroplasty. Clin Orthop Relat Res. 2011;469(6):1651–9.
45. Hart AJ, Sabah SA, Bandi AS, Maggiore P, Tarassoli P, Sampson B, AS J. Sensitivity and specificity of blood cobalt and chromium metal ions for predicting failure of metal-on-metal hip replacement. J Bone Joint Surg Br. 2011;93(10):1308–13.
46. Brodner W, Bitzan P, Meisinger V, Kaider A, Gottsauner-Wolf F, Kotz R. Serum cobalt levels after metal-on-metal total hip arthroplasty. J Bone Joint Surg Am. 2003;85-A(11):2168–73.
47. Savarino L, Padovani G, Ferretti M, Greco M, Cenni E, Perrone G, Greco F, Baldini N, Giunti A. Serum ion levels after ceramic-on-ceramic and metal-on-metal total hip arthroplasty: 8-year minimum follow-up. J Orthop Res. 2008;26(12):1569–76.
48. Daniel J, Ziaee H, Pynsent PB, McMinn DJ. The validity of serum levels as a surrogate measure of systemic exposure to metal ions in hip replacement. J Bone Joint Surg Br. 2007;89(6):736–41.
49. MacDonald SJ, Brodner W, Jacobs JJ. A consensus paper on metal ions in metal-on-metal hip arthroplasties. J Arthroplasty. 2004;19(8 Suppl 3):12–6.
50. De Smet K, De Haan R, Calistri A, Campbell PA, Ebramzadeh E, Pattyn C, Gill HS. Metal ion measurement as a diagnostic tool to identify problems with metal-on-metal hip resurfacing. J Bone Joint Surg Am. 2008;90 Suppl 4:202–8.

Results of the Long-Term Follow-Up Study After the Metasul Metal-on-Metal Cementless Total Hip Arthroplasty

14

Keiji Haraguchi, Junichirou Koyanagi, Kosuke Tsuda, and Keiju Fujiwara

14.1 Introduction

The contemporary metal-on-metal total hip arthroplasty (THA) with a large femoral head has been used expecting the positive effects on stability and durability. However, increased revision rates because of adverse reactions to metal debris (ARMD) for a relatively short postoperative period have been reported worldwide [4, 7, 8]. Large-diameter metal-on-metal bearings have declined, accordingly.

On the other hand, concerning the second-generation metal-on-metal THA with a relatively small 28 mm head, some successful long-term results were reported [2, 3, 12, 13]. However, complications related to ARMD were not thoroughly investigated. We retrospectively reviewed the results of the more than 10-year follow-up after the Metasul metal-on-metal cementless THA to validate the continued use for the metal-on-metal bearing couples.

14.2 Methods

Between 1997 and 2002, 87 patients (97 hips) underwent the Metasul® (Zimmer Inc., Warsaw, IN) metal-on-metal cementless THA. The acetabular cups used were the APR cup (Zimmer Inc., Warsaw, IN) and the Converge cup (Zimmer Inc., Warsaw, IN). The APR cup was the early type, which had the unreliable liner-locking mechanism. The Converge cup was the later type, in which the liner-locking mechanism was improved to have enough reliability. The Metasul inlay (Zimmer Inc., Warsaw, IN) was the polyethylene-sandwiched metal liner. The femoral

K. Haraguchi, MD, PhD (✉) • J. Koyanagi, MD, PhD • K. Tsuda, MD, PhD
K. Fujiwara, MD, PhD
Department of Orthopaedic Surgery, Osaka General Medical Center,
3-1-56 Bandaihigashi, Sumiyoshi-ku, Osaka 558-5885, Japan
e-mail: k-haraguchi@gh.opho.jp

K. Knahr (ed.), *Tribology in Total Hip and Knee Arthroplasty*,
DOI 10.1007/978-3-642-45266-6_14, © EFORT 2014

component used was the Alloclassic SL stem (Zimmer Inc., Warsaw, IN), and the femoral head used was a 28 mm-diameter head. The femoral head and the metal liner were made of high-carbon wrought-forged cobalt-chromium alloy. The head-neck ratio of the implants was 2.0.

Operations were performed through the posterolateral approach in the lateral decubitus position. Thirteen surgeons with 2–15 years of surgical experience operated in this study. The cementless acetabular cup was fixed with two to three supplemental screws after line to line reaming. The target angle of the cup inclination was 45°. However, that of the cup anteversion was variable by the surgeons and not consistent. The combined anteversion technique [1, 16] was not used.

Seven patients died of unrelated cause to arthroplasty. Twelve patients were lost before the 10-year follow-up. These 19 patients (19 hips) maintained well-functioning hips. Seventeen patients (18 hips) were revised. Of them, two patients died of unrelated cause to arthroplasty after revision. The remaining 51patients (60 hips) with more than 10-year follow-up were the subject of the clinical evaluation. The average age was 59.9 years (34–74 years), and the average follow-up period was 12.3 years (10–15 years). The preoperative diagnoses were osteoarthritis in 53 hips, inflammatory arthritis in five hips, and osteonecrosis of the femoral head in two hips.

Clinical evaluation was performed by using the Merle D'Aubigné and Postel hip scores preoperatively and the latest follow-up from the medical records. The presence of the palpable pseudotumor was also investigated.

Radiographic evaluation was performed for 68 patients (78 hips) excluding those who were lost and died with well-functioning THA. Osseointegration, osteolysis, and cup orientation were evaluated using the anteroposterior and lateral X-rays of the affected hip. The cup orientation was evaluated by measurement of radiographic inclination and anteversion of the cup [11]. The cup orientation was defined as in the safe zone when the radiographic inclination of the cup was between 30 and 50 and the radiographic anteversion of the cup was between 5 and 25 [9].

The reasons for reoperation were also investigated. Survival rates were calculated for all 87 patients using the Kaplan-Meier method.

14.3 Results

The average Merle D'Aubigné and Postel hip scores were improved from 8.5 (pain 2.1, mobility 4.0, walk 2.4) preoperatively to 16.3 (pain 5.8, mobility 5.4, walk 5.1) at the latest follow-up. No patient without reoperation complained of the mass around the operated hip.

Radiographically, except for two cups loosened and revised, all of the other femoral and acetabular components were osseointegrated at the latest follow-up. Osteolysis was seen for seven hips. Three of them were revised, and six of them were implanted with the APR cup. Femoral osteolysis was seen in only one hip implanted with the APR cup.

The radiographic inclination and anteversion of the cup (average ± standard deviation) were 45.6° ± 5.9° (34.8–62.5) and 18.7° ± 11.2° (0–42.3), respectively. Fifty

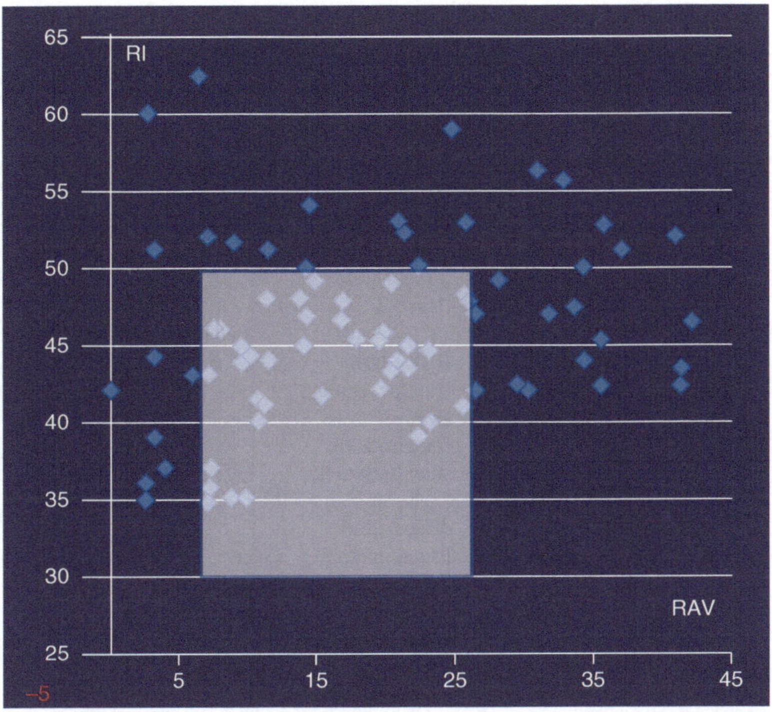

Fig. 14.1 Scattergram of the cup orientation. The safe zone for the cup orientation was shown as the area surrounded with a square. *RI* radiographic inclination of the cup, *RAV* radiographic anteversion of the cup

percent of the cups without reoperation and only one-third of the cups with reoperation were in the safe zone (Fig. 14.1).

The reasons for reoperation were examined for the patients using the APR cup and for those using the Converge cup separately (Table 14.1). The main reasons for reoperation of the APR cup were the liner dissociation between the liner and the metal shell, and pelvic osteolysis. In Case 2, the extracted liner showed concentric abrasive backside wear of the polyethylene (Fig. 14.2). Histological specimens of the osteolytic lesion showed giant cells that phagocytized polyethylene particles.

On the other hand, patients using the Converge cup showed pseudotumor formation and pain. One patient with pseudotumor complained of leg edema (Case 12). CT revealed that the mass located anterior to the hip joint was indenting the femoral vessels. Another patient with pseudotumor (Case 13) complained of a large mass around the buttock and the proximal thigh. Histological specimens of the pseudotumors (Case 12, 13) showed extensive necrosis of the soft tissue. We considered these two cases as ARMD. Neck impingement was confirmed as notch formation on the stem neck against the metal portion of the Metasul liner intraoperatively in all of the eight hips using the Converge cup. Pain was induced by extension and external rotation of the hip motion, which produced prosthetic impingement. In

Table 14.1 List of reoperated patients

Case	Duration to revision (years)	Cup	Main reasons for reoperation	Related matters	Impingement	Safe zone
1	3.6	APR	Infection		–	○
2	6.7	APR	Pelvic lysis	Liner dissociation	+	×
3	7.4	APR	Recurrent dislocation		+	×
4	7.7	APR	Liner dissociation		+	×
5	8.5	APR	Pain	Liner dissociation	–	○
6	9.1	APR	Pelvic lysis		–	○
7	12.3	APR	Cup loosening		–	○
8	12.4	APR	Femoral fracture with stem loosening		–	×
9	12.7	APR	Liner dissociation		+	×
10	13.6	APR	Pseudotumor	Liner dissociation	–	○
11-1	5.7	Converge	Recurrent dislocation	Pain	+	×
12	6.0	Converge	Pseudotumor	Leg edema	+	×
13	7.9	Converge	Pseudotumor		+	×
14	8.0	Converge	Infection	Pseudotumor	+	×
11-2	8.3	Converge	Pain		+	○
15	8.7	Converge	Pain		+	×
16	9.8	Converge	Pelvic lysis		+	×
17	11.4	Converge	Cup loosening		+	×

total, only 33 % of the cups were in the safe zone, and 67 % of the necks showed impingement.

Survival rates (95 % confidence interval) were 94.9 % (80.9–98.7) defined with the endpoint as revision for aseptic loosening (Fig. 14.3) and 71.2 % (56.1–81.3) defined with the endpoint as any reoperation (Fig. 14.4). Survival rates were dropped by the reasons unrelated to mechanical loosening.

14.4 Discussion

Survival rates at more than 10 years after the Metasul metal-on-metal THA were reported previously by some authors [2, 3, 12, 13]. The reported survival rates at 10–16 years were 92.2–94.4 %. In this study, however, the survival rates at 15 years defined with the endpoint as revision for aseptic loosening were 94.9 %; the survival rates at 15 years defined with the endpoint as any reoperation decreased to 71.2 %. Concerning the reasons for revision, liner dissociation and recurrent dislocation

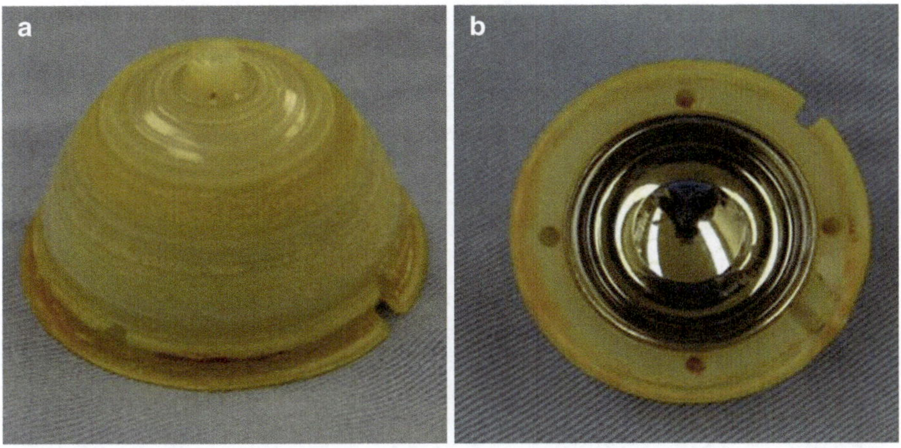

Fig. 14.2 (**a**, **b**) Photos of the extracted Metasul liner in a case with pelvic osteolysis. (**a**) Backside view. Severe concentric abrasive wear of the polyethylene was seen. (**b**) Bearing side view. Deformation of the rim of the liner was seen. Bearing surface was glossy and no visible wear was observed

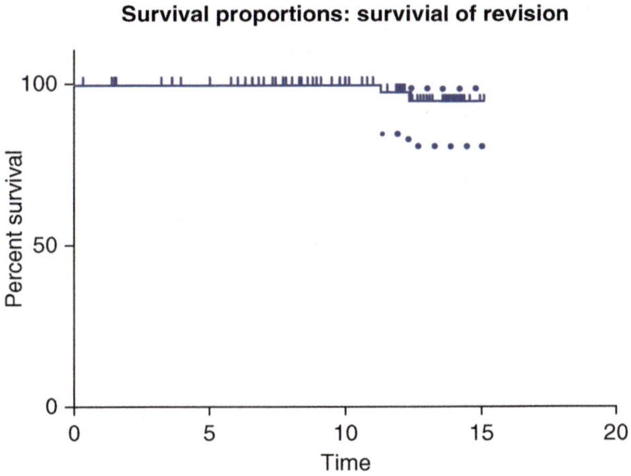

Fig. 14.3 Survival curves using the Kaplan-Meier method. *Dotted line* shows 95 % confidence intervals. The endpoint was defined with revision for aseptic loosening

were reported to be the common reasons [2, 12, 13]; however, pelvic osteolysis and pseudotumor were uncommon in the previous study [5].

In this study, five revisions were performed for the reasons associated with liner dissociation of the APR Cup, and three revisions were performed for those associated with pelvic osteolysis. Usrey et al. indicated that head-neck ratio less than 2.0 showed high risk of prosthetic impingement and resultant backside wear [15]. The head-neck ratio of the implants used was 2.0. The backside wear of the polyethylene of the Metasul liner was supposed to be one of the causes of the pelvic osteolysis of the APR cup. Another possible reason for pelvic osteolysis was metallosis induced

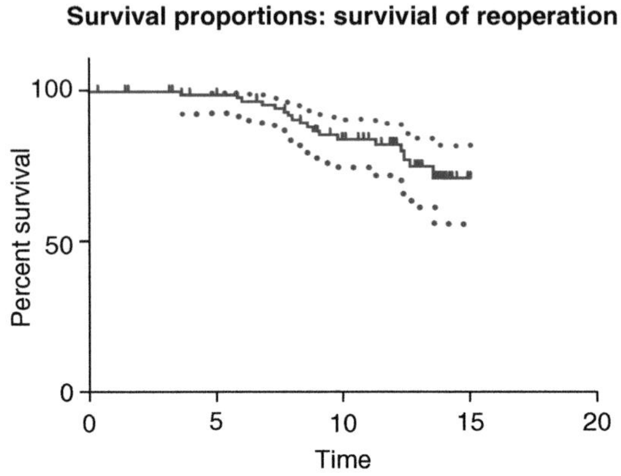

Fig. 14.4 Survival curves using the Kaplan-Meier method. *Dotted line* shows 95 % confidence intervals. The endpoint was defined with any reoperations

by impingement. Two patients with pseudotumor were considered to be the cases with ARMD, and the incidence was 2.1 %.

The most critical points were that only 33 % of the cups were in the safe zone, and 67 % of the necks showed impingement in revision cases. Malik et al. reported that prosthetic impingement and the resultant liner dissociation could occur after the Metasul metal-on-metal THA with proper cup alignment [10].

In this study, the operations were performed by 13 surgeons with several years of surgical experience for the period of 6 years. The importance of the cup orientation and combined anteversion for hard-on-hard bearings [6, 14] was not well recognized at that time. The target for the cup orientation could not be controlled. The metal-on-metal implant with low head-neck ratio with improper cup alignment was considered to be the critical factor.

In conclusion, the second-generation metal-on-metal cementless THA also encountered ARMD in 2.1 %. Prosthetic impingement caused by improper cup orientation was the critical factor for the longevity of the second-generation metal-on-metal THA with a 28 mm head. We concluded that there is little benefit for the continued use of metal-on-metal bearings in THA.

References

1. Amuwa C, Dorr LD. The combined anteversion technique for acetabular component anteversion. J Arthroplasty. 2008;23(7):1068–70.
2. Dastane M, Wan Z, Deshmane P, et al. Primary hip arthroplasty with 28-mm Metasul articulation. J Arthroplasty. 2011;26(4):662–4.
3. Eswaramoorthy V, Moonot P, Kalairajah Y, et al. The Metasul metal-on-metal articulation in primary total hip replacement: clinical and radiological results at ten years. J Bone Joint Surg Br. 2008;90(10):1278–83.
4. Graves SE, Rothwell A, Tucker K, et al. A multinational assessment of metal-on-metal bearings in hip replacement. J Bone Joint Surg Am. 2011;93 Suppl 3:43–7.
5. Holloway I, Walter WL, Zicat B, et al. Osteolysis with a cementless second generation metal-on-metal cup in total hip replacement. Int Orthop. 2009;33(6):1537–42.

6. Langton DJ, Jameson SS, Joyce TJ, et al. The effect of component size and orientation on the concentrations of metal ions after resurfacing arthroplasty of the hip. J Bone Joint Surg Br. 2008;90(9):1143–51.
7. Langton DJ, Jameson SS, Joyce TJ, et al. Early failure of metal-on-metal bearings in hip resurfacing and large-diameter total hip replacement: a consequence of excess wear. J Bone Joint Surg Br. 2010;92(1):38–46.
8. Langton DJ, Joyce TJ, Jameson SS, et al. Adverse reaction to metal debris following hip resurfacing: the influence of component type, orientation and volumetric wear. J Bone Joint Surg Br. 2011;93(2):164–71.
9. Lewinnek GE, et al. Dislocations after total hip-replacement arthroplasties. J Bone Joint Surg Am. 1978;60(2):217–20.
10. Malik A, Dorr LD, Long WT. Impingement as a mechanism of dissociation of a metasul metal-on-metal liner. J Arthroplasty. 2009;24(2):323.e13–e16.
11. Murray DW. The definition and measurement of acetabular orientation. J Bone Joint Surg Br. 1993;75(2):228–32.
12. Randelli F, Banci L, D'Anna A, et al. Cementless metasul metal-on-metal total hip arthroplasties at 13 years. J Arthroplasty. 2012;27(2):186–92.
13. Saito S, Ishii T, Mori S, et al. Long-term results of metasul metal-on-metal total hip arthroplasty. Orthopedics. 2010;11:33(8).
14. Sugano N, Nishii T, Miki H, et al. Mid-term results of cementless total hip replacement using a ceramic-on-ceramic bearing with and without computer navigation. J Bone Joint Surg Br. 2007;89(4):455–60.
15. Usrey MM, Noble PC, Rudner LJ, et al. Does neck/liner impingement increase wear of ultrahigh-molecular-weight polyethylene liners? J Arthroplasty. 2006;21(6 Suppl 2):65–71.
16. Widmer KH, Zurfluh B. Compliant positioning of total hip components for optimal range of motion. J Orthop Res. 2004;22(4):815–21.

15 Clinical and Radiological Results Following Revision Surgery of Metal-on-Metal Articulation in Total Hip Arthroplasty

Peter Radakovits and Karl Knahr

15.1 Introduction

In the 1950s, metal-on-metal (MoM) articulations started being used in total hip arthroplasty (THA). Poor clinical results due to loosening and mechanical failure led to the discontinuation of MoM and the use of metal-on-polyethylene (MoP) and ceramic-on-polyethylene (CoP) articulating partners. Both MoP and CoP had high failure rates due to osteolysis and bone destruction induced by wear particles. In the 1980s, the second generation of MoM, with improved materials, design factors, and manufacturing technique, was introduced. Today there are many different MoM designs with various metallurgies available. These differences have led to variable clinical performance.

A review of international literature and national registries shows that there is a higher revision rate for MoM articulations in THA, but there is disagreement about the factors which are responsible for these higher revision rates [3, 10, 21, 22]. Although MoM articulations produce less wear than every other combination of articulation partners except ceramic-on-ceramic (CoC), several published studies have found the wear of MoM articulations tends to be more aggressive on the soft tissue surrounding the hip joint [8, 24]. Hypersensitive reactions of the soft tissue are described, and a lot of clinical data report the appearance of pseudotumors and adverse reaction to metal debris (ARMD) [2, 4, 8, 19, 20, 24, 25]. An ARMD is often associated with elevated serum levels of metal ions measured in vivo.

National registries as well as many published studies show that there is evidence correlating large-diameter femoral heads to higher rates of revision surgery [18, 20–22]. Furthermore, there seems to be a consensus about the importance of the concentration of carbon in the cobalt chromium molybdenum alloy. The data

P. Radakovits (✉) • K. Knahr
Department of Orthopedic, Orthopedic Hospital Vienna Speising GmbH,
Speisinger Strasse 109, Vienna 1130, Austria
e-mail: peter.radakovits@oss.at

K. Knahr (ed.), *Tribology in Total Hip and Knee Arthroplasty*,
DOI 10.1007/978-3-642-45266-6_15, © EFORT 2014

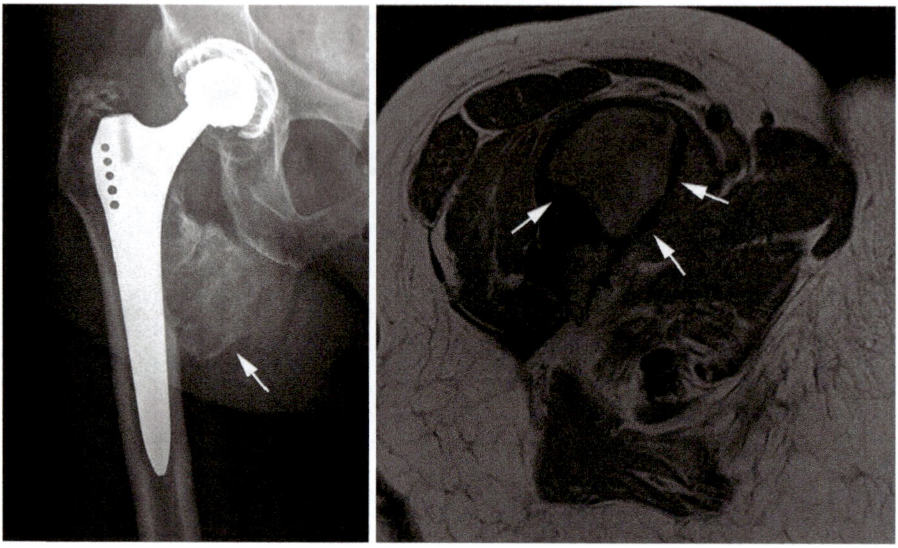

Fig. 15.1 Pseudotumor and ARMD 6.2 years after THA with MoM articulation

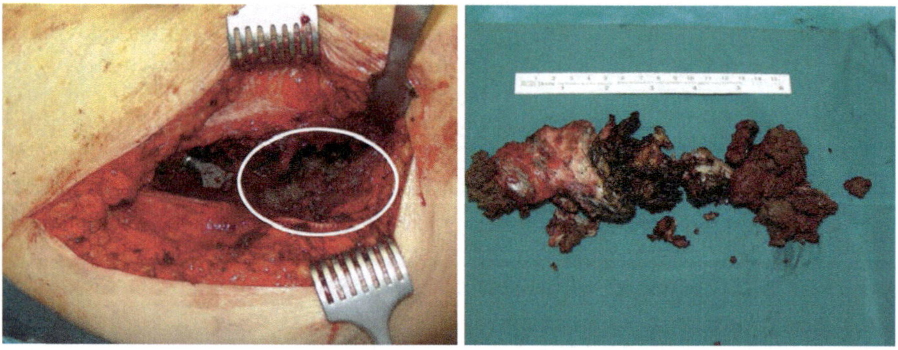

Fig. 15.2 Total synovectomy and resection of the pseudotumor

from several clinical studies show high success rates for high-carbon (>0.2 wt%) alloys and poor performance for low-carbon alloys [12, 15–17, 23].

Revision surgeries of MoM articulations were done for the following reasons: progressive osteolysis, aseptic loosening of implant, nonspecific (groin) pain, adverse reaction to metal debris (ARMD) with pseudotumors, or elevated levels of serum cobalt and chromium (Figs. 15.1 and 15.2) [6, 9].

International literature concerning the results of MoM articulation revisions in THA shows elevated infection rates [11]. There are also reports documenting metal ions' rapid decrease of elevated serum levels to almost normal levels through revision surgery [1, 5]. As there are less data surrounding the clinical outcome of MoM articulation revisions, our intention was to evaluate the clinical and radiological outcome of revised MoM articulation in THA.

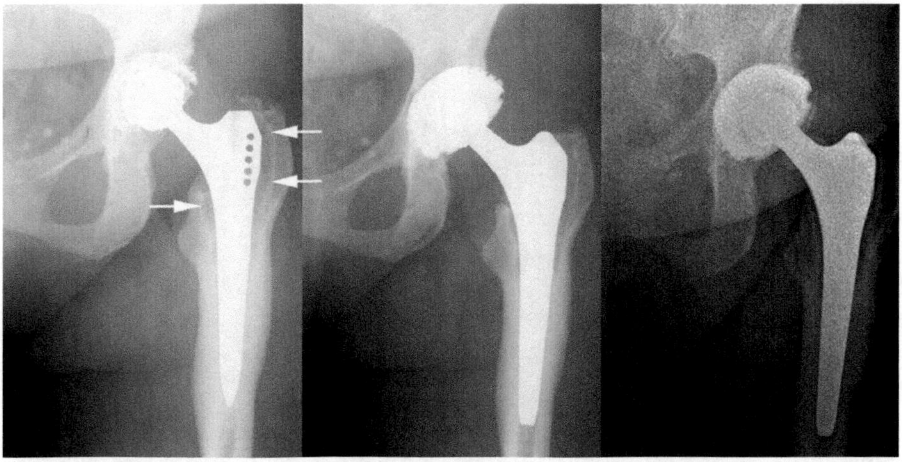

Fig. 15.3 Progressive osteolysis 4.2 years after THA with MoM articulation – exchange of THA – no progression of osteolysis or radiolucent lines 10.9 years after revision surgery

15.2 Material and Method

Between 1996 and 2008, we revised 39 patients (39 THAs) with 28 mm MoM articulation in our department – 27 women and 12 men. Only five of them had their first surgery in our institution. The average age at the time of the revision surgery was 60.2 (35.6–83.3) years, and the revision was performed an average of 5.1 (0.8–13.3) years after the implantation of the MoM articulation. Twenty-two low-carbon and 17 high-carbon MoM articulations were revised in our study group.

In 24 cases, revision surgery was done because of progressive osteolysis and/or aseptic loosening of components. Fourteen patients underwent revision because of nonspecific groin pain, and one patient was revised due to recurrent dislocation because of adverse reaction to metal debris.

Before surgery we evaluated standard x-rays and serum levels to check for infection (complete blood count, CRP), and if necessary, we also made MRI or CT scans to know more about the current condition of osseous and soft tissue in relation to pseudotumor, ARMD, bone loss/osteolysis, and infection. Periprosthetic joint infections with MoM articulations were excluded from our study sample.

All revision surgeries were done in supine position with a modified lateral approach (Bauer/Hardinge). In every case we did a total synovectomy of the hip joint with resection of the pseudotumor and at the very least exchanged the endoprosthesis' liner and head.

Often more was required: in 13 cases we needed to exchange the cup, in three surgeries we had to change the stem, and in eight revisions it was necessary to change the whole prosthesis (cup and stem) (Figs. 15.3 and 15.4). We took at least one specimen of synovial tissue for histological examination and at least three samples for bacteriological cultures during each revision.

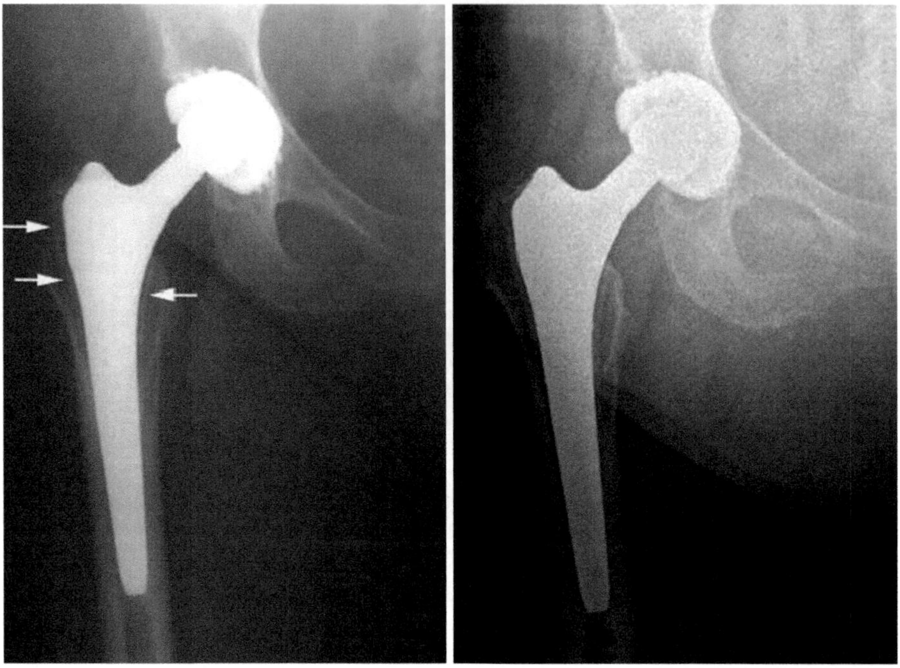

Fig. 15.4 Increasing pain and radiolucent lines at the prox. stem (Zones I and VII) 2.1 years after THA with MoM articulation – no progression of radiolucent lines 8.5 years after revision surgery with total synovectomy and exchange of head and liner

To evaluate the outcome of revised MoM articulations, a retrospective, consecutive, single-center study was conducted, examining standard x-rays and serum cobalt and chromium levels, as well as clinical examination utilizing the Harris hip score, WOMAC score, and SF-36.

15.3 Results

Twenty-seven patients were available for a follow-up, averaging 8.4 (3.3–14.3) years after revision surgery. The mean age of follow-up patients was 68.5 (43.9–82.9) years. Of the remaining 12, four patients were deceased with no further revision surgery and eight patients were lost to follow-up.

The mean Harris hip score increased from 58.9 to 87.2 points at the time of the latest follow-up (Fig. 15.5). This improvement was highly significant ($p < 0.001$).

Using SF-36, we compared our sample group with normal data for 70-year-olds (Fig. 15.6). We found an enhancement in general health and positive results in other categories, although only the categories role physical, social functioning, bodily pain, role emotional, and mental health were significant ($p < 0.05$).

Using the WOMAC score, we compared our sample set with normative data referring to pain, function, and stiffness of the operated hip joint (Fig. 15.7). The results are consistently good but only significant for pain and stiffness ($p < 0.05$).

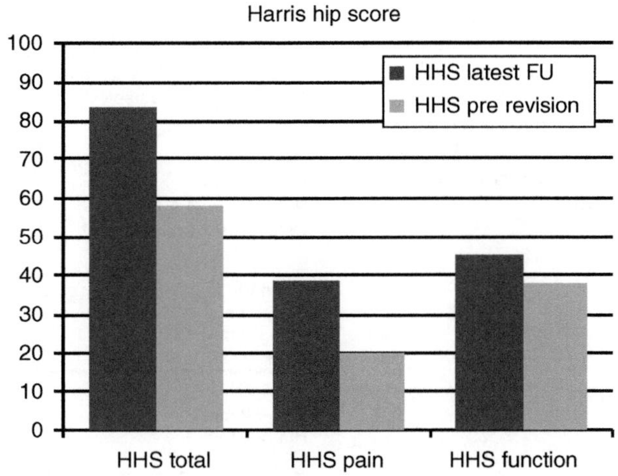

Fig. 15.5 HHS

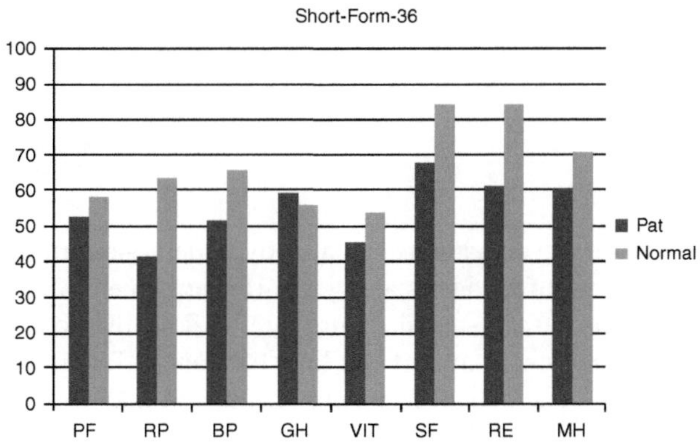

Fig. 15.6 SF-36

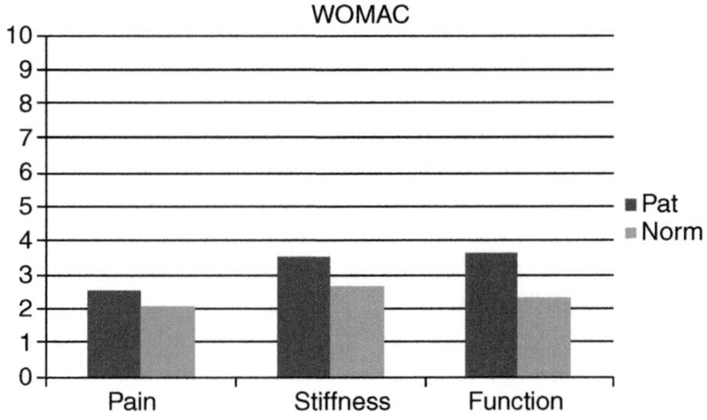

Fig. 15.7 WOMAC

All the serum cobalt and chromium levels we examined at the latest follow-up were in the normal range (cobalt <0.5 μg/l, chromium <5 μg/l).

For our radiological analysis, standard x-rays were scanned for radiolucent lines (RLL), osteolysis, and loosening of component (Fig. 15.8). All x-rays showed stable components with no progression of osteolysis at the time of the latest follow-up.

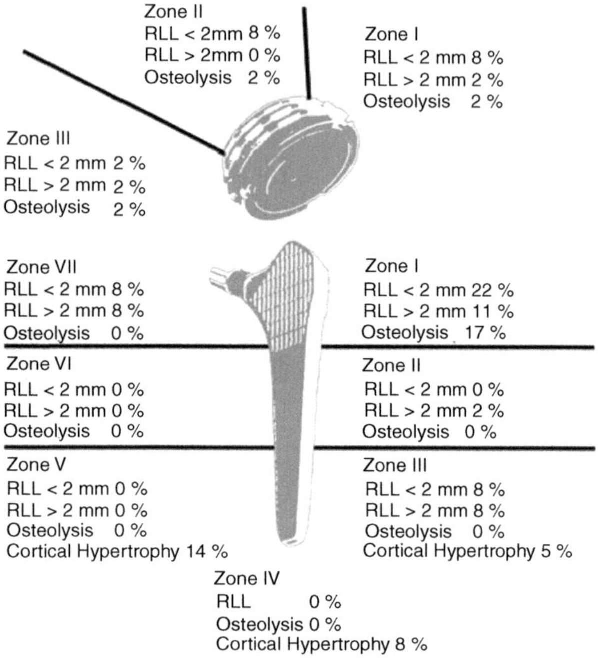

Fig. 15.8 Radiological analysis with evaluation of radiolucent lines (*RLL*), osteolysis, and cortical bone reaction in acetabular zones according to DeLee and femoral zones according to Gruen

However, seven patients had already undergone further revision surgery for reasons other than infection, meaning a re-revision rate of 22.6 % in our sample.

In one case, re-revision surgery was done due to aseptic loosening of the stem – first revision was a head and liner exchange. Two patients had aseptic loosening of the cup – one patient had a cup, head, and liner exchange during the first revision, and the other patient had a head and liner exchange. Two patients had recurrent dislocations – one of them underwent a cup, head, and liner exchange, and the other patient had a further revision surgery in another hospital. In two cases we had to perform a re-revision surgery because of cup breakage: one patient had a stem, head, and liner exchange due to previous osteolysis/aseptic loosening, and the cup breakage was a consequence of the osteolysis around the original cup (Fig. 15.9) – the second patient had a high-impact trauma.

15.4 Discussion

In this retrospective study on revisions of metal-on-metal articulations in total hip arthroplasty, clinical results were largely positive. We did not see any progression of osteolysis or bone resorption after revision surgery in our radiological analysis. In most of our sample cases affected by osteolysis because of ARMD, we observed bony consolidation around the endoprosthesis after revision surgery. Obviously our

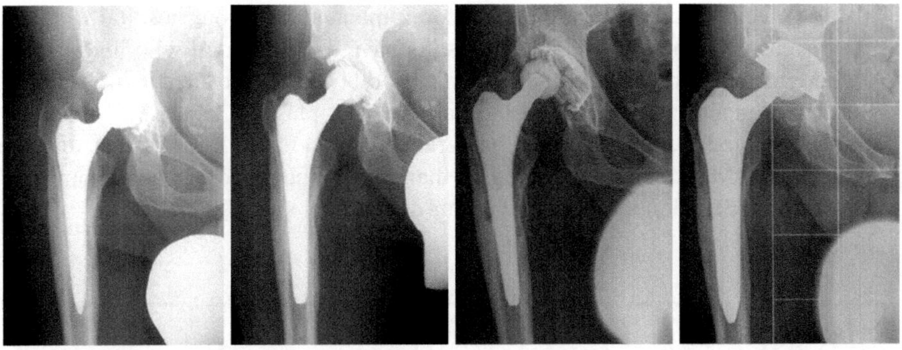

Fig. 15.9 Osteolysis and loosening of the stem 8.8 years after THA with MoM articulation; revision surgery with exchange of stem, head, and liner; breakage of the original cup 3.2 years after revision; consolidation of the bone with remission of osteolysis 5.4 years after re-revision surgery with exchange of THA

sample group is inhomogeneous with a mismatch between women and men; we are with international literature stating that female patients with MoM articulations have a higher risk for revision surgery, especially in hip resurfacing [13].

It must be noticed that these 39 revision surgeries were done over a period of 12 years from 1996 to 2008 and that we revised different total hip arthroplasty systems from different companies, meaning we performed revision surgeries on low-carbon hip systems as well as high-carbon total hip arthroplasties. Many studies show that low-carbon MoM articulations produce significantly more wear than high-carbon articulations, which leads to more aggressive soft tissue reactions (ARMD) with pseudotumor, osteolysis, and component loosening [12, 17, 23].

At the time of the latest follow-up, serum specimens did not show increased levels of cobalt or chromium. This is in accordance with international literature, where elevated serum levels rapidly decrease – in the first weeks, almost normal serum levels were reached [1, 5]. We did not check serum metal ion levels before revision surgery in our study, so we cannot report on a decrease of potentially elevated cobalt and chromium serum levels.

Furthermore there seem to be unknown, patient-specific factors that are responsible for failure of MoM articulations in THA [7, 14].

Conclusion

Aseptic loosening, progressive osteolysis, nonspecific groin pain, and ARMD often occur in THA with MoM articulations. In our consecutive, retrospective, single-center study, we achieved an improvement in patients' quality of life through revision surgery that, at the very least, exchanged the metal-on-metal articulation and provided a total synovectomy with resection of the pseudotumor. We recommend short-term clinical and radiological examination of THAs with MoM articulation, and we advise early revision surgery in the case of progressive osteolysis or painful hip joints.

We avoid metal-on-metal articulation implantations at our hospital for these very reasons. Although very good results have been reported with high-carbon MoM articulations with 28 and 32 mm femoral heads, there are a lot of excellent articulation alternatives for use in total hip arthroplasty, e.g., ceramic on cross-linked polyethylene or ceramic-on-ceramic. Considering the fact that revision rates of MoM articulations are higher than every other tribological combination, we have not used metal-on-metal in our department since 2006.

References

1. Ball ST, Severns D, Linn M, Meyer RS, Swenson FC. What happens to serum metal ion levels after a metal-on-metal bearing is removed? J Arthroplasty. 2013;28(8):53–5.
2. Bisschop R, Boomsma MF, Van Raay JJ, Tiebosch AT, Maas M, Gerritsma CL. High prevalence of pseudotumors in patients with a Birmingham hip resurfacing prosthesis: a prospective cohort study of hundred and twenty-nine patients. J Bone Joint Surg Am. 2013;95(17): 1554–60.
3. Bjorgul K, Novicoff WN, Andersen ST, Ahlund OR, Bunes A, Wiig M, Brevig K. High rate of revision and a high incidence of radiolucent lines around Metasul metal-on-metal total hip replacements: results from a randomized controlled trial of three bearings after seven years. Bone Joint J. 2013;95-B(7):881–6.
4. Daniel J, Holland J, Quigley L, Sprague S, Bhandari M. Pseudotumors associated with total hip arthroplasty. J Bone Joint Surg Am. 2012;94(1):86–93.
5. Ebreo D, Khan A, El-Meligy M, Armstrong C, Peter V. Metal ion levels decrease after revision for metallosis arising from large-diameter metal-on-metal hip arthroplasty. Acta Orthop Belg. 2011;77(6):777–81.
6. Grammatopoulos G, Pandit H, Kwon YM, Gundle R, McLardy-Smith P, Beard DJ, Murray DW, Gill HS. Hip resurfacing revised for inflammatory pseudotumour have a poor outcome. J Bone Joint Surg Br. 2009;91(8):1019–24.
7. Hart AJ, Matthies A, Henckel J, Ilo K, Skinner J, Noble PC. Understanding why metal-on-metal hip arthroplasties fail: a comparison between patients with well-functioning and revised Birmingham hip resurfacing arthroplasties AAOS exhibit selection. J Bone Joint Surg Am. 2012;94(4):e221–10.
8. Hart AJ, Satchithananda K, Liddle AD, Sabah SA, McRobbie D, Henckel J, Cobb JP, Skinner JA, Mitchell AW. Pseudotumors in association with well-functioning metal-on-metal hip prostheses: a case-control study using three-dimensional computed tomography and magnetic resonance imaging. J Bone Joint Surg Am. 2012;94(4):317–25.
9. Hauptfleisch J, Pandit H, Grammatopoulos G, Gill HS, Murray DW, Ostlere S. A MRI classification of periprosthetic soft tissue masses (pseudotumours) associated with metal-on-metal resurfacing hip arthroplasty. Skeletal Radiol. 2012;41(2):149–55.
10. Jameson SS, Baker PN, Mason J, Rymaszewska M, Gregg PJ, Deehan DJ, Reed MR. Independent predictors of failure up to 7.5 years after 35 386 single-brand cementless total hip replacements: a retrospective cohort study using National Joint Registry data. Bone Joint J. 2013;95-B(6):747–57.
11. Judd KT, Noiseux N. Concomitant infection and local metal reaction in patients undergoing revision of metal-on-metal total hip arthroplasty. Iowa Orthop J. 2011;31:59–63.
12. Korovessis P, Petsinis G, Repanti M, Repantis T. Metallosis after contemporary metal-on-metal total hip arthroplasty. Five to nine-year follow-up. J Bone Joint Surg Am. 2006; 88(6):1183–91.

13. Liu F, Gross TP. A safe zone for acetabular component position in metal-on-metal hip resurfacing arthroplasty: winner of the 2012 HAP PAUL award. J Arthroplasty. 2013;28(7):1224–30.
14. Matthies AK, Skinner JA, Osmani H, Henckel J, Hart AJ. Pseudotumors are common in well-positioned low-wearing metal-on-metal hips. Clin Orthop Relat Res. 2012;470(7):1895–906.
15. Migaud H, Putman S, Combes A, Berton C, Bocquet D, Vasseur L, Girard J. Metal-on-metal bearing: is this the end of line? We do not think so. HSS J. 2012;8(3):262–9.
16. Migaud H, Putman S, Krantz N, Vasseur L, Girard J. Cementless metal-on-metal versus ceramic-on-polyethylene hip arthroplasty in patients less than fifty years of age. J Bone Joint Surg Am. 2011;93(2):137–42.
17. Milosev I, Trebse R, Kovac S, Cör A, Pisot V. Survivorship and retrieval analysis of Sikomet metal-on-metal total hip replacements at a mean of seven years. J Bone Joint Surg Am. 2006;88(6):1173–82.
18. Munro JT, Masri BA, Duncan CP, Garbuz DS. High complication rate after revision of large-head metal-on-metal total hip arthroplasty. Clin Orthop Relat Res. 2013. [Epub ahead of print].
19. Nawabi DH, Hayter CL, Su EP, Koff MF, Perino G, Gold SL, Koch KM, Potter HG. Magnetic resonance imaging findings in symptomatic versus asymptomatic subjects following metal-on-metal hip resurfacing arthroplasty. J Bone Joint Surg Am. 2013;95(10):895–902.
20. Nawabi DH, Nassif NA, Do HT, Stoner K, Elpers M, Su EP, Wright T, Potter HG, Padgett DE. What causes unexplained pain in patients with metal-on-metal hip devices? A retrieval, histologic and imaging analysis. Clin Orthop Relat Res. 2013. [Epub ahead of print].
21. No authors listed. Australian Orthopedic Association National Joint Replacement Registry: hip and knee arthroplasty annual report. 2012.
22. No authors listed. National Joint Registry for England and Wales: 9th annual report. 2012.
23. Repantis T, Vitsas V, Korovessis P. Poor mid-term survival of the low-carbide metal-on-metal Zweymüller-plus total hip arthroplasty system: a concise follow-up, at a minimum of ten years, of a previous report. J Bone Joint Surg Am. 2013;95(6):e331–4.
24. Wiley KF, Ding K, Stoner JA, Teague DC, Yousuf KM. Incidence of pseudotumor and acute lymphocytic vasculitis associated lesion (ALVAL) reactions in metal-on-metal hip articulations: a meta-analysis. J Arthroplasty. 2013;28(7):1238–45.
25. Williams DH, Greidanus NV, Masri BA, Duncan CP, Garbuz DS. Prevalence of pseudotumor in asymptomatic patients after metal-on-metal hip arthroplasty. J Bone Joint Surg Am. 2011;93(23):2164–71.

16 Evaluation of Different Consensus Statements on Thresholds for Metal Ions in Metal-on-Metal Total Hip Arthroplasties

Christiaan P. van Lingen, Harmen B. Ettema, and Cees C.P.M. Verheyen

16.1 Introduction

The introduction of large-head metal-on-metal (MoM) hip replacements projected promising results initially. Low wear in laboratory mechanical tests, no relevant risk of material fracture, a high design variability, and an expected increased range of motion seemed to justify the application of MoM bearings in both hip resurfacing and large-head stemmed hip replacement [1–3].

Nevertheless, wear and corrosion of these implants could potentially lead to a release of metal products into surrounding tissue and body fluids as well as internal organs. Metal accumulation may result in local "adverse reactions to metal debris" (ARMD) [4] and potentially induce systemic adverse effects (i.e. toxicity, teratogenicity and carcinogenicity) [5–8].

Recent reports on pseudotumor formation and high failure rates of hip resurfacing and MoM total hip arthroplasty have initiated a discussion about the systemic biological effects of MoM implants [9–18]. Since these safety concerns have been raised, several health authorities and scientific societies in different countries have published recommendations for the use and monitoring of MoM implants [19–24].

Until recently, there were no guidelines on what constitutes an unacceptably high level of ions in blood for patients receiving orthopedic implants. At the moment, there is no general international consensus on the threshold and follow-up on metal ion levels [16]. Collecting several consensus statements regarding thresholds for metal ions in MoM arthroplasty could render a promising insight into this complex concept.

C.P. van Lingen, MD (✉) • H.B. Ettema, MD, PhD • C.C.P.M. Verheyen, MD, PhD
Department of Orthopaedic Surgery and Traumatology,
Isala klinieken, Zwolle, The Netherlands
e-mail: c.c.p.m.verheyen@isala.nl

K. Knahr (ed.), *Tribology in Total Hip and Knee Arthroplasty*,
DOI 10.1007/978-3-642-45266-6_16, © EFORT 2014

16.2 Metal Ion Analysis

Metal ion determination of body fluids can be performed in whole blood, serum, and urine with different techniques. An analysis in whole blood or serum is preferable, since urine requires a 24-hour collection and the levels seem to be more variable to variation in hydration of the individual [25]. There is no evidence that either serum or whole blood is superior [26, 27]. The use of whole blood seems more practical without an extra laboratory process which can introduce pollution and may be favored for practical reason depending on local preference. Smolders et. al. proposed a conversion formula between whole blood and serum ion levels [27].

Determination of metal ion levels in whole blood and serum is performed under the rules of internal and external quality control [28]. Inductively coupled plasma mass spectrometry (ICP-MS) or graphite furnace atomic absorption spectrometry (GF-AAS) methods are valid, the former being more precise and has lower detection limits [29].

16.3 Reference Values

Results of metal concentrations measurements are often presented in different units to describe the metal concentration. The units ("parts per billion") nmol/L and g/L have been established. The unit "ppb" is outdated, and its use is discouraged. The unit "ppb" is more or less interchangeable with "ug/L." In the unit "nmol/L," the individual molar mass of the element is taken into account. This unit can be converted into the most common concentration μg/L. For cobalt 1 μg/L equals 17 nmol/L and 1 μg/L chromium equals 19 nmol/L.

Cobalt and chromium are considered as essential trace elements, which play an important role in metabolism, but can be toxic in high concentrations. Trace elements cobalt and chromium are present in low concentrations in the healthy organism. Normal renal function is needed to excrete the excess of cobalt and chromium. The reference value for a healthy individual is less than 0.5 μg/L [30].

Factors that influence cobalt levels are, besides renal impairment, also the use of nutritional supplements, certain medication (cobalt chloride for anemia) and other metal implants.

It is well recognized that implantation of a MoM prosthesis results in increased blood levels of metal ions, especially cobalt and chromium. After their run-in phases (the first 12 months), the cobalt levels stabilize in a well-functioning implant to concentrations <2 μg/L [31–34]. The systemic concentrations of cobalt and chromium metal correlate well with the linear and volumetric wear of the bearing surfaces [2, 5]. Various causes can lead to wear of the bearing interface, which causes the systemic concentrations of cobalt and chromium to increase measurably. These include, for example, implant design and higher edge loading conditions such as an increased inclination of the cup and a smaller femoral head [14, 35]. Moreover, the head-neck junction where the tapered femoral neck (male taper, trunnion) connects to the femoral head adds an additional metal interface which can be another source of wear [14].

16.4 Interpretation of Ion Levels

Since safety concerns on MoM implants have risen, several health authorities and scientific societies and organizations as well as research groups have published recommendations for the use and follow-up of these implants.

Recommendations regarding the need for metal ion analysis and ion levels are controversial, and there is in fact no international consensus whether chromium and/or cobalt should even be monitored [28].

Threshold levels for ions levels for orthopedic implants are provided by several institutions during the past 5 years though. Median ion levels and acceptable ranges corresponding with well or insufficiently functioning MoM implants are reported [30, 36, 46] (Fig. 16.1).

More recent studies provide a more precise threshold level for cobalt in unilaterally operated patients with additional information regarding sensitivity and specificity [9, 10, 13, 14, 37–39, 47]. These are listed in Table 16.1. Endpoints differ considerably between these studies. The specificity for predicting a poor clinical result in these studies is sometimes high but sensitivity is uniformly low. Metal ions only seem to adequately predict the presence of volumetric wear and a metal ion trend may be more predictive for malfunctioning bearing than a single measurement [50]. Taking into account these observations, institutional

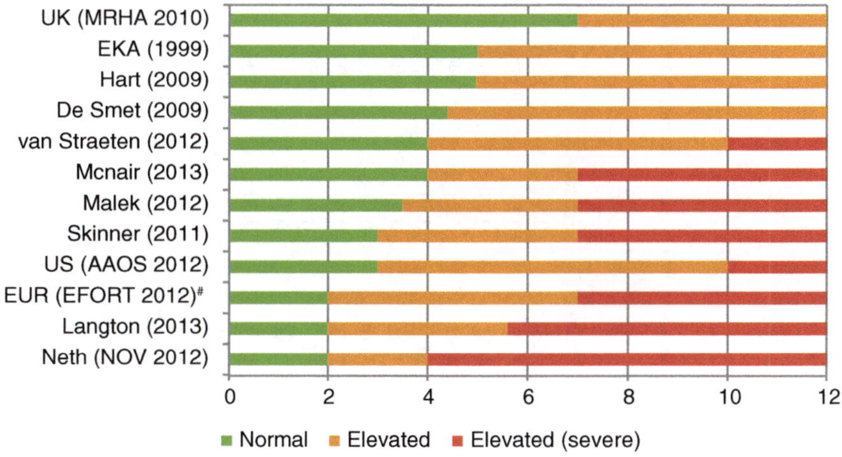

Fig. 16.1 Graph showing values of cobalt threshold levels provided by several institutions. #Defined a range of 2–7 μg/L, where they expect a future threshold value for clinical concern when appropriate evidence becomes available to develop a precise cutoff level [21, 23, 36–45]

Table 16.1 Different threshold levels and their endpoints in literature [48]

Metal ion	Threshold	Sensitivity	Specificity	Positive predictive value	Negative predictive value	Unilateral/ bilateral	Endpoint	Reference
Cobalt/chromium	7.00	0.52	0.89	0.65[b]	0.82[b]	Unilateral	Failure prosthesis	Hart et al. [37]
	4.97	0.63	0.86	n.s[a]	n.s			
Cobalt	4.00	0.25	0.95	n.s	n.s	Unilateral	Clinical radiological problems	Van der Straeten et al. [38]
Chromium	4.60	0.22	0.96	n.s	n.s			
Cobalt	5.00	0.39	0.91	n.s	n.s	Bilateral		
Chromium	7.40	0.43	0.93	n.s	n.s			
Cobalt/chromium	7.00	0.57	0.65	0.52	0.69	Unilateral	ARMD	Malek et al. [39]
Cobalt/chromium	3.50	0.86	0.27	0.44	0.74			
Cobalt	7.00	0.61	0.58	0.4	0.6	Unilateral	Tissue destruction	Griffin et al. [49]
Chromium	7.00	0.31	0.76	0.38	0.63			
Cobalt	4.50	0.90	0.94	0.99	0.71	Unilateral	Wear rate ≥2 mm^3	Sidaginamale et al. [41]
Chromium	7.85	0.86	0.94	0.98	0.63			

[a]Not specified
[b]Calculated with data from article

recommendations for a certain safe cutoff level or threshold for further investigation become questionable. Other studies also show that there is not enough evidence for precise threshold levels of metal ions as a trigger for intervention or to predict adverse systemic effects for an individual patient [19, 21, 24, 28].

The American Conference of Governmental Industrial Hygienist (ACGIH) established a Biological Exposure Index for cobalt of 1 μg/L in blood at the end of the workweek of occupationally exposed workers [51]. For the general population, the diet is the main source of exposure to cobalt, dietary intake is variable with reported values of 5 and 50 μg/day [30].

In 2012 the UK MHRA adopted 7 μg/L for their medical device alert. Above this level additional investigations are recommended which include cross-sectional imaging (MDA-UK). In their January 2013 safety communication on MoM hip implants, the FDA did not define a threshold level as a trigger for revision or any other medical intervention [52]. The AAOS defines three groups in a stratification scheme. The cutoff points mentioned in this scheme are for the low-risk group metal ion level of <3 ppb, in the medium risk group 3–10 ppb, and in the high-risk group >10 ppb.

In their consensus statement on management of MoM bearings, the European Federation of National Associations of Orthopaedics and Traumatology (EFORT), the European Hip Society (EHS), the Arbeitsgemeinschaft Endoprothetik (AE) and the Deutsche Arthrose Hilfe (DAH) use two cobalt levels: levels without clinical concern <2 μg/L and a threshold value for clinical concern which is expected to be within the range of 2–7 μg/L. The Dutch Orthopaedic Association (NOV) advice on MoM hip implants in 2011 showed four cutoff points: normal <2 μg/L, slightly elevated 2–4 μg/L, elevated above 4 μg/L and extremely elevated >20 μg/L [21]. The Agence francaise de securité sanitaire des produits de santé, France, does not use ion levels in their advice but emphasizes clinical and radiological follow-up [19].

At the moment, there is no evidence that cobalt concentrations below 2 μg/L are associated with metal-related health problems. According to the European multidisciplinary consensus, this is a threshold representing a level without clinical concern [28].

Conclusions

There exists no obvious consensus in the current literature on threshold levels for metal ions and how to interpret them, but certain trends are observed. At the moment, there are no clear guidelines on how to interpret metal ion levels nor is enough data available for bilateral MoM implants. Whether a threshold in the range of 2–7 μg/L will be determined to differentiate between a well-functioning prosthesis and clinical concern remains to be seen. Moreover, it is still largely unclear whether a maximal acceptable level can be determined above which revision surgery should be considered. There is still insufficient support for values such as the >20 μg/L level as suggested by some authors [38]. Metal ion levels should be repeated and their development over time considered. Rather than a single diagnostic tool, metal ions should be considered in the entire context of the clinical and radiological findings.

References

1. Amstutz HC, Beaule PE, Dorey FJ, Le Duff MJ, Campbell PA, Gruen TA. Metal-on-metal hybrid surface arthroplasty: two to six year follow-up study. J Bone Joint Surg Am. 2004;86:28–39.
2. Amstutz HC, Le Duff MJ, Campbell PA, Gruen TA, Wisk LE. Clinical and radiographic results of metal-on-metal hip resurfacing with a minimum ten-year follow-up. J Bone Joint Surg Am. 2010;92:2663–71.
3. McMinn DJW, Daniel J, Ziaee H, Pradhan C. Indications and results of hip resurfacing. Int Orthop. 2011;35:231–7.
4. Langton DJ, Joyce TJ, Jameson SS, Lord J, Van Orsouw M, Holland JP, Nargol AV, De Smet KA. Adverse reaction to metal debris following hip resurfacing: the influence of component type, orientation and volumetric wear. J Bone Joint Surg Br. 2011;93:164–71.
5. Freeman MA, Swanson SA, Heath JC. Study of the wear particles produced from cobalt-chromium-molybdenum-manganese total joint replacement prostheses. Ann Rheum Dis. 1969;28(5 Suppl):29.
6. Ladon D, Doherty A, Newson R, Turner J, Bhamra M, Case CP. Changes in metal levels and chromosome aberrations in the peripheral blood of patients after metal-on-metal hip arthroplasty. J Arthroplasty. 2004;19(8 Suppl 3):78–83.
7. Papageorgiou I, Yin Z, Ladon D, Baird D, Lewis AC, Sood A, Newson R, Learmonth ID. Genotoxic effects of particles of surgical cobalt chrome alloy on human cells of different age in vitro. Mutat Res. 2007;619:45–58.
8. Tsaousi A, Jones E, Case CP. The in vitro genotoxicity of orthopaedic ceramic (Al_2O_3) and metal (CoCr alloy) particles. Mutat Res. 2010;697:1–9.
9. Kwon YM, Ostlere SJ, McLardy-Smith P, Athanasou NA, Gill HS, Murray DW. "Asymptomatic" pseudotumors after metal-on-metal hip resurfacing arthroplasty. Prevalence and metal ion study. J Arthroplasty. 2011;26:511–8.
10. Kwon YM, Thomas P, Summer B, Pandit H, Taylor A, Beard D, Murray DW, Gill HS. Lymphocyte proliferation responses in patients with pseudotumors following metal-on-metal hip resurfacing arthroplasty. J Orthop Res. 2010;28:444–50.
11. Matthies AK, Skinner JA, Osmani H, Henckel J, Hart AJ. Pseudotumors are common in well-positioned low-wearing metal-on-metal hips. Clin Orthop Relat Res. 2012;470: 1895–906.
12. Bosker BH, Ettema HB, Boomsma MF, Kollen BJ, Maas M, Verheyen CC. High incidence of pseudotumor formation after large-diameter metal-on-metal total hip replacement. A prospective cohort study. J Bone Joint Surg Br. 2012;94:755–61.
13. Langton DJ, Jameson SS, Joyce TJ, Gandhi JN, Sidaginamale R, Mereddy P, Lord J, Nargol AV. Accelerating failure rate of the ASR total hip replacement. J Bone Joint Surg Br. 2011;93:1011–6.
14. Langton DJ, Jameson SS, Joyce TJ, Hallab NJ, Natu S, Nargol AV. Early failure of metal-on-metal bearings in hip resurfacing and large-diameter total hip replacement: a consequence of excess wear. J Bone Joint Surg Br. 2010;92:38–46.
15. Meyer H, Mueller T, Goldau G, Chamaon K, Ruetschi M, Lohmann CH. Corrosion at the cone/taper interface leads to failure of large-diameter metal-on-metal total hip arthroplasties. Clin Orthop Relat Res. 2012;470:3101–8.
16. Cohen D. How safe are metal-on-metal implants? BMJ. 2012;344:e1410.
17. Godlee F. Serious risks from metal-on-metal hip implants. http://www.bmj.com/content/344/bmj.e1539. Checked Sept 2013.
18. Torjesen I. Lifelong checks are needed for patients fitted with dangerous hip implants. BMJ. 2012;344:e1545.
19. Afssaps, Agence francaise de securité sanitaire des produits de santé. Prothèses de hanche ASR du fabricant DePuy rappelées en juillet 2010. Recommandations de l'Afssaps.2012. http://ansm.sante.fr/content/download/39685/518877/version/3/file/pi-120229-protheses-DePuy.pdf. Checked Sept 2013.

20. BHS. BHS statements on large diameter metal on metal bearing total hip replacements. 2012. http://www.britishhipsociety.com/uploaded/BHSMOMTHR.pdf. Checked Sept 2013.
21. Dutch Orthopaedic Association. The use of metal-on-metal hip replacements: more strict advice to NOV members, 17 January 2012. http://www.orthopeden.org/uploads/UT/Eh/UTEhC1OA0-mRSJTfROfA/Advice-NOV-on-the-use-of-MoM-hip-replacements-17-01-2012.pdf. Checked Sept 2013.
22. Lombardi A, Barrack R, Berend K, et al. The Hip Society: algorithmic approach to diagnosis and management of metal-on-metal arthroplasty. J Bone Joint Surg Br. 2012;94(11 Suppl):14–8.
23. MHRA. Medical device alert. All metal-on-metal (MoM) hip replacements. 25 June 2012. http://www.mhra.gov.uk/home/groups/dtsbs/documents/medicaldevicealert/con155767.pdf. Checked Sept 2013.
24. Health Products and Food Branch Inspectorate HC. Important safety information regarding metal-on-metal hip implant surgery. 11 Apr 2012. http://www.hc-sc.gc.ca/dhp-mps/altformats/pdf/medeff/advisories-avis/prof/2012/metalimplanthpc-cps-eng.pdf. Checked Sept 2013.
25. MacDonald SJ, Brodner W, Jacobs JJ. A consensus paper on metal ions in metal-on-metal hip arthroplasties. J Arthroplasty. 2004;19:12–6.
26. Walter LR, Marel E, Harbury R, Wearne J. Distribution of chromium and cobalt ions in various blood fractions after resurfacing hip arthroplasty. J Arthroplasty. 2008;23(6):814–21. doi:10.1016/j.arth.2007.07.003.
27. Smolders JMH, Bisseling P, Hol A, Van Der Straeten C, Schreurs BW, van Susante JLC. Metal ion interpretation in resurfacing versus conventional hip arthroplasty and in whole blood versus serum. How should we interpret metal ion data? Hip Int. 2011;21:587–95.
28. Hannemann F, Hartmann A, Schmitt J, Lützner J, Seidler A, Campbell P, Delaunay CP, Drexler H, Ettema HB, García-Cimbrelo E, Huberti H, Knahr K, Kunze J, Langton DJ, Lauer W, Learmonth I, Lohmann CH, Morlock M, Wimmer MA, Zagra L, Günther KP. European multidisciplinary consensus statement on the use and monitoring of metal-on-metal bearings for total hip replacement and hip resurfacing. Orthop Traumatol Surg Res. 2013;99(3):263–71. doi:10.1016/j.otsr.2013.01.005.
29. Sampson B, Hart A. Clinical usefulness of blood metal measurements to assess the failure of metal-on-metal hip implants. Ann Clin Biochem. 2012;49:118–31.
30. Minoia C, Sabbiomo E, Apostoli P, Pietra R, Pozzoli L, Gallorini M, Nicolaou G, Alessio L, Capodaglio E. Trace element reference values in tissues from inhabitants of the European community. A study of 46 elements in urine, blood and serum of Italian subjects. Sci Total Environ. 1990;95:89–105.
31. Rieker CB, Köttig P. In vivo tribological performance of 231 metal-on-metal hip articulations. Hip Int. 2002;12:73–6.
32. Antoniou J, Zukor DJ, Mwale F, Minarik W, Petit A, Huk OL. Metal ion levels in the blood of patients after hip resurfacing: a comparison between twenty-eight and thirty-six-millimeter-head metal-on-metal prostheses. J Bone Joint Surg Am. 2008;90 Suppl 3:142–8.
33. Back DL, Young DA, Shimmin AJ. How do serum cobalt and chromium levels change after metal-on-metal hip resurfacing? Clin Orthop. 2005;438:177–81.
34. Moroni A, Savarino L, Hoque M, Cadossi M, Baldini N. Do ion levels in hip resurfacing differ from metal-on-metal that midterm? Clin Orthop. 2011;469(1):180–7.
35. Wagner M, Wagner H. Medium-term results of a modern metal-on-metal system in total hip replacement. Clin Orthop Relat Res. 2000;379:123–33.
36. De Smet K, Campbell P, Van Orsouw M, et al. Interpretation of metal ion levels after metal-on-metal hip resurfacing. 2010 Annual Meeting AAOS. New Orleans; 2010.
37. Hart AJ, Sabah SA, Bandi AS, et al. Sensitivity and specificity of blood cobalt and chromium metal ions for predicting failure of MoM hip replacement. J Bone Joint Surg Br. 2011;93:1308–13.
38. van der Straeten C, Grammatopoulos G, Gill HS, Calistri A, Campbell P, De Smet KA. The 2012 Otto Aufranc Award: the interpretation of metal ion levels in unilateral and bilateral hip resurfacing. Clin Orthop Rel Res. 2013;471:377–85.

39. Malek IA, King A, Sharma H, Malek S, Lyons K, Jones S, John A. The sensitivity, specificity and predictive values of raised plasma metal ion levels in the diagnosis of adverse reaction to metal debris in symptomatic patients with a metal-on-metal arthroplasty of the hip. J Bone Joint Surg Br. 2012;94(8):1045–50.
40. Skinner J, Kay P. Commentary: metal on metal hips. BMJ. 2011;342:d3009. doi:10.1136/bmj.d3009.
41. Sidaginamale RP, Joyce TJ, Lord JK, Jefferson R, Blain PG, Nargol AV, Langton DJ. Blood metal ion testing is an effective screening tool to identify poorly performing metal-on-metal bearing surfaces. Bone Joint Res. 2013;2(5):84–95.
42. Macnair RD, Wynn-Jones H, Wimhurst JA, Toms A, Cahir J. Metal ion levels not sufficient as a screening measure for adverse reactions in metal-on-metal hip arthroplasties. J Arthroplasty. 2013;28(1):78–83.
43. AAOS Metal-on-Metal: 2012 Update, http://ww.aaos.org/news/aaosnow/may12/cover2.asp.
44. Consensus statement "Current Evidence on the Management of Metal-on-Metal Bearings." http://www.iss.it/binary/riap2/cont/2012_05_10_MoM_Consensus_statement.pdf.
45. Deutsche Forschungsgemeinschaft. Expositionsäquivalente für Krebserzeugende Arbeitsstoffe. Weinheim: VCH Verlag Weinheim; 1992.
46. De Smet K, De Haan R, Calistri A, et al. Metal ion measurement as a diagnostic tool to identify problems with metal-on-metal hip resurfacing. J Bone Joint Surg Am. 2008;90 Suppl 4:202–8.
47. Triclot P. Total hip replacement with metal-on-metal bearing system with a high content in carbon. Results at minimum 12 years of a consecutive series. Rev Chir Orthop Trauma. 2009;95S:85–91.
48. Kretzer JP, Van Der Straeten C, Sonntag R, Müller U, Streit M, Moradi B, Jäger S, Reinders J. Metal ion concentrations in patients with metal-metal bearings in prostheses. Orthopade. 2013;42(8):622–8. doi:10.1007/s00132-012-2035-3.
49. Griffin WL, Fehring TK, Kudrna JC, Schmidt RH, Christie MJ, Odum SM, Dennos AC. Are metal ion levels a useful trigger for surgical intervention? J Arthroplasty. 2012;27(8 Suppl):32–6.
50. Smolders JM, Hol A, van Susante JL. Metal ion trend may be more predictive for malfunctioning metal-on-metal implants then a single measurement. Hip Int. 2013;23(5):434–40. doi:10.5301/hipint.5000066.
51. Catalani S, Rizzetti MC, Padovani A, Apostoli P. Neurotoxicity of cobalt. Hum Exp Toxicol. 2012;31(5):421–37. doi:10.1177/0960327111414280. Epub 2011.
52. FDA. FDA safety communication: metal-on-metal hip implants. 2013. http://www.fda.gov/medicaldevices/safety/alertsandnotices/ucm335775.htm.

Association Between Histological Findings and Whole Blood Metal Ion Levels with Pseudotumor Characteristics Indentified in MRI

17

Aleksi Reito, Petra Elo, Jorma Pajamäki, Timo Puolakka, and Antti Eskelinen

17.1 Introduction

Clinical manifestation of adverse soft tissue complications related to metal-on-metal (MoM) implants is variable [1–4]. Intracapsular findings include metallosis, synovitis, synovial hypertrophy, effusion, and capsular necrosis [2, 5, 6]. In some patients adverse reaction to metal debris (ARMeD) may manifest as an aggressive pseudotumor. Microscopic findings may include massive perivascular lymphocyte infiltration with fibrin exudates or even synovial necrosis. This type of histological reaction has been termed ALVAL (aseptic lymphocytic vasculitis-associated lesion), and it has been proposed to be a specific type of reaction seen around MoM hips [7]. The term ARMeD has been proposed as an umbrella term to include all previously described adverse wear related to soft tissue complications [8].

In earlier studies reporting on histological findings of patients who had been revised due to suspected pseudotumor, ALVAL has been a frequent finding. Several authors, however, have stated that histological diagnosis of ALVAL is not pathognomic for pseudotumor [1, 9]. However, it is still unknown to what extent ALVAL is seen in hips diagnosed with pseudotumor compared to hips with intracapsular ARMeD. It is also unknown whether different PTs (cystic versus solid) posses different histological findings.

We hypothesized that an ALVAL-type reaction would lead to pseudotumor formation and non-pseudotumor-type ARMeD would be related to excess wear and macrophage-dominated foreign body reaction in synovia. Our secondary aim was to establish any correlation between MR imaging characteristics and histological features of pseudotumors and blood metal ion levels.

A. Reito, MD (✉) • P. Elo, MD, PhD • J. Pajamäki, MD, PhD
T. Puolakka, MD, PhD • A. Eskelinen, MD, PhD
Coxa Hospital for Joint Replacement Ltd, Tampere, Finland
e-mail: aleksi.reito@uta.fi

K. Knahr (ed.), *Tribology in Total Hip and Knee Arthroplasty*,
DOI 10.1007/978-3-642-45266-6_17, © EFORT 2014

17.2 Methods

ASR (DePuy, Warsaw, In, USA) MoM hip replacements were used in 1,036 operations (887 patients) at our institution between March 2004 and December 2009. ASR hip resurfacing devices were implanted in 415 patients (497 hips) and 471 patients (537 hips) received an ASR XL THR. MHRA announced a medical device alert regarding the ASR hip replacements in September 2010 [10]. After the announcement, we established a screening program to identify possible articulation-related complications in patients with these implants.

The screening was initiated at a mean of 4.0 years postoperatively. All patients received an Oxford Hip Score (OHS) questionnaire and were clinically examined (including Harris Hip Score) by a physiotherapist at our outpatient clinic. Anteroposterior and lateral radiograph of the hip and anteroposterior pelvic radiograph were taken prior to each visit. Each patient was also referred for WB Cr and Co ion concentration measurements. All patients were primarily referred for magnetic resonance imaging (MRI) using metal artifact reduction sequence (MARS). If MRI was contraindicated for medical reasons or if the patient suffered from claustrophobia, an ultrasonography was used.

According to our screening protocol, MRI findings have been classified prospectively using the Norwich classification. For investigational purposes, all hips revised until May 2012 were reclassified retrospectively using a modified Imperial classification [9]. We divided Imperial Class 1 into separate classes of 1A and 1B: Thin-walled fluid collections with walls mainly in apposition were classified as 1A. Thin-walled fluid collections with walls mainly not in apposition, on the other hand, were classified as 1B.

Revision surgery was considered if (1) there was a clear pseudotumor observed on cross-sectional imaging regardless of symptoms or whole blood metal ion levels; or (2) the patient had elevated whole blood metal ion levels and hip symptoms despite a normal finding on cross-sectional imaging; or (3) the patient had a continuously symptomatic hip or progressive symptoms regardless of imaging findings or metal ion levels. Symptoms included hip pain, discomfort, sense of instability, and/or impaired function of the hip and sounds from the hip (clacking, squeaking). Whole blood metal ion levels were regarded as being elevated if either chromium or cobalt exceeded 5 ppb.

Diagnosis of adverse reactions to metal debris was based on perioperative findings. Failure was classified as being secondary to adverse reactions to metal debris if the following criteria were met: (1) There was presence of metallosis or macroscopic synovitis in the joint; and/or (2) a pseudotumor was found during revision; and/or (3) a moderate to high amount of perivascular lymphocytes along with tissue necrosis and/or fibrin deposition was seen in the histopathologic sample; and (4) perioperatively there was no evidence of component loosening or periprosthetic fracture. Furthermore, infection was ruled out by multiple (at least five) bacterial cultures obtained during revision surgery.

In each revision operation, one to three samples have been retrieved for histological analysis. Analysis has been semiquantitative in respect to the amount of synovial fibrin (none, focal, moderate, extensive), macrophages, and perivascular lymphocytes (PVLs) (absent, mild, moderate, high). We introduced using ALVAL score in the histological analysis 9 months after the start-up of the protocol, and hence ALVAL score was not available for all samples [11].

Kendall's tau (τ) coefficient is used to investigate correlation between ranked categorical variables (tau-b for squared consistency tables, tau-c for rectangular tables). Differences in mean values among several categories were studied using ANOVA, and differences in medians were studied using Kruskal-Wallis test.

17.3 Results

In total, 92 revised hips in 92 unilateral patients had full clinical data and were included in the study (Table 17.1). ALVAL score was available in 64 cases. PT was diagnosed in 59 cases preoperatively (Tables 17.2 and 17.3).

Table 17.1 Demographics of the patients

Sex	Males	32
	Females	60
Implant type	THA	63
	HR	29
Age at the primary operation	Mean (SD, range)	56.2 years (10.8, 15–75)
Time to revision	Mean (SD, range)	4.5 years (1.4, 1.4–7.6)
Femoral diameter	Mean (range)	48.9 mm (43–59)
Acetabular inclination	Mean (SD, range)	50.3° (8.0°, 31.6°–73.6°)

Table 17.2 Classification of MRI findings

0 (No PT)	33
1A	9
1B	13
2A	13
2B	22
3	2

Table 17.3 Distribution of MRI signal intensities

T1 weighted	Pseudocapsule	Hypo	28
		Iso	8
		Unclassified	1
	Core	Hypo	11
		Iso	14
		Hyper	10
		Variable	1
		Unclassified	1
T2 weighted	Pseudocapsule	Hypo	35
		Iso	1
		Unclassified	1
	Core	Hypo	1
		Iso	3
		Hyper	23
		Variable	9
		Unclassified	1

Table 17.4 Correlation of histological analysis and ALVAL subscores

	Amount of fibrin	Amount of macrophages	Amount of PVLs
Synovial lining score	.733, $p<0.001$	–	–
Inflammatory infiltrate	–	−.324, $p=0.003$	.887, $p<0.001$

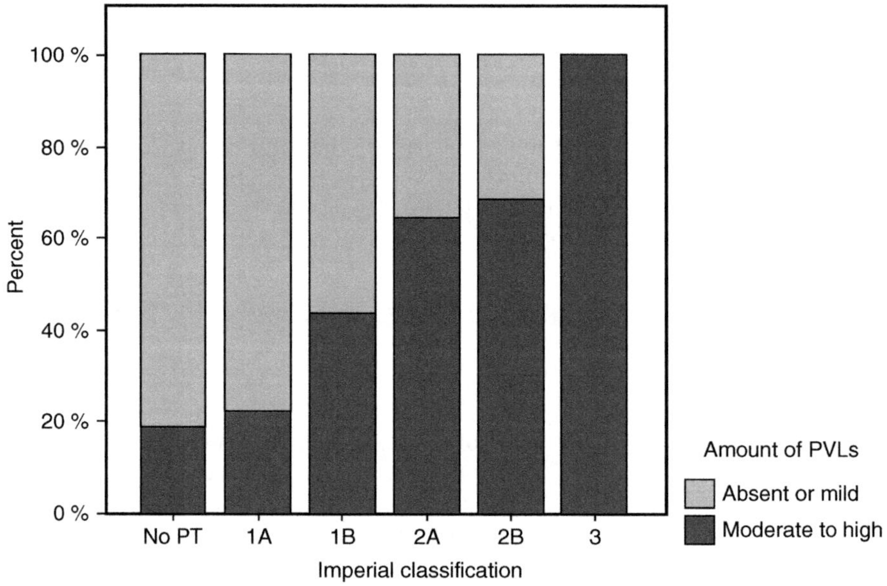

Fig. 17.1 Correlation between PVLs and severity of MRI finding

In order to validate our semiquantitative analysis of histological samples, we investigated the correlation between the amount of fibrin, macrophages, and PVLs with the ALVAL subscores (Table 17.4). Strong correlation was seen in amounts of fibrin and PVLs. A moderate correlation was seen in the amount of macrophages. It must be noted that inflammatory infiltrate score increases with increasing amount of PVLs, whereas macrophages are only noted in the lowest inflammatory infiltrate scores.

17.3.1 Histological Features and PT Classification

Both amount ($\tau=.313$, $p<0.001$) and presence (absence or mild vs. moderate to high) ($\tau=.494$, $p<0.001$) of PVLs correlated positively with the severity of MRI finding (Fig. 17.1). Macrophage infiltration correlated negatively, but weakly with the MRI finding ($\tau=-.246$, $p=0.015$). Fibrin deposition showed no correlation with MRI finding ($\tau=.106$, $p=0.153$).

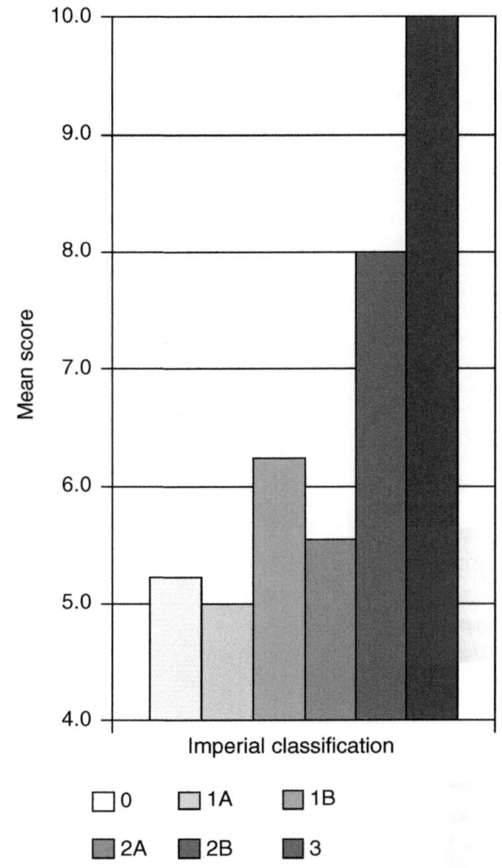

Fig. 17.2 Mean ALVAL score in respect to MRI finding

Total ALVAL score was associated with severity of MRI finding (means $p<.001$, medians $p=.007$) (Fig. 17.2). Total ALVAL score also showed significant correlation with MRI finding ($\tau=.280$, $p=.002$).

Severity of MRI finding was not associated with increased synovial lining score (means $p=.23$, medians $p=.18$); however, there was a positive correlation with synovial lining score and severity of the MRI finding ($\tau=.203$, $p=.021$) (Fig. 17.3).

High inflammatory infiltrate score was associated with severity of MRI finding (means $p<.001$, medians $p=.002$) (Fig. 17.4). Inflammatory infiltrate score also showed significant correlation with MRI finding ($\tau=.317$, $p<.001$).

High tissue organization score was associated with severity of MRI finding (means $p=.022$, medians $p=.031$) (Fig. 17.5). Tissue organization score also showed significant correlation with MRI finding ($\tau=.311$, $p<.003$).

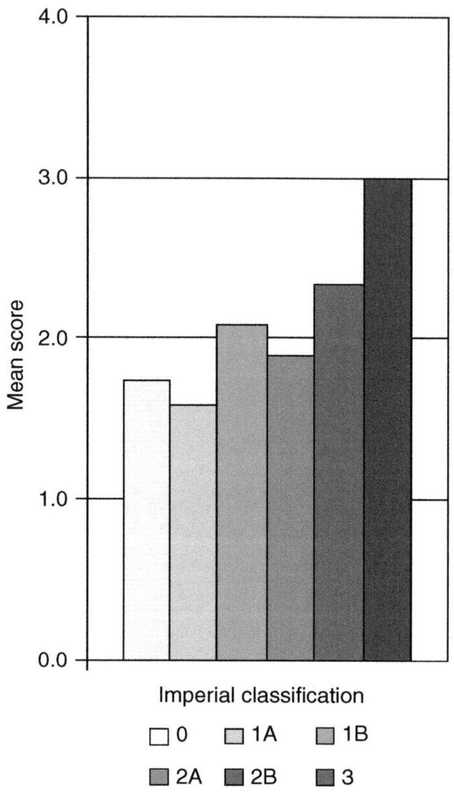

Fig. 17.3 Mean synovial lining score in respect to MRI finding

17.3.2 Histological Features and Pseudotumor Characteristics

No significant differences in histological findings nor in ALVAL subscores were observed between different T1-weighted pseudocapsule or core signals in hips with PT. There was a trend of higher ALVAL scores in hips with hyperintense T1-weighted core signal (Table 17.5).

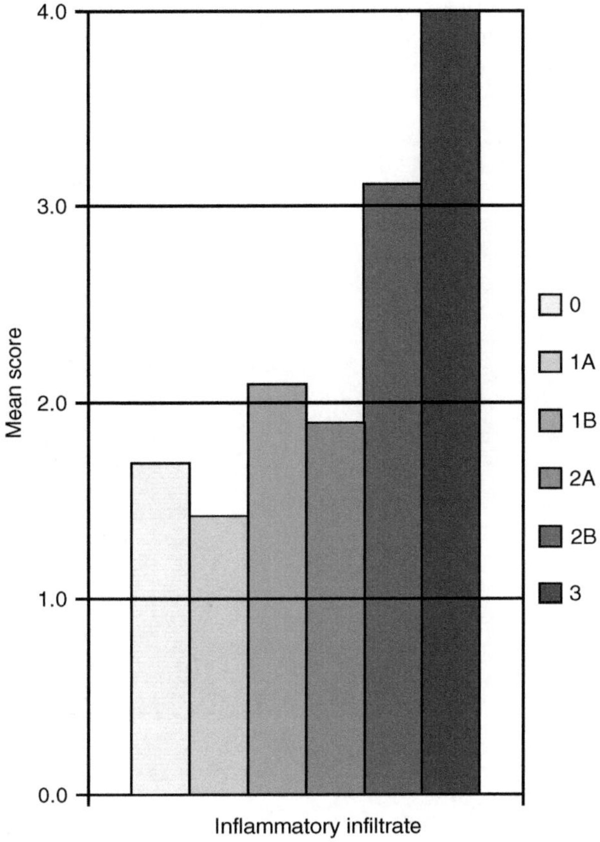

Fig. 17.4 Inflammatory infiltrate score in respect to MRI finding

However, T2-weighted hyperintense (typical fluid) core signal was associated both with increased macrophage infiltration ($p = .006$) (Fig. 17.6) and with decreased fibrin deposition ($p = .003$) (Fig. 17.7) when compared to PTs with variable T2 core signal. Further, PTs with variable T2-weighted (atypical fluid) core signal had significantly higher ALVAL score as well as higher score in two subcategories (Table 17.6).

Fig. 17.5 Tissue organization score in respect to MRI finding

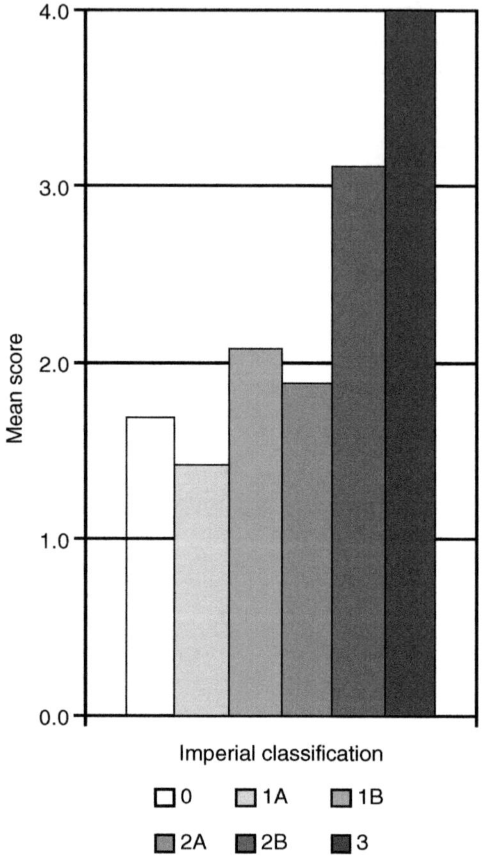

Table 17.5 T1-weighted core signal with mean and median values for total ALVAL score

Total ALVAL score	Means, $p=.066$	Medians, $p=.052$
Hypointense	5.5	5.0
Isointense	5.9	5.5
Hyperintense	7.6	8.0

17.3.3 Pseudotumor Characteristics and WB Metal Ion Levels

No differences were seen in WB metal ion levels between different MRI findings (Cr, $p=.16$; Co, $p=.38$). However, patients with PT with hyperintense T1-weighted core signal had significantly higher median WB Co and Cr levels compared to patients with other signal intensities (Table 17.7).

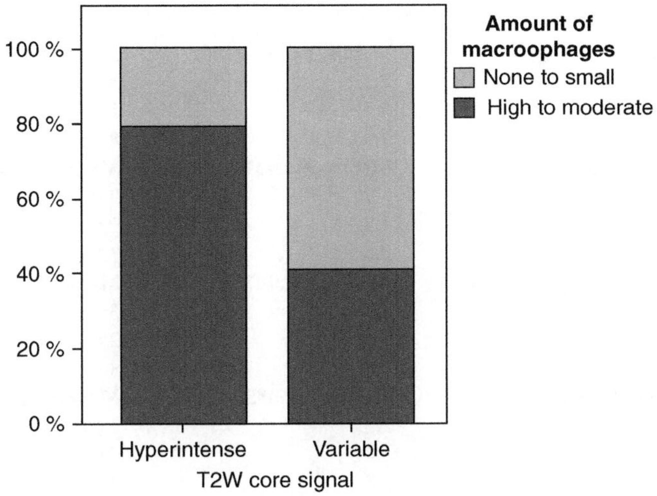

Fig. 17.6 T2-weighted core signal and amount of macrophages seen in the synovial sample

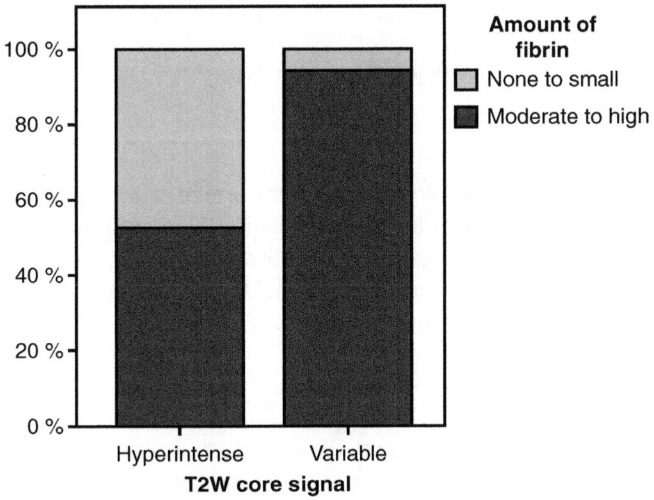

Fig. 17.7 T2-weighted core signal and amount of fibrin seen in the synovial

Table 17.6 Comparison of ALVAL (sub)score with different T2-weighted core signal intensities

ALVAL score	**Means, $p = .006$**	**Median, $p = .01$**
Isointense	8.3	8.0
Hyperintense	5.5	5.0
Variable	7.9	8.0
Synovial lining score	**Means, $p = .022$**	**Medians, $p = .026$**
Isointense	2.7	3.0
Hyperintense	1.8	2.0
Variable	2.6	3.0
Inflammatory infiltrate score	**Means, $p = .007$**	**Medians, $p = .011$**
Isointense	3.3	3.0
Hyperintense	1.9	2.0
Variable	2.8	3.0
Tissue organization	**Means, $p = .085$**	**Medians, $p = .091$**
Isointense	2.3	2.0
Hyperintense	1.8	2.0
Variable	2.6	3.0

Table 17.7 Median WB cobalt and chrome values for different T1-weighted signal intensities

	Median WB chrome	Median WB cobalt
Hypointense	4.1 ppb (1.8–10.3)	8.45 ppb (1.1–29.5)
Isointense	4.8 ppb (1.1–46.19)	9.7 ppb (0.9–95.49)
Hyperintense	25.4 ppb (5.0–93.9)	72.1 ppb (2.0–224.7)

Conclusion

We found that several histological features correlated with severity of MRI finding and thus with the Imperial PT classification. The most important finding was that the amount and presence of PVLs correlated positively with MRI finding. This suggests that extracapsular ARMeD, i.e., pseudotumor, represents a lymphocyte-dominated immune response. Furthermore, the higher the amount of PVLs, the more severe the PT, either PT with atypical fluid or solid contents. Higher total ALVAL score was seen in hips with a solid PT or a PT presenting with thick walls and atypical fluid signal. This is partly due to high inflammatory infiltrate score. But also the high tissue organization score is most likely contributing to this. High tissue organization score indicates tissue necrosis, and therefore our results suggest that in addition to PVLs, necrosis is associated with more severe MRI findings.

Several significant correlations were seen between PT characteristics and histological features. Hyperintense core signal in T1-weighted images is known to indicate atypical fluid content. Hart et al. suggested that in a PT, hyperintense T1-weighted core signal might represent high metal ion content or proteinaceous material [9]. Our results support this. PTs with atypical fluid signal in T2-weighted images had significantly higher total ALVAL score and tissue organization score. Moreover, there was a trend for higher total ALVAL score in hips with atypical fluid content in T1-weighted images. Thus, proteinaceous material could represent necrotic mass inside the PT adjacent to lymphocytic infiltration in synovia.

Table 17.8 Suggestions for three subclasses for ARMeD based on our results

Class A	Intracapsular ARMeD (No PT in MRI)		Macrophage-dominated immune response	Intact synovial lining	Low to moderate ALVAL score	Moderately elevated WB metal ion levels
Class B1	Extracapsular ARMeD	PT with typical fluid signal (hyperintense T2-weighted core signal)	Macrophage-dominated immune response	Intact synovial lining	Low to moderate ALVAL score	Moderately elevated WB metal ion levels
Class B2		PT with atypical fluid signal (hyperintense T1-weighted/ variable T2-weighted core signal intensity)	Lymphocyte-dominated immune response	Synovial destruction	High ALVAL score	Very high WB metal ion levels

Additionally, we detected significantly higher WB metal ion levels in these patients indicating increased wear. Previously it has been suggested that typical adverse reaction in MoM hips presenting with massive PVL infiltration would be caused by hypersensitivity rather than increased wear [11]. Since patients with atypical fluid signal had significantly higher WB metal ion levels, our findings do not support this hypothesis. Furthermore, in a recent study it was shown that high tissue metal content was associated to PVL infiltration [12].

Another specific feature was seen in PTs with hyperintense signal in T2-weighted images. Hyperintense signal intensity indicates a PT with typical fluid content, i.e., a cystic PT. In these lesions, inflammatory cell response was mainly macrophage dominated indicating increased wear. Higher WB metal ion levels were not however seen in these hips with cystic core signal. Moreover, these hips evinced low total ALVAL score along with low synovial lining and inflammatory infiltrate score indicating absence of PVLs and synovial destruction. Hips without extracapsular PT evinced similar findings indicating that hips with intracapsular ARMeD have similar characteristics compared to hips with cystic PT.

We analyzed perioperative histological and pre-revision cross-sectional findings and WB metal ion levels in patients revised due to ARMeD. We were mainly able to identify two different manifestations of ARMeD (Table 17.8). Lymphocyte-dominated immune response along with more severe tissue necrosis is associated with thick-walled PTs with atypical fluid signal. Cystic PTs and intra-articular ARMeD present with macrophage-dominated immune response and more intact synovial lining. Higher WB metal ions are seen in the former group. Further studies are warranted to investigate the etiopathogenesis and prognosis of different types of ARMeD seen in the MRI in order to clarify the clinical implications of our findings.

However, our results suggest that it may be possible to differentiate between these two manifestations of ARMeD based on MRI findings.

References

1. Hayter CL, Gold SL, Koff MF, Perino G, Nawabi DH, Miller TT, et al. MRI findings in painful metal-on-metal hip arthroplasty. AJR Am J Roentgenol. 2012;199:884–93.
2. De Smet K, De Haan R, Calistri A, Campbell PA, Ebramzadeh E, Pattyn C, et al. Metal ion measurement as a diagnostic tool to identify problems with metal-on-metal hip resurfacing. J Bone Joint Surg Am. 2008;90:202–8.
3. Chang EY, McAnally JL, Van Horne JR, Statum S, Wolfson T, Gamst A, et al. Metal-on-metal total hip arthroplasty: do symptoms correlate with MR imaging findings? Radiology. 2012;265:848–57.
4. Hauptfleisch J, Pandit H, Grammatopoulos G, Gill HS, Murray DW, Ostlere S. A MRI classification of periprosthetic soft tissue masses (pseudotumours) associated with metal-on-metal resurfacing hip arthroplasty. Skeletal Radiol. 2012;41:149–55.
5. Nishii T, Sakai T, Takao M, Yoshikawa H, Sugano N. Ultrasound screening of periarticular soft tissue abnormality around metal-on-metal bearings. J Arthroplasty. 2012;27:895–900.
6. Browne JA, Bechtold CD, Berry DJ, Hanssen AD, Lewallen DG. Failed metal-on-metal hip arthroplasties: a spectrum of clinical presentations and operative findings. Clin Orthop Relat Res. 2010;468:2313–20.
7. Willert HG, Buchhorn GH, Fayyazi A, Flury R, Windler M, Koster G, et al. Metal-on-metal bearings and hypersensitivity in patients with artificial hip joints. A clinical and histomorphological study. J Bone Joint Surg Am. 2005;87:28–36.
8. Langton DJ, Jameson SS, Joyce TJ, Hallab NJ, Natu S, Nargol AV. Early failure of metal-on-metal bearings in hip resurfacing and large-diameter total hip replacement: a consequence of excess wear. J Bone Joint Surg Br. 2010;92:38–46.
9. Hart AJ, Satchithananda K, Liddle AD, Sabah SA, McRobbie D, Henckel J, et al. Pseudotumors in association with well-functioning metal-on-metal hip prostheses: a case–control study using three-dimensional computed tomography and magnetic resonance imaging. J Bone Joint Surg Am. 2012;94:317–25.
10. Medicines and Healthcare Products and Regulation Agency. Medical Device Alert: ASR™ hip replacement implants manufactured by DePuy International Ltd (MDA/2010/069). 2010: http://www.mhra.gov.uk/home/groups/dts-bs/documents/medicaldevicealert/con093791.pdf.
11. Campbell P, Ebramzadeh E, Nelson S, Takamura K, De Smet K, Amstutz HC. Histological features of pseudotumor-like tissues from metal-on-metal hips. Clin Orthop Relat Res. 2010;468:2321–7.
12. Lohmann CH, Meyer H, Nuechtern JV, Singh G, Junk-Jantsch S, Schmotzer H, et al. Periprosthetic tissue metal content but not serum metal content predicts the type of tissue response in failed small-diameter metal-on-metal total hip arthroplasties. J Bone Joint Surg Am. 2013;95:1561–8.

Part V

Improvements of Polyethylene – Have We Reached the Goal?

Evolution of UHMWPE: Do We Need Antioxidants?

18

Orhun K. Muratoglu and Ebru Oral

18.1 Introduction

Periprosthetic osteolysis is primarily caused by particulate debris created through wear of UHMWPE components used in total joint arthroplasty [15], resulting in bone resorption around implants and in most cases leading to revision surgery (Fig. 18.1). Osteolysis was a major problem until the advancement of highly cross-linked UHMWPEs in the mid-1990s. The clinical use of highly cross-linked UHMWPE in total hips has been tried as early as the 1970s by a number of clinicians in the United Kingdom [2, 3], in South Africa [12, 14], and in Japan [27–29]. The success of these early, experimental highly cross-linked UHMWPE formulations was not appreciated until much later when the long-term clinical follow-up data became available [45]; therefore, the widespread clinical use of these experimental formulations did not materialize. In the mid-1990s, with the growing concern of periprosthetic osteolysis, combined research efforts of many centers around the world resulted in the development of the more contemporary, first-generation highly cross-linked UHMWPE formulations [22, 25]. These efforts were greatly helped by the more sophisticated understanding of the interplay between kinematics and wear of the load-bearing surfaces [6] and adverse effects of trapped free radicals on oxidative stability of gamma-sterilized UHMWPE components [8]. The more clinically relevant hip and knee simulator wear testing was instrumental in preclinical testing. Accelerated aging was also used to better understand potential material changes in the long term.

First-generation highly cross-linked UHMWPE was introduced for use in acetabular liners in the late 1990s, followed by its use in tibial knee inserts in the

O.K. Muratoglu, PhD (✉) • E. Oral, PhD
Harris Orthopaedic Laboratory, Massachusetts General Hospital,
55 Fruit St. GRJ 113, Boston, MA 02114, USA
e-mail: omuratoglu@partners.org

K. Knahr (ed.), *Tribology in Total Hip and Knee Arthroplasty*,
DOI 10.1007/978-3-642-45266-6_18, © EFORT 2014

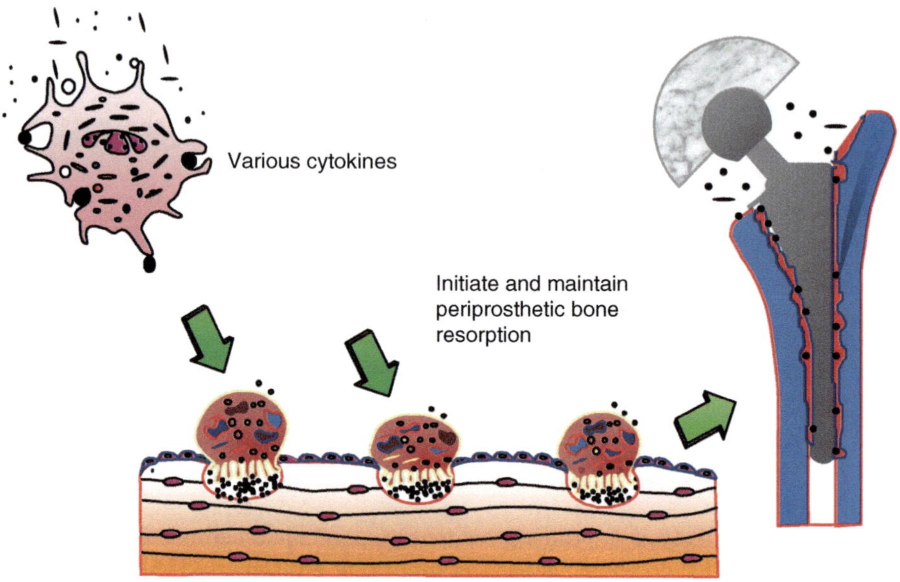

Fig. 18.1 Particulate debris generated by the wear of UHMWPE components initiates an adverse biological response that results in the resorption of bone around the implants, also known as periprosthetic osteolysis

mid-2000s. Clinical follow-up studies are showing excellent outcomes in total hips [19, 20]. In one study, Karrholm and coworkers [16] followed 21 patients with bilateral total hips for 10 years (Fig. 18.2). The patients were randomized to receive conventional polyethylene on one side and highly cross-linked polyethylene on the contralateral side with 28 mm femoral heads. The extent of femoral head penetration into the acetabular liner was quantified by the use of radiostereometric analysis (RSA). After the first year of bedding in, the rate of femoral head penetration, which indicates the wear rate, was markedly lower with the hips that were treated using the highly cross-linked polyethylene acetabular liners in comparison with those that were treated using conventional polyethylene.

The primary aim in the development of the highly cross-linked polyethylene was to reduce the rate of osteolysis by reducing wear. There are now a number of reports from different centers showing significantly reduced rate of osteolysis in patients treated with highly cross-linked polyethylene acetabular liners [19, 20]. In one study, Mall et al. [21] followed 48 patients treated with highly cross-linked polyethylene and 50 patients treated with conventional polyethylene with a minimum follow-up of 5 years. They detected osteolysis in 2 % of the cases in the highly cross-linked polyethylene cohort in comparison with 24 % of the cases in the conventional polyethylene cohort. In another study, Bragdon et al. [5] reported on 768 patients that were treated with highly cross-linked polyethylene acetabular liners and showed no osteolysis up to 13 years of follow-up.

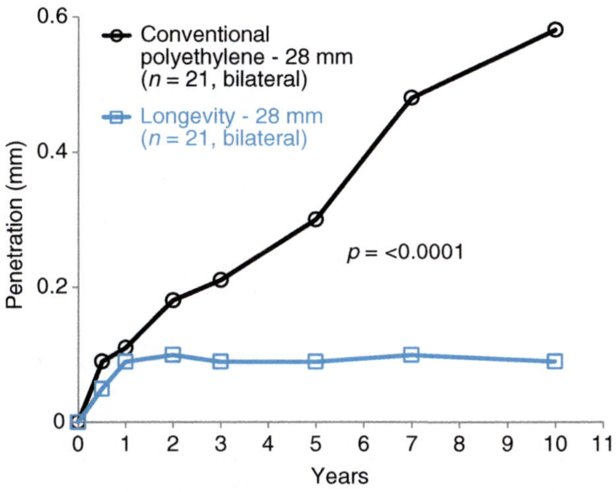

Fig. 18.2 Karrholm et al. [16] followed 21 patients with bilateral total hip replacements. The patients were randomized to receive either a conventional polyethylene or an irradiated and melted (electron beam radiation dose of 100 kGy) polyethylene acetabular liner together with 28 mm cobalt chromium femoral heads. They used radiostereometric analysis (RSA) to determine the femoral head penetration into the acetabular liners in vivo. The penetration during the first year is primarily due to creep and bedding-in along with wear. Subsequently, the penetration is mostly due to the wear of the polyethylene. With the highly cross-linked polyethylene acetabular liners, they showed significantly reduced rate of wear (slope of the line after the first year) in comparison with the conventional polyethylene liners

18.2 Radiation Cross-Linking and First-Generation Materials

Cross-linking of UHMWPE or polyethylene can be achieved by the use of ionizing radiation or chemical means, such as by the use of peroxides. The contemporary highly cross-linked polyethylenes are exclusively cross-linked by ionizing radiation. Polyethylene is a semicrystalline material, with crystalline domains embedded within an amorphous matrix (Fig. 18.3). When the polyethylene is subjected to ionizing radiation, such as gamma or electron beam, carbon-hydrogen bonds are broken and free radicals are generated. The free radicals in the amorphous phase have sufficient mobility to react with each other to form cross-links. However, the ones formed in the crystalline domains are not as mobile and they remain trapped (Fig. 18.4). In the long term, oxygen can diffuse throughout the implant and react with these trapped free radicals. The outcome of this reaction, i.e., oxidation, is not desirable as the primary consequence is the embrittlement of the polymer through recrystallization. The embrittlement is often manifested in the form of pitting and delamination and sometimes fracture of the components.

The adverse effects of exposure to ionizing radiation on the long-term mechanical properties were first recognized with gamma-in-air-sterilized conventional polyethylene components [41, 43]. This understanding was later applied to the development of the first-generation highly cross-linked polyethylenes. Subsequent

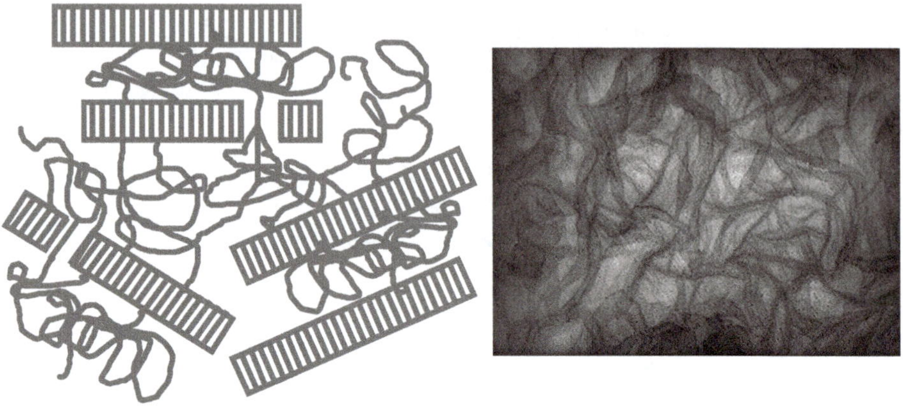

Fig. 18.3 UHMWPE is a semicrystalline material. On the left is a schematic showing crystalline domains embedded in the amorphous matrix. On the right is a transmission electron micrograph of UHMWPE showing dark regions stained with osmium tetroxide making the crystalline domains visible within the amorphous matrix

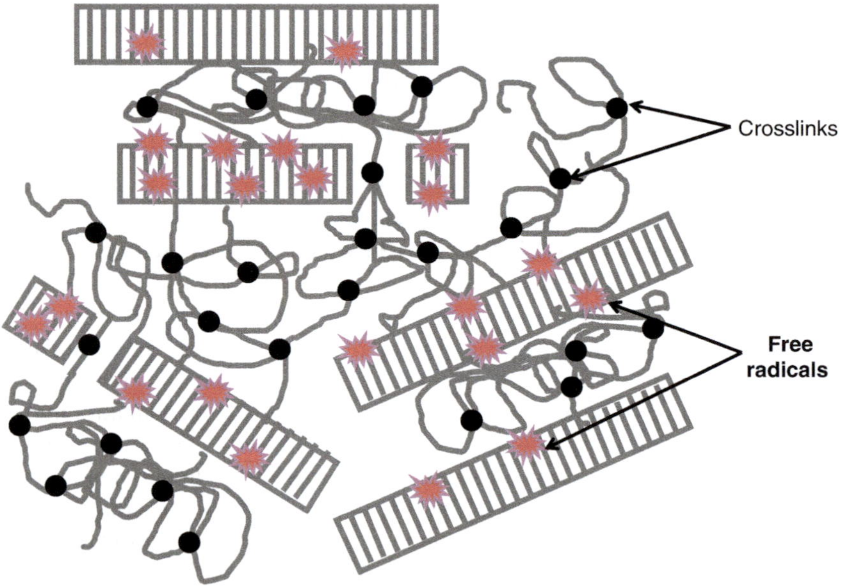

Fig. 18.4 Irradiation of UHMWPE breaks carbon-hydrogen bonds and creates free radicals in the amorphous and crystalline domains. The free radicals in the amorphous phase recombine with each other to form cross-links, while the ones in the crystalline domains remain trapped because of the substantially lower mobility of the molecules incorporated into the crystals. The trapped free radicals are the precursors to the well-known oxidation-induced embrittlement of gamma-sterilized UHMWPE components

to irradiation, polyethylene was subjected to melting or annealing to improve its oxidative stability. Melting eliminates the crystals and allows the trapped free radicals to react with each other. Postirradiation melting has been the gold standard for

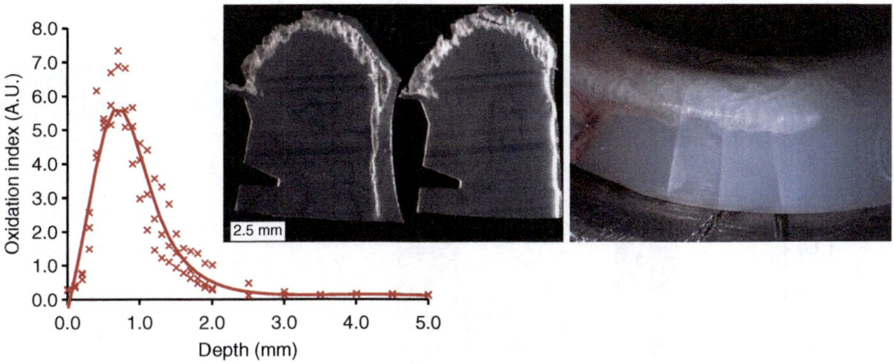

Fig. 18.5 An example of an irradiated and annealed UHMWPE acetabular liner that was also terminally gamma sterilized in inert gas after 10 years of in vivo service shows high levels of subsurface oxidation. Impingement of the femoral neck onto the rim of the component caused subsurface and radial cracks as shown on the right-hand side. Thin sections microtomed around the locking mechanism and the rim of the component showed marked embrittlement, manifested by the formation of subsurface "white banding" as shown in the middle photograph (reference)

first-generation highly cross-linked polyethylenes in terms of long-term oxidative stability [7]. Surgically explanted irradiated and melted components show very low oxidation levels. Postirradiation annealing heats the polymer below its melting point and reduces the number of trapped free radicals. The analysis of long-term surgically explanted irradiated and annealed components shows high levels of oxidation [11, 17]. One example of an irradiated and annealed acetabular liner that was also terminally gamma sterilized in nitrogen is shown in Fig. 18.5. This component was in vivo for 10 years. The analysis after explantation showed a 45-fold increase in oxidation level and fourfold decrease in cross-link density.

18.3 Oxidation Mechanisms

The oxidation reactions of residual free radicals created by ionizing radiation are well understood and well documented [1, 10]. However, a more recent study showed that the stability of highly cross-linked polyethylene components decreases markedly after exposure to synovial fluid and loading during in vivo service [24]. For instance, irradiated and melted polyethylene components show no detectable oxidation after shelf storage in air for 10 years or longer. However, when an irradiated and melted polyethylene component is retrieved from a patient after 2 months of in vivo service or longer, it shows high levels of oxidation within 2 years of shelf storage in air. Two potential mechanisms that could be responsible for the in vivo changes in oxidative stability were proposed: (1) absorbed lipids and (2) cyclic loading. Costa et al. [9] have found that lipids readily diffuse into polyethylene components in vivo from the synovial fluid. They identified a number of lipids, among which was squalene. Squalene was the most abundant lipid found in their surgically retrieved polyethylene components. Subsequent studies analyzed the potential adverse effects of

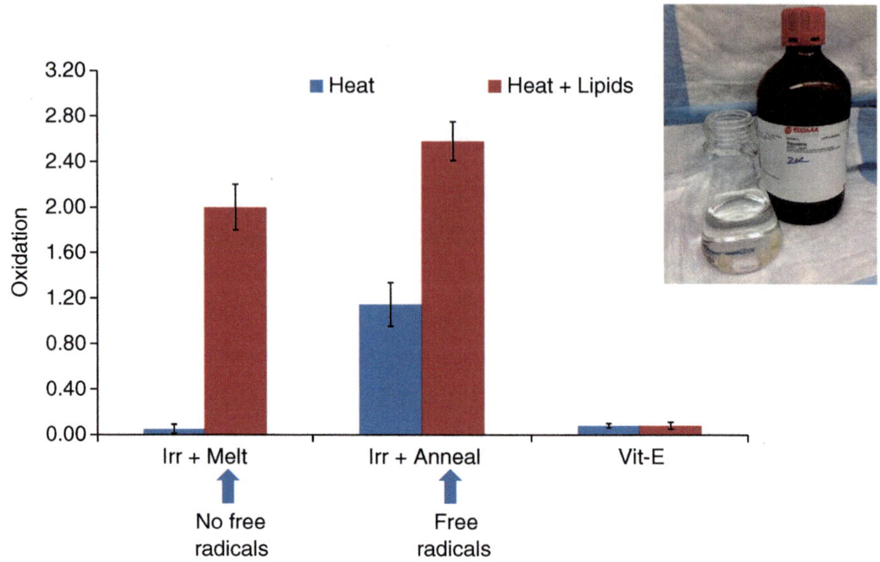

Fig. 18.6 Oral et al. [31] investigated the effect of absorbed lipids (squalene) on oxidative stability by subjecting UHMWPE test samples to accelerated aging in a pressure vessel under 5 atm of pure oxygen at 70 °C for 2 weeks. In the presence of lipids, the oxidative stability of polyethylene was compromised except when vitamin E was present

absorbed squalene on oxidative stability of polyethylene and found an increased level of oxidation during accelerated aging when squalene was previously doped into the test samples [31] (Fig. 18.6). The effect of cyclic loading on oxidative stability has also been reported by a number of research groups studying levels of oxidation in surgically explanted total hip and total knee polyethylene components. Medel et al. [23] showed higher oxidation levels in loaded regions of explanted tibial knee inserts in comparison with the parts of the same components that were not loaded in vivo. In a preclinical study, the extent of oxidation increased with the presence of cyclic load during accelerated aging [26] (Fig. 18.7).

18.4 The Role of Antioxidants in Highly Cross-Linked Polyethylene

The outcomes with the first-generation highly cross-linked polyethylene have been exceptional during the first decade of clinical use. The long-term performance of these devices in the second and the third decades of use is still unknown. The irradiated and annealed polyethylene components are showing elevated levels of oxidation in vivo; the material property changes associated with this oxidation are likely to compromise the long-term performance of these devices. With the irradiated and melted polyethylene components, while the oxidation due to residual free radicals

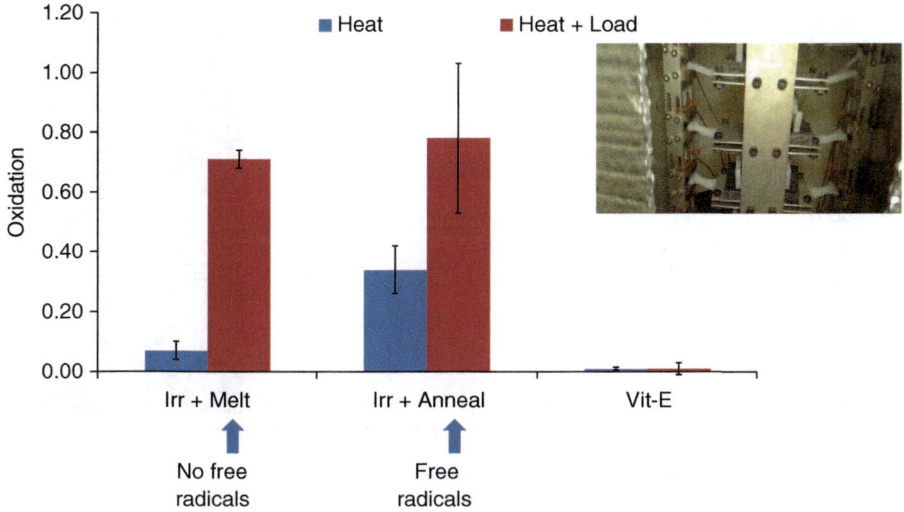

Fig. 18.7 Nabar et al. [26] investigated the effect of cyclic loading (bending) on oxidative stability by subjecting UHMWPE test samples to accelerated aging in air at 80 °C for 5 weeks. Cyclic load further compromised the oxidative stability of polyethylene except when vitamin E was present

created by radiation cross-linking is not a concern, the more recently proposed in vivo oxidation mechanisms could potentially alter the long-term performance of these devices. Therefore, the addition of antioxidants is beneficial in protecting the highly cross-linked polyethylene against long-term oxidation and its potential undesirable effects on in vivo performance during the second and third decades.

Vitamin E is the most widely used antioxidant to stabilize highly cross-linked polyethylene. The mechanism by which vitamin E protects the material is through scavenging of free radicals. As a result, if vitamin E is present in the polyethylene during radiation cross-linking, it also interferes with the cross-linking process [32, 33, 40]. When a vitamin E/polyethylene blend is irradiated, not only the cross-linking efficiency is reduced, but also the vitamin E is depleted in the blend. Several methods have been developed to overcome these adverse effects: (1) diffusing vitamin E into polyethylene after irradiation [38, 39], (2) blending vitamin E into polyethylene and irradiating at an elevated temperature [36], and (3) blending vitamin E into polyethylene, irradiating, and mechanically annealing.

In the presence of vitamin E, the wear behavior of highly cross-linked polyethylene is not altered. The material still has excellent wear resistance. In addition, even though the polymer is not melted after irradiation and it contains detectable residual free radicals, the antioxidant protects it against oxidation in the long term [18, 37, 42]. There are several other advantages of the antioxidants in highly cross-linked polyethylene: (1) Vitamin E prevents the oxidation caused by absorbed squalene during accelerated aging (Fig. 18.6); (2) vitamin E prevents the oxidation caused by cyclic loading during accelerated aging (Fig. 18.7); (3) when vitamin E is present, postirradiation melting is not needed; as a result, mechanical properties are not

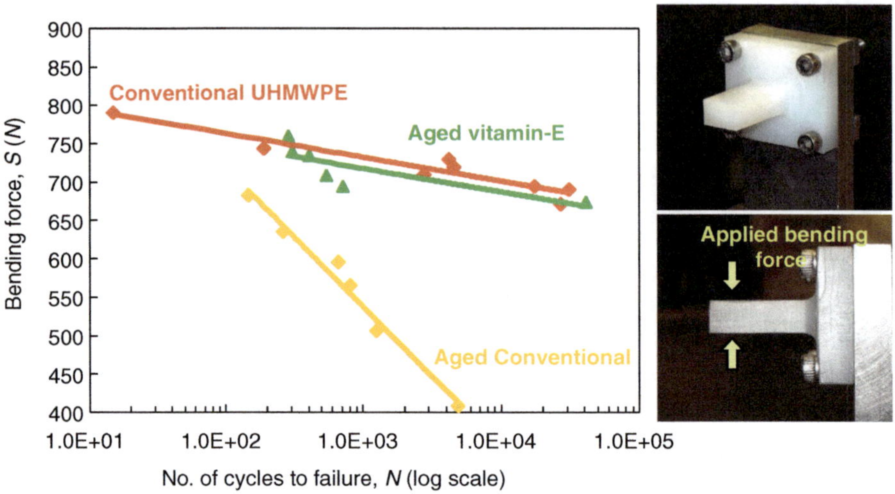

Fig. 18.8 Oral et al. [35] studied the effect of accelerated aging in air at 80 °C for 5 weeks on fatigue life of conventional polyethylene and vitamin E-stabilized highly cross-linked polyethylene using cantilever test samples. Conventional polyethylene was gamma sterilized in nitrogen; therefore, it contained residual free radicals. Conventional polyethylene oxidized after accelerated aging and demonstrated loss of fatigue life, while the vitamin E-stabilized highly cross-linked polyethylene retained its fatigue life even after accelerated aging

compromised as they would be in irradiated and melted polyethylene components [30]; (4) similarly, in the presence of vitamin E, as postirradiation melting is not needed, fatigue resistance of the material is not compromised as it would be in irradiated and melted polyethylene components [30, 34, 38] (Fig. 18.8); and (5) finally, there is evidence of reduced functional biological activity of particulate debris when vitamin E is present in the polymer [44] (Fig. 18.9).

Vitamin E-stabilized highly cross-linked polyethylene components have been in clinical use for over 5 years in total hips; their use in total knees is more recent. Clinical follow-up studies in total hip patients are showing excellent outcomes. In one study where patients received vitamin E-stabilized highly cross-linked polyethylene, acetabular liners together with 38 mm cobalt chromium femoral heads, which were followed by the RSA technique, show very low wear [13] (Fig. 18.10). Not only the reported wear rate is lower with vitamin E-stabilized highly cross-linked polyethylene but also the extent of creep deformation is lower in comparison with the first-generation highly cross-linked polyethylene (Fig. 18.10). As the first-generation irradiated and melted polyethylene components have lower crystallinity as a result of the melting step, they also have lower resistance against creep deformation. In contrast, with the vitamin E stabilization, melting is not needed to improve oxidative stability. The benefits of avoiding melting include increasing the strength of the material, increasing the fatigue resistance of the material, and also increasing the resistance against creep deformation. The findings from the RSA studies corroborate improved creep resistance in vivo in patients.

	Sham	Vitamin E	Virgin	*P*-value
Topographical osteolysis score	0.00 ± 0.00	1.63 ± 0.88	3.83 ± 1.98	$p < 0.001$
Osteoclast quantification	0.00 ± 0.00	3.80 ± 5.20	8.00 ± 6.30	$p = 0.028$

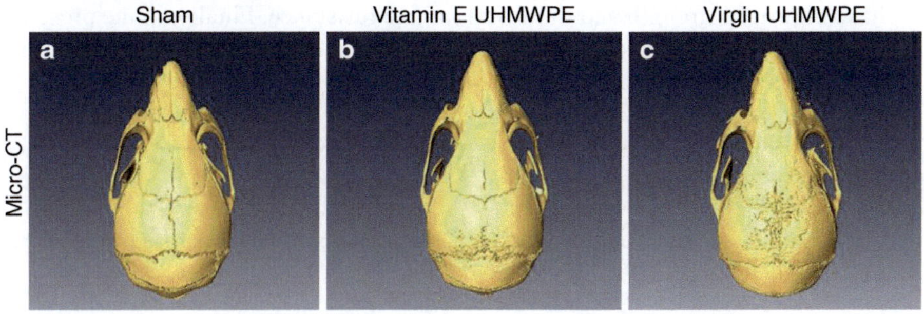

Fig. 18.9 Bichara et al. [4] reported on the functional biological activity of submicron-sized particulate debris fabricated from virgin UHMWPE (100 kGy irradiated and melted) and vitamin E-stabilized highly cross-linked UHMWPE. They used a murine calvaria model and compared to sham control (**a**). The animals that were implanted with vitamin E-containing particulate debris (**b**) showed substantially less bone resorption in comparison with the virgin particles without vitamin E (**c**)

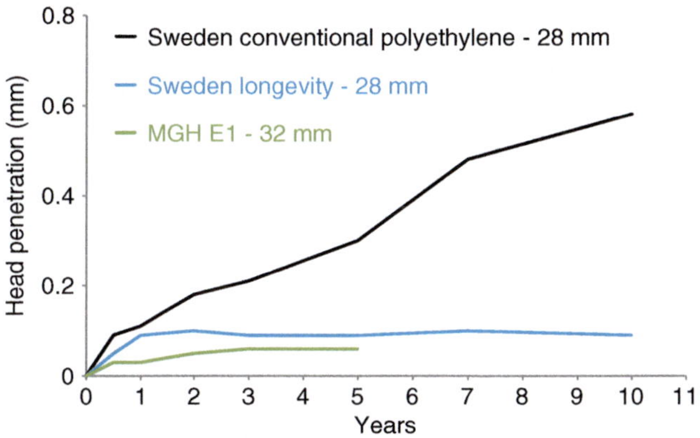

Fig. 18.10 Femoral head penetration as a function of in vivo service in patients with total hips where vitamin E-stabilized highly cross-linked acetabular liners were used in conjunction with 38 mm femoral heads are compared to data from Fig. 18.1. The wear rate (slope of the line after the first year) is significantly reduced with vitamin E-stabilized highly cross-linked UHMWPE acetabular liners in comparison with conventional polyethylene and is similar to the first-generation irradiated and melted (longevity 28 mm) polyethylene

Conclusions

Radiation cross-linking substantially improves the wear resistance of polyethylene components used in total joints. Thermal treatment following radiation cross-linking is necessary to improve the oxidative stability. Melting is more efficient in improving the long-term stability in comparison with annealing. The first-decade outcomes with the first-generation highly cross-linked polyethylenes are good; to ensure that these outcomes continue well into the second and the third decade, antioxidants have been introduced. With the antioxidants, the oxidative stability of the material will be ensured in the longer term; in addition, the components fabricated with vitamin E-stabilized cross-linked polyethylene have improved strength and improved fatigue resistance. Finally, in the presence of vitamin E, particulate debris appears to be less biologically active in causing periprosthetic osteolysis.

References

1. Al-Malaika S. Autoxidation. In: Scott G, editor. Atmospheric oxidation and antioxidants. Amsterdam: Elsevier Science Publishers B.V; 1993. p. 45–82.
2. Atkinson JR, Cicek RZ. Silane crosslinked polyethylene for prosthetic applications. Part I. Certain physical and mechanical properties related to the nature of the material. Biomaterials. 1983;4:267–75.
3. Atkinson JR, Cicek RZ. Silane crosslinked polyethylene for prosthetic applications. Part II. Creep and wear behavior and a preliminary molding test. Biomaterials. 1984;5:326–35.
4. Bichara DA, Malchau E, Hylleholt N, Cakmak S, Muratoglu OK. Particles from Vitamin-E diffused highly cross-linked UHMWOE induce less osteolysis compared to highly cross-linked virgin UHMWPE in a murine calvaria model. In: Transactions of the 60th annual meeting of the Orthopedic Research Society. New Orleans, LA: Orthopaedic Research Society, 2014.
5. Bragdon CR, Doerner M, Martell JM, Jarrett BT, Palm H, Malchau H. The 2012 John Charnley Award winner: clinical multi-centric studies of the wear performance of highly cross-linked re-melted polyethylene in THR. Clin Orthop Relat Res. 2013;471:393–402.
6. Bragdon CR, O'Connor DO, Lowenstein JD, Jasty M, Biggs SA, Harris WH. A new pin-on-disk wear testing method for simulating wear of polyethylene on cobalt-chrome alloy in total hip arthroplasty. J Arthroplasty. 2001;16(5):658–65.
7. Collier J, Currier B, Kennedy FE, Currier JH, Timmins GS, Jackson SK, Brewer RL. Comparison of cross-linked polyethylene materials for orthopaedic applications. Clin Orthop Relat Res. 2003;414:289–304.
8. Collier J, Sutula L, Currier B, John H, Wooding R, Williams I, Farber K, Mayor M. Overview of polyethylene as a bearing material: comparison of sterilization methods. Clin Orthop. 1996;333:76–86.
9. Costa L, Bracco P, del Prever EB, Luda MP, Trossarelli L. Analysis of products diffused into UHMWPE prosthetic components in vivo. Biomaterials. 2001;22(4):307–15.
10. Costa L, Jacobson K, Bracco P, Brach del Prever EM. Oxidation of orthopaedic UHMWPE. Biomaterials. 2002;23:1613–24.
11. Currier B, Mayor M, Currier J, Lyford K, Collier J. Crossfire™ retrievals-what can we learn? In: Transactions of the 51st annual meeting of the Orthopaedic Research Society. Washington, D.C: Orthopaedic Research Society; 2005. p. 1182.
12. DuPlessis T, Grobbelaar C, Marais F. The improvement of polyethylene prostheses through radiation crosslinking. Radiat Phys Chem. 1977;9:647–52.
13. Greene M, Sillesen N, Nebergall A, Rubash H, Kwon Y-M, Bragdon C, Malchau H. RSA evaluation of vitamin E diffused highly crosslinked polyethylene and acetabular and femoral component stability. In: Annual meeting of the American academy of orthopaedic surgeons. Chicago: American Academy of Orthopaedic Surgeons; 2013. p. 560.

14. Grobbelaar CJ, DuPlessis TA, Marais F. The radiation improvement of polyethylene prostheses. J Bone Joint Surg. 1978;60-B(3):370–4.
15. Harris WH. Osteolysis and particle disease in hip replacement. A review. Acta Orthop Scand. 1994;65(1):113–23.
16. Karrholm J, Digas G, Thanner J, Herberts P. Five to seven years experience with highly cross-linked PE. In: Transactions of the 24th SICOT Meeting. Hong Kong: Societe International de Orthopedique et de Traumatologie, 2008.
17. Kurtz S, Austin M, Azzam K, Sharkey P, MacDonald D, Medel F, Hozack W. Mechanical properties, oxidation and clinical performance of retrieved highly crosslinked Crossfire liners after intermediate-term implantation. J Arthroplasty. 2010;25(4):614–25.
18. Kurtz S, Dumbleton J, Siskey R, Wang A, Manley M. Trace concentrations of vitamin E protect radiation crosslinked UHMWPE from oxidative degradation. J Biomed Mater Res. 2008;90A:549–63.
19. Kurtz S, Gawel H, Patel J. History and systematic review of wear and osteolysis outcomes for first-generation highly crosslinked polyethylene. Clin Orthop Relat Res. 2011;469:2262–77.
20. Leung SB, Egawa H, Stepniewski A, Beykirch S, Engh Jr CA, Engh Sr CA. Incidence and volume of pelvic osteolysis at early follow-up with highly cross-linked and noncross-linked polyethylene. J Arthroplasty. 2007;22(6 Suppl 2):134–9.
21. Mall N, Nunley R, Zhu J, Maloney W, Barrack R, Clohisy J. The incidence of acetabular osteolysis in young patients with conventional versus highly crosslinked polyethylene. Clin Orthop Relat Res. 2011;469:372–81.
22. McKellop H, Shen F-W, Lu B, Campbell P, Salovey R. Development of an extremely wear resistant ultra-high molecular weight polyethylene for total hip replacements. J Orthop Res. 1999;17(2):157–67.
23. Medel FJ, et al. Gamma inert sterilization: a solution to polyethylene oxidation? J Bone Joint Surg. 2009;91:839–49.
24. Muratoglu O, Wannomae K, Rowell S, Micheli B, Malchau H. Ex vivo stability loss of irradiated and melted UHMWPE. J Bone Joint Surg Am. 2010;92:2809–16.
25. Muratoglu OK, Bragdon CR, O'Connor DO, Jasty M, Harris WH. A novel method of cross-linking ultra-high-molecular-weight polyethylene to improve wear, reduce oxidation, and retain mechanical properties. Recipient of the 1999 HAP Paul Award. J Arthroplasty. 2001;16(2):149–60.
26. Nabar S, Wannomae K, Muratoglu O. Environmental stress cracking of contemporary and alpha-tocopherol doped UHMWPEs. In: Transactions, 54th annual meeting of the Orthopaedic Research Society. San Francisco: Orthopaedic Research Society; 2008. p. 1684.
27. Oonishi H, Clarke I, Masuda S, Amino H. Study of retrieved acetabular sockets made from high-dose, cross-linked polyethylene. J Arthroplasty. 2001;16(8 suppl):129–33.
28. Oonishi H, Clarke IC, Yamamoto K, Masaoka T, Fujisawa A, Masuda S. Assesment of wear in extensively irradiated UHMWPE cups in simulator studies. J Biomed Mater Res A. 2004;68(52).
29. Oonishi H, Takayama Y, Tsuji E. Improvement of polyethylene by irradiation in artificial joints. Radiat Phys Chem. 1992;39(6):495–504.
30. Oral E, Christensen S, Malhi A, Wannomae K, Muratoglu O. Wear resistance and mechanical properties of highly crosslinked UHMWPE doped with vitamin E. J Arthroplasty. 2006;21(4):580–91.
31. Oral E, Ghali B, Neils A, Muratoglu O. A new mechanism of oxidation in UHMWPE caused by squalene absorption. J Biomed Mater Res. 2012;100B:742–51.
32. Oral E, Godleski Beckos C, Malhi A, Muratoglu O. The effects of high dose irradiation on the cross-linking of vitamin E-blended UHMWPE. Biomaterials. 2008;29:3557–60.
33. Oral E, Greenbaum ES, Malhi AS, Harris WH, Muratoglu OK. Characterization of irradiated blends of alpha-tocopherol and UHMWPE. Biomaterials. 2005;26(33):6657–63.
34. Oral E, Malhi A, Muratoglu O. Mechanisms of decrease in fatigue crack propagation resistance in irradiated and melted UHMWPE. Biomaterials. 2006;27:917–25.

35. Oral E, Malhi A, Wannomae K, Muratoglu O. Highly cross-linked UHMWPE with improved fatigue resistance for total joint arthroplasty. J Arthroplasty. 2008;23(7):1037–44. Winner of the 2006 'HAP' Paul Award.
36. Oral E, Neils A, Rowell S, Lozynsky A, Muratoglu O. Increasing irradiation temperature maximizes vitamin E grafting and wear resistance of UHMWPE. J Biomed Mater Res B Appl Biomater. 2013;101B(3):436–40.
37. Oral E, Rowell SL, Muratoglu OK. The effect of alpha-tocopherol on the oxidation and free radical decay in irradiated UHMWPE. Biomaterials. 2006;27:5580–7.
38. Oral E, Wannomae KK, Hawkins NE, Harris WH, Muratoglu OK. A-tocopherol doped irradiated UHMWPE for high fatigue resistance and low wear. Biomaterials. 2004;25(24):5515–22.
39. Oral E, Wannomae KK, Rowell SL, Muratoglu OK. Diffusion of vitamin E in ultra-high molecular weight polyethylene. Biomaterials. 2007;28(35):5225–37.
40. Parth M, Aust N, Lederer K. Studies on the effect of electron beam radiation on the molecular structure of ultra-high molecular weight polyethylene under the influence of alpha-tocopherol with respect to its application in medical implants. J Mater Sci Mater Med. 2002;13(10):917–21.
41. Premnath V, Harris W, Jasty M, Merrill E. Gamma sterilization of UHMWPE articular implants: an analysis of the oxidation problem. Ultra high molecular weight poly ethylene. Biomaterials. 1996;17:1741–53.
42. Rowell S, Oral E, Muratoglu O. Comparative oxidative stability of a-tocopherol blended and diffused UHMWPEs at 3 years of real-time aging. J Orthop Res. 2011;29:773–80.
43. Sutula L, et al. The Otto Aufranc Award. Impact of gamma sterilization on clinical performance of polyethylene in the hip. Clin Orthop. 1995;319:28–40.
44. Teramura S, Russell S, Ingham E, Fisher J, Tomita N, Fujiwara K, Tipper J. Reduced biological response to wear particles from UHMWPE containing vitamin E. In: Transactions of the 55th annual meeting of the Orthopaedic Research Society. Las Vegas: Ortopaedic Research Society; 2009. p. 2377.
45. Wroblewski B, Siney P, Fleming P. Low-friction arthroplasty of the hip using alumina ceramic and cross-linked polyethylene: a 17-year follow-up report. J Bone Joint Surg Br. 2005; 87B:1220–1.

What Happens to the Vitamin E in a Vitamin-Stabilised HXLPE?

19

Daniel Delfosse, Reto Lerf, and Christian Adlhart

19.1 Introduction

Today many of the second-generation highly cross-linked polyethylenes (HXLPE) use vitamin E (chemical name: α-tocopherol; see Fig. 19.1) as antioxidant to further enhance the longevity of the implant [1–3]. There are two main technologies how to add the vitamin E to the polyethylene: by infusion or by blending. Depending on the manufacturing and sterilisation process and the chosen level of cross-linking, the vitamin E will thus be subjected to different amounts of high energy irradiation.

While several studies mention some sort of "grafting" of the vitamin E to the polyethylene [4–8], little is known about the specific chemical reactions of the α-tocopherol molecule under high energy irradiation. This is mainly due to the fact that the reactions between α-tocopherol and long chains of polyethylene create macromolecules in a solid that cannot be easily characterised even by modern analytical technology. It would be helpful, however, to understand and quantify the chemical reactions occurring between α-tocopherol and polyethylene so as to give definite answers to the following questions:

Where does the vitamin E go in a HXLPE? Is there a danger of leaching out? Is the activity of the vitamin E as an oxygen and free radical scavenger undisturbed? Will the HXLPE remain protected against oxidation for a long time?

The aim of this research is to characterise what happens to the α-tocopherol when it is subjected to different levels of irradiation (for cross-linking and/or for

D. Delfosse (✉) • R. Lerf
Innovation and Technology Group, Mathys Ltd Bettlach,
Bettlach CH-2544, Switzerland
e-mail: daniel.delfosse@mathysmedical.com; reto.lerf@mathysmedical.com

C. Adlhart
Institute of Chemistry and Biological Chemistry, Zurich University of Applied Sciences ZHAW, Wädenswil CH-8820, Switzerland
e-mail: adas@zhaw.ch

K. Knahr (ed.), *Tribology in Total Hip and Knee Arthroplasty*,
DOI 10.1007/978-3-642-45266-6_19, © EFORT 2014

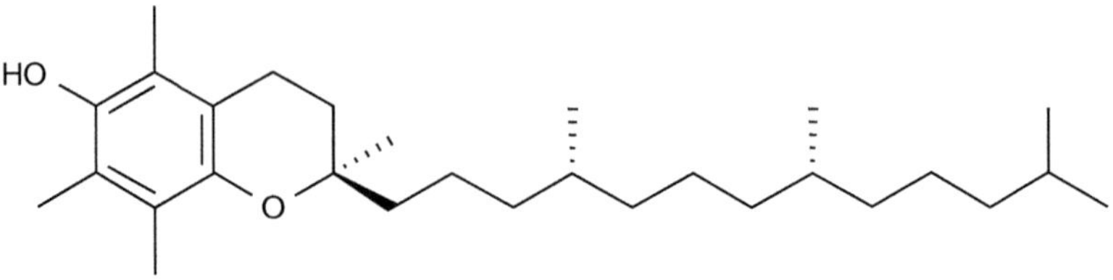

Fig. 19.1 Chemical structure of the α-tocopherol molecule

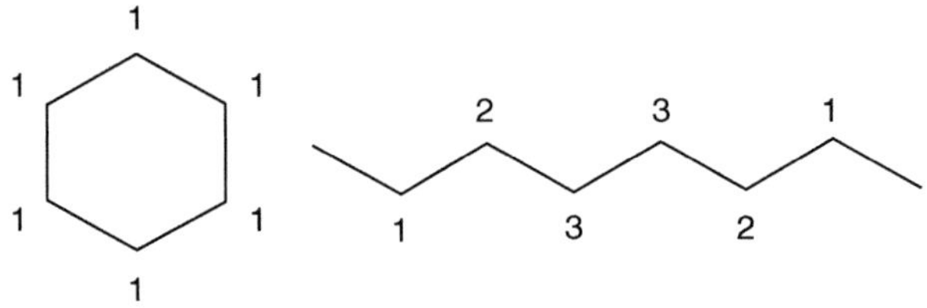

Fig. 19.2 Chemical structure of cyclohexane (*left*) and n-octane (*right*)

γ-sterilisation) in an environment of hydrocarbons. Based on the findings it will be possible to conclude how mobile the α-tocopherol molecule remains and if there is a potential danger of leaching out.

19.2 Methods

In a laboratory-scale experiment, 0.1 % α-tocopherol was blended with model hydrocarbons small enough to carry out a thorough chemical characterisation by means of gas chromatography-mass spectrometry (GC-MS), high-performance liquid chromatography (HPLC), matrix-assisted laser desorption/ionisation time-of-flight mass spectrometry (MALDI-TOF-MS) and nuclear magnetic resonance (NMR) before and after irradiation with dose levels corresponding to γ-sterilisation and cross-linking. Solutions of 100 ml cyclohexane or n-octane containing 0.1 wt.% a-tocopherol were γ-irradiated at a dose of 0.0 (blank), 27.5 and 97.9 kGy at BBF Sterilisationsservice (Kernen-Rommelshausen, Germany). The specific methods for sample preparation and chemical characterisation are described in detail by Badertscher et al. [9].

The novelty of this research lies in the fact that small hydrocarbon molecules were used to represent the much longer hydrocarbon chains that make up the polyethylene materials used in orthopaedics. These small hydrocarbons are liquids that can be chemically characterised in great detail to gain insight into the possible chemical reactions occurring between hydrocarbons and α-tocopherol when subjected to γ-irradiation. Even though the applicability of liquid model hydrocarbons for UHMWPE is limited due to different mobility of the antioxidant and the hydrocarbon radicals, the general reaction mechanisms are comparable.

As model materials, cyclohexane and n-octane were selected (Fig. 19.2). The n-octane can be thought of as a very small polyethylene molecule, consisting of only eight carbon atoms instead of some 250,000 typical for UHMWPE GUR1020. These eight atoms make up for three separate preferred chemical reaction sites, i.e. at atoms 2, 3 and 4, labelled 1, 2 and 3 in Fig. 19.2 (these three reaction sites are also identical to atoms 7, 6 and 5, respectively), and 1 less preferred reaction site at atom 1 or 8. In the cyclohexane on the other hand, all six potential reaction sites are chemically identical (therefore all labelled as 1 in Fig. 19.2). In theory when using cyclohexane, for each distinct chemical reaction between α-tocopherol and cyclohexane, a separate molecule will result and can subsequently be identified.

Laboratory-scale samples of HXLPE were prepared by mixing UHMWPE powder GUR 1020 and two different concentrations of vitamin E (0.1 wt-% and 1.0 wt-%). The samples were sintered and cross-linked with 96.5 kGy, following the recipe for the vitamys material (Mathys Ltd Bettlach, Switzerland) with a nominal cross-linking dose of 100 kGy [10]. Additionally, commercially available HXLPE prepared by "infusion" (E1-Poly, Ringloc-X liner size 66/36, Biomet, Warsaw IN, USA) and by "blending" (vitamys, RM Pressfit vitamys size 66/36, Mathys Ltd Bettlach, Switzerland) were analysed by spectroscopy (FTIR) for vitamin E content and homogeneity. In all samples, 0.3 mm sections were cut in two directions perpendicular to each other by a microtome HM 350 (Microm GmbH, Germany). The spectra of all sections were recorded by a Bio-Rad FTS-45 (Bio-Rad Laboratories, United Kingdom) in transmission with an aperture size of 1 × 1 cm at a resolution of 4 cm^{-1}. The vitamin E index (VEI) was calculated as the ratio of the area of a characteristic vitamin E peak (1,275–1,245 cm^{-1}) to the polyethylene reference peak (1,985–1,850 cm^{-1}). The relative vitamin E index (RVEI) was calculated by subtracting the background of a pure UHMWPE.

In order to assess the stability of the formed chemical bond between α-tocopherol and polyethylene, the laboratory-scale samples and commercial HXPLE materials were subjected to a chemical extraction by putting them in heptane for 48 h at 98 °C. This treatment is a very effective method to extract all free, i.e. not chemically bound, α-tocopherol from the samples.

19.3 Results

The γ-irradiated samples of the 0.1 % α-tocopherol solution in cyclohexane were analysed by GC-MS and MALDI-TOF-MS. The total ion current of the GC chromatogram showed only a few significant peaks, namely, the α-tocopherol peak at 15.92 min and one additional peak at 21.12 min (Fig. 19.3, lower curve), thus confirming that only one major chemical reaction had occurred between the two partners. To assess the chemical structure of the molecule responsible for the second peak, a reference material for the suspected 6-O-cyclohexyl-α-tocopherol ether was used (synthetically accessible from a-tocopherol and cyclohexanol following the Mitsunobu reaction [11, 12]). As expected, the GC-MS analysis of the 6-O-cyclohexyl-α-tocopherol ether resulted in a peak at 21.12 min (Fig. 19.3, upper curve).

The results of the laboratory-scale experiment clearly show that the α-tocopherol is chemically "grafted" to cyclohexane exclusively by a phenolic ether bond. The

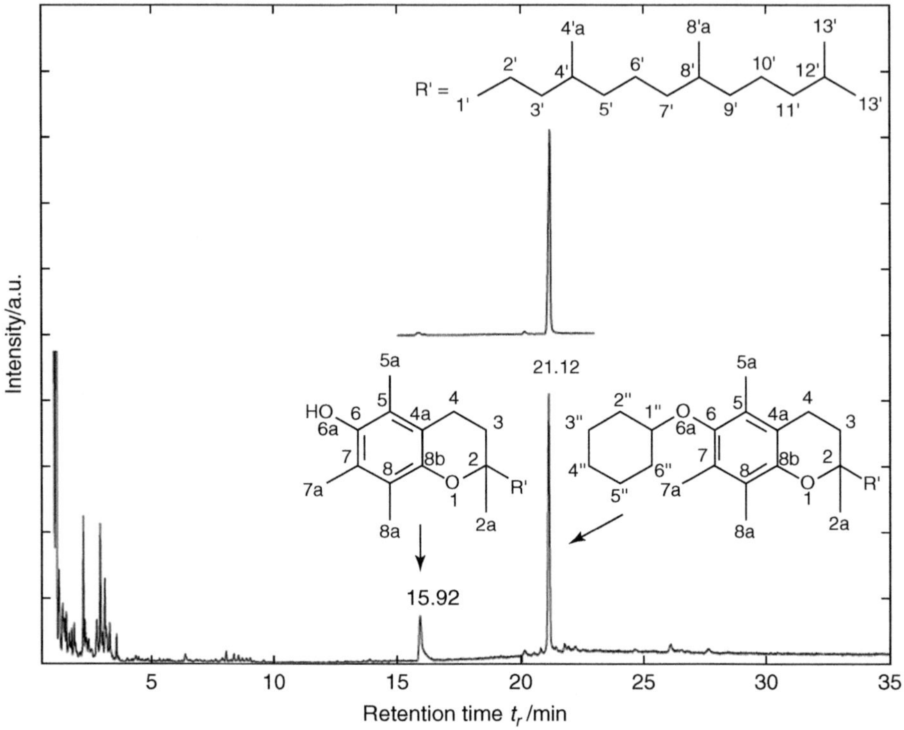

Fig. 19.3 GC-MS chromatogram of the reaction products of 0.1 % α-tocopherol in cyclohexane after γ-irradiation with a dose of 97.9 kGy

degree of ether formation was found to be strongly correlated with the irradiation dose. For the cyclohexane, 34 %, resp. 68 % of α-tocopherol was transformed into 6-0-cyclohexyl-α-tocopherol ether after irradiating with 27.5, resp. 97.9 kGy.

For the n-octane, assuming only one distinct chemical reaction to take place, three different but chemically equivalent ether products were expected. As shown in Fig. 19.4, in addition to the α-tocopherol peak at 15.92 min, three major peaks were detected at 19.79, 20.15 and 20.86 min. The corresponding molecules are shown beside the peaks (labelled as 2d, 2c and 2b). In addition, a small peak was detected at 22.42 min, corresponding to the non-preferred chemical reaction with atom 1 or 8 of the n-octane. The resulting molecule is labelled as 2a.

Again, the degree of ether formation increased with increasing irradiation dose. For the n-octane, 31 %, resp. 74 %, of α-tocopherol was transformed into ether products after irradiating with 27.5, resp. 97.9 kGy.

The homogeneity of the vitamin E distribution in commercial HXLPE depends largely on the manufacturing method. An "infused" HXLPE will possess a vitamin E distribution that is generated by a typical diffusion process, whereas a "blended" HXLPE will have more homogeneous vitamin E content. This difference can be clearly seen in Fig. 19.5. It also shows that an "infused" HXLPE will generally contain a larger amount of vitamin E than a "blended" HXLPE to guarantee a sufficient vitamin E content throughout the whole part.

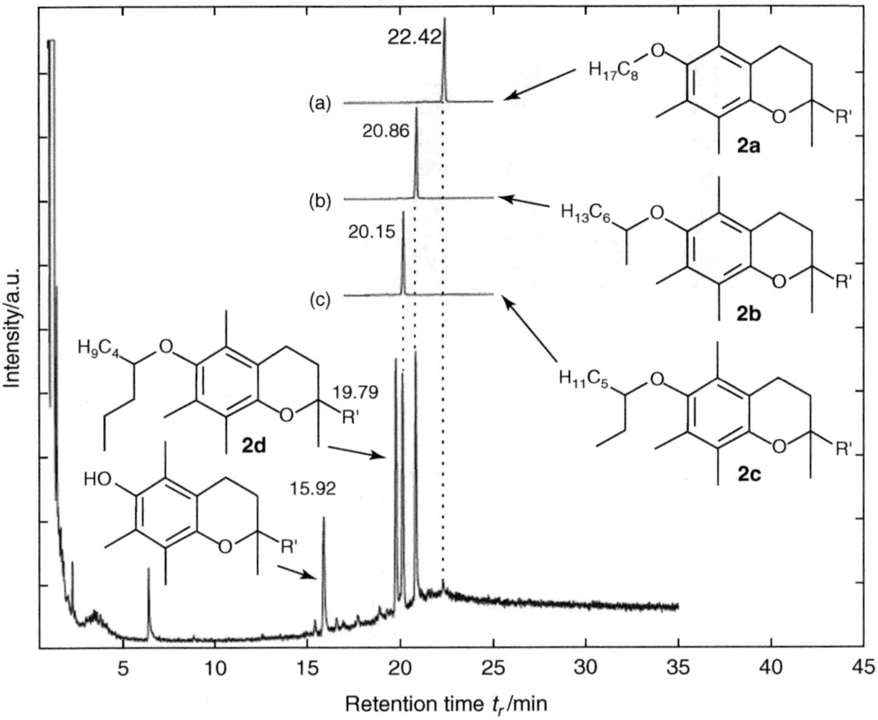

Fig. 19.4 GC-MS chromatogram of the reaction products of 0.1 % α-tocopherol in n-octane after γ-irradiation with a dose of 97.9 kGy. "2a", "2b" and "2c" mark the three different, but chemically equivalent ether products, while "2d" marks the non-preferred ether product

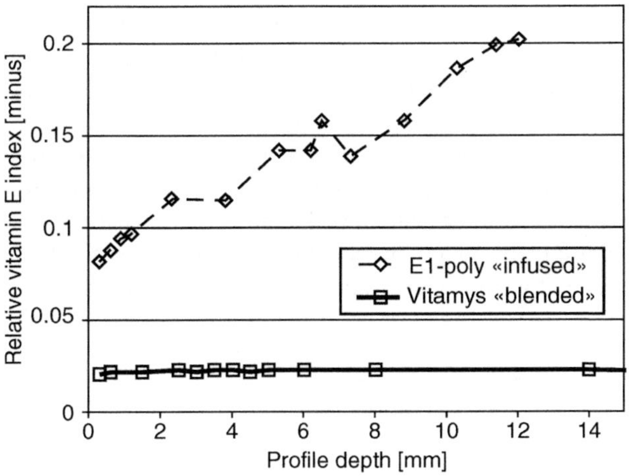

Fig. 19.5 Concentration profile (as relative vitamin E index) through the cross-section of two commercial HXLPE materials (E1-poly, Biomet and vitamys, Mathys Ltd Bettlach)

With laboratory-scale samples, it was shown that the heptane elution process is a highly efficient method for extracting vitamin E. In all nonirradiated samples, independent of the vitamin E content, close to 100 % of the vitamin E was extracted (Fig. 19.6). This is not surprising as without irradiation, the α-tocopherol molecule is not chemically

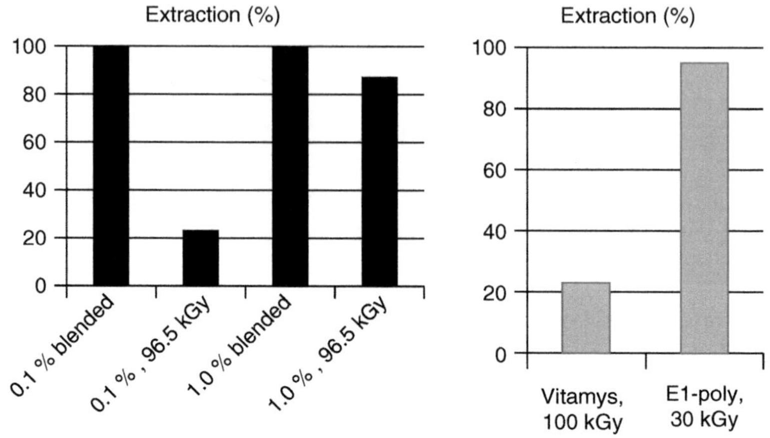

Fig. 19.6 Relative vitamin E index of laboratory (*left*) and commercial (*right*) HXLPE materials (E1-poly, Biomet and vitamys, Mathys Ltd Bettlach) before and after extraction

bound to the polyethylene. However, after a cross-linking dose of 96.5 kGy, complete extraction was no longer possible. For samples containing 0.1 % α-tocopherol, 23 % were extracted, leaving 77 % of the original vitamin E content inside the cross-linked material, i.e. 0.08 %. For samples containing 1.0 % α-tocopherol, 87 % were extracted, leaving only 13 % of the original vitamin E, i.e. 0.13 %. The phenolic reaction between α-tocopherol and polyethylene seems to depend not only on the dose of irradiation but also on the total amount of α-tocopherol molecules present.

The extraction of vitamin E from the commercial HXLPE showed a good correlation to the laboratory experiment. For the E1-poly (mean vitamin E content approximately 0.5 %, infused, γ-sterilised at 25–30 kGy), 5 % of the vitamin E appeared to be "grafted", i.e. could not be extracted. For the vitamys material (vitamin E content 0.1 %, blended, cross-linked at 100 kGy, gas plasma sterilised), 77 % of the vitamin E remained, correlating well with the 77 % of the laboratory sample and the 68 and 74 % phenolic reaction of 0.1 % α-tocopherol in cyclohexane and n-octane. Once more, the higher the initial vitamin E content and the lower the irradiation dose, the more vitamin E could be extracted. It is however good to know that even in a (highly unlikely) worst-case scenario of elution, both commercial materials would still retain enough vitamin E to guarantee a high oxidation resistance. For the E1-poly, the remaining vitamin E content would be approximately 0.02 % and for the vitamys approximately 0.08 %.

19.4 Discussion

In the introduction we raised a number of questions that may be clinically relevant. These questions are individually addressed here:

1. Where does the vitamin E go in a HXLPE?

   The α-tocopherol is readily soluble in polyethylene. It can be blended before sintering or it can be introduced afterwards by an infusion process. Once the material is subjected to γ-irradiation, a dose-dependent amount of α-tocopherol will be chemically bound ("grafted") to the polyethylene chains by an ether formation. The chemical reaction is a so-called phenolic ether formation between the OH group of the α-tocopherol (top left in Fig. 19.1) and a free radical of the polyethylene chain. Grafting of α-tocopherol on UHMWPE upon irradiation by formation of phenolic ethers also explains both the observed loss of the phenolic OH group and the reduced amount of extractable α-tocopherol.

2. Is there a danger of leaching out?
   All α-tocopherol that is not "grafted" can be extracted out of the HXLPE material given a suitable method such as heptane extraction. In a natural human joint, however, the implant is surrounded by synovial fluid, consisting mainly of water. In this environment, it is very unlikely that the fat-soluble vitamin E is extracted. Evidently the maximum amount that may theoretically leach out of an implant is limited by the total amount of α-tocopherol it contains. For a RM Pressfit vitamys hip cup (Mathys Ltd Bettlach, Switzerland), weighing some 50 g, the total amount of the 0.1 % α-tocopherol added is 50 mg, much lower than the maximum recommended daily intake of vitamin E (approximately 300–500 mg for adults).
3. Is the activity of the vitamin E as an oxygen and free radical scavenger undisturbed?
   Yes, the second-generation HXLPE (protected by addition of an antioxidant) have an excellent resistance against oxidation before and after cross-linking and/or γ-sterilisation [1–3, 13]. This property persists even when the cross-linked material is subjected to elution processes. We now know why, because at least some of the α-tocopherol is "grafted" to the polyethylene structure and can no longer leach out.
4. Will the HXLPE remain protected against oxidation for a long time?
   Yes, the excellent oxidation resistance of "vitamin-doped" HXLPE has been shown repeatedly with different mechanical and tribological tests using artificial ageing protocols to simulate the in vivo oxidation behaviour [1–3, 13].

The second-generation HXLPE materials are also highly wear resistant, equivalent to the first-generation HXLPE. They keep this property, however, even when subjected to artificial ageing. To show the difference of wear behaviour between the different materials, hip simulator testing of conventional UHMWPE, first- and second-generation HXLPE, was carried out before and after ageing.

All hip simulator tests were performed according to ISO 14242-1:2012 at RMS Foundation, Switzerland, using a servo-hydraulic six-station hip simulator (EndoLab, Thansau/Rosenheim, Germany) at a temperature of 37 ± 1 °C, simulating all three in vivo angular displacements, flexion/extension, abduction/adduction and internal/external rotation of a gait cycle, applying a maximum load of 3.0 kN. As articulation partners 28 or 32 mm CoCr heads were used against UHMWPE GUR 1020 (RM Pressfit cup, size 50/28, Mathys Ltd Bettlach), vitamys (RM Pressfit vitamys cup, size 50/28, Mathys Ltd Bettlach) and Durasul (Alpha hooded liners, size KK/32, Zimmer GmbH, Switzerland). Artificial ageing was carried out at 70 °C and 5 bar oxygen according to ASTM F2003-02. It is generally accepted that artificial ageing of 15, 30 and 60 days corresponds to an oxidative loading equivalent of approximately 10, 20 and 40 years inside the human body.

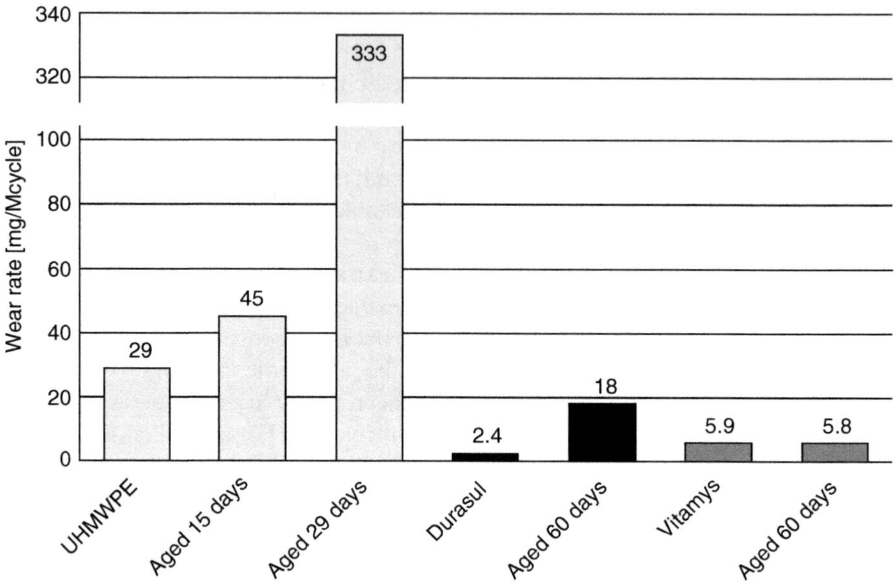

Fig. 19.7 Wear rates of hip simulator testing with conventional UHMWPE and first- and second-generation HXLPE materials (Durasul, Zimmer and vitamys, Mathys Ltd Bettlach) before and after accelerated ageing

The results of the hip simulator tests are shown in Fig. 19.7. As expected, both HXLPE materials show much lower wear than the conventional γ-sterilised UHMWPE in the unaged condition. The measured wear rates were 29 ± 3 mg/Mcycles for the UHMWPE, 5.9 ± 1.0 mg/Mcycles for vitamys and 2.4 ± 2.3 mg/Mcycles for Durasul. After 15 and 29 days artificial ageing, the measured wear rates of the conventional UHMWPE had increased considerably to45 ± 5 and 333 ± 18 mg/Mcycles. Hip simulator testing was not possible after 60 days of ageing due to the resulting brittleness of the UHMWPE samples. For the HXLPE, however, even after 60 days of artificial ageing, the measured wear rates were still reasonably low with 18 ± 3 mg/Mcycles for Durasul and even completely unaffected with 5.8 ± 1.0 mg/Mcycles for vitamys. These results give us a well-founded hope that the second-generation HXLPE will remain protected against oxidation and continue to perform as well as right after implantation for a very long time in vivo.

Conclusion

The α-tocopherol was proven to chemically bind exclusively by an ether formation. This "grafting" explains both the observed loss of the phenolic group and the reduced amount of extractable α-tocopherol. It also indicates why the activity of the vitamin E as an oxygen and free radical scavenger remains undisturbed.

Both commercially available vitamin E-doped HXLPE studied will – even in a worst-case scenario of elution – retain enough antioxidant to remain protected against oxidation for a very long time in vivo, probably for life.

References

1. Lerf R, Zurbrügg D, Delfosse D. Use of vitamin E to protect cross-linked UHMWPE from oxidation. Biomaterials. 2010;31:3643–8.
2. Bracco P, Oral E. Vitamin E stabilised UHMWPE for total joint implants. Clin Orthop Relat Res. 2011;469:2286–93.
3. Oral E, Muratoglu OK. Vitamin E diffused, highly crosslinked UHMWPE: a review. Int Orthop. 2011;35:215e–23.
4. Al-Malaika S, Ashley H, Issenhuth S. The antioxidant role of α-tocopherol in polymers, I. The nature of transformation products of α-tocopherol formed during melt processing of LDPE. J Polym Sci A. 1994;32:3099–113.
5. Al-Malaika S. Perspectives in stabilisation of polyolefins. Adv Polym Sci. 2004;169:121–50.
6. Mallégol J, Carlsson DJ, Deschênes L. Antioxidant effectiveness of vitamin E in HDPE and tetradecane at 32°C. Polym Degrad Stab. 2001;73:269–80.
7. Wolf C, Muratoglu OK. Radiation grafting of vitamin E to ultrahigh molecular weight polyethylene. ORS annual meeting, Long Beach, CA; 2011. p. 1178
8. Lerf R, Zurbrügg D, Delfosse D. Homogeneity and grafting of Small and large quantities of vitamin E in ultrahigh molecular weight polyethylene. Abstracts of 5th UHMWPE international meeting. Philadelphia; 2011. p. 25
9. Badertscher RP, Lerf R, Delfosse D, Adlhart C. Grafting of a-tocopherol upon γ-irradiation in UHMWPE probed by model hydrocarbons. Polym Degrad Stab. 2012;97:2255–61.
10. Lidgren L, Bengtsson P, Sjövall P, Wesslen B. A method for the preparation of UHMWPE doped with an antioxidant and an implant made thereof. European Patent EP1161489, priority date 17 Feb 1999.
11. Swamy KCK, Kumar NNB, Balaraman E, Kumar KVPP. Mitsunobu and related reactions: advances and applications. Chem Rev. 2009;109:2551–651.
12. Elson KE, Jenkins ID, Loughlin WA. The Hendrickson reagent and the Mitsunobu reaction: a mechanistic study. Org Biomol Chem. 2003;1:2958–65.
13. Oral E, Christensen SD, Malhi AS, Wannomae KK, Moratoglu OK. Wear resistance and mechanical properties of highly cross-linked, ultrahigh-molecular weight polyethylene doped with vitamin E. J Arthroplasty. 2006;21:580–91.

HXLPE with Vitamin E in Isoelastic Monoblock Pressfit Cup: 2-Year Follow-Up with Clinical and Radiological Scores

20

Philipp Rehbein, Y. Abtroun, M. Beck, J. Baines, A. de Gast, A. Steenmeijer, G. French, R. Becker, A. Pijnenburg, Karl Knahr, L. Hollmann, and N. Helmy

20.1 Introduction

Elective joint replacement for the hip joint with implantation of a hip joint endoprosthesis is a common and successful surgery with good register and study data. In addition to the qualitative assessment of these studies and registry data, the

P. Rehbein (✉) • Y. Abtroun
Orthopädische Klinik, St. Josefs-Hospital, Wiesbaden, 65189, Germany
e-mail: prehbein@joho.de, http://www.joho.de

M. Beck
Clinic for Orthopaedic Surgery, Luzerner Kantonsspital, Lucerne, Switzerland

J. Baines
Department of Orthopaedic, Golden Jubilee National Hospital, Clydebank, UK

A. de Gast
Department of Orthopaedic, Diakonessenhuis Utrecht/Zeist, Utrecht, The Netherlands

A. Steenmeijer
Department of Orthopaedic, Ziekenhuis Bronovo, Den Haag, The Netherlands

G. French
Department of Orthopaedic, Ormiston Orthopaedics Manukau, Manukau, New Zealand

R. Becker
Department of Orthopaedics and Traumatology, Städtisches Klinikum Brandenburg GmbH, Brandenburg, Germany

A. Pijnenburg
Department of Orthopaedic, Ziekenhuis Amstelland, Amstelveen, The Netherlands

K. Knahr
Orthopädisches Spital Wien-Speising GmbH, Speisinger Strasse 109, 1130 Vienna, Austria

L. Hollmann
Department of Orthopaedic, Streekziekenhuis Koningin Beatrix, Winterswijk, The Netherlands

N. Helmy
Department of Orthopaedic, Bürgerspital Solothurn, Solothurn, Switzerland

K. Knahr (ed.), *Tribology in Total Hip and Knee Arthroplasty*,
DOI 10.1007/978-3-642-45266-6_20, © EFORT 2014

material properties of mobile pairings play a significant role next to the surgical approaches, anchoring techniques (cementless versus cemented) and implant designs (straightstem prosthesis, short-stem prosthesis, hip resurfacement).

For the mobile couplings in recent years the following combinations of pairings increasingly came to clinical application: ceramic on ceramic, polyethylene of different generations on ceramic or metal on metal. In the cementless acetabular implant technique, isoelastic monoblock pressfit cups are evaluated differently compared to metal-backed cups with modular inlays. An isoelastic cup is an "all-poly" monoblock cup. The anchorage is cementless and primary stability is achieved with a pressfit mechanism. The contact surface to the bone particles is a titanium particle-coated surface (Fig. 20.1).

Both for the isoelastic monoblock cups of the older generation and the new generation, there exists a good study database. Ihle et al. [3] could show long-term results for 20 years that the isoelastic pressfit cup of classic polyethylene has a long survival rate. After about 18 years, however, abrasion and its side effects were the most common reasons for revision of material. Wyss et al. [7] examined 5-year results of an uncemented isoelastic pressfit cup (made from UHMWPE) and found that the migration rates and wear rates were far for this cup under the predictive criteria for implant failure. In addition to these studies, a register database is available as well.The "New Zealand Arthroplasty Register" [5] demonstrated for the isoelastic RM pressfit cup with 4,046 cases and 9,770 observed component years a revision rate of 0.56 per 100 component years.

In addition to these good clinical data, there are also some studies that described different in vitro behavior of highly cross-linked polyethylene (HXLPE) doped with vitamin E. Banche et al. [1] could present the thesis that vitamin E-enriched UHMWPE has the potential to reduce bacterial adhesion mechanism with an investigation of the adhesion potential of staphylococci. Also biomechanical in vitro studies with highly cross-linked polyethylene (HXLPE) enriched with vitamin E show a valid database. For this group of authors, Beck et al. [2] showed that highly cross-linked polyethylene (HXLPE) enriched with vitamin E not only has a generally better abrasion resistance compared to UHMWPE but that it is biomechanically significantly superior to UHMWPE especially in the state of an aging simulation. Besides these results in the same study, it could be demonstrated as well that the in vivo wear rate of highly cross-linked polyethylene (HXLPE) with cross-linking doses above 90 kGy does not differ at different head sizes (28 versus 36 mm), while with cross-linking doses below 90 kGy, a larger head diameter of 36 mm shows higher wear rates compared to a head diameter of 28 mm.

The focus of this study is whether these important in vitro findings on highly cross-linked polyethylene (HXLPE) enriched with vitamin E are also visible in clinical use. The goal of this study is therefore the inclusion and assessment of a patient population for elective total hip replacement with the use of a cementless "all-poly" monoblock pressfit cup, which is manufactured with highly cross-linked polyethylene (HXLPE) and doped with vitamin E (Fig. 20.2).

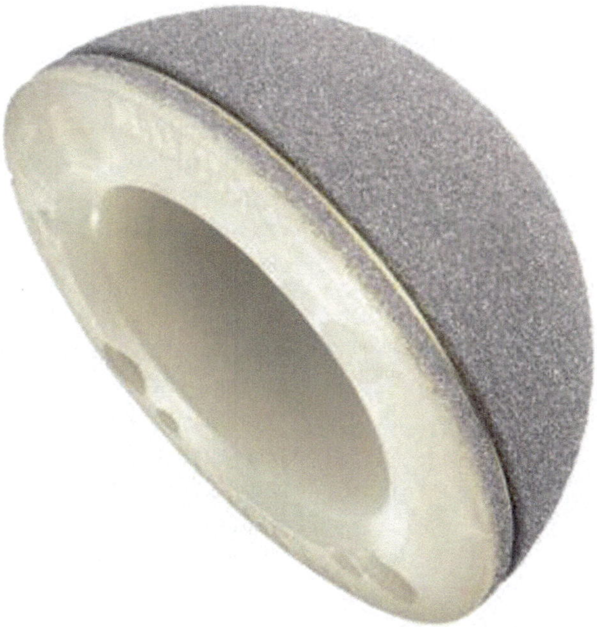

Fig. 20.1 The RM Pressfit vitamys® cup

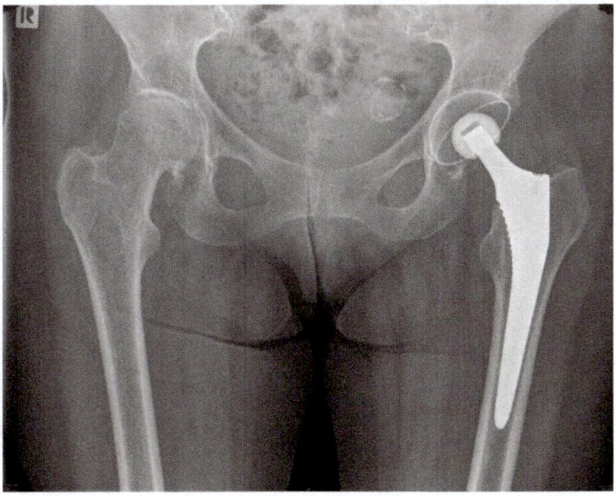

Fig. 20.2 Native X-ray of cementless THR with RM Pressfit vitamys® cup

20.2 Material and Methods

The study design is a prospective follow-up multicenter surveillance study. Ten Hospitals in Europe and one clinic in New Zealand were included in the study. The follow-up protocol includes the evaluation of the Harris hip score (HHS) and the visual analog scales (VAS) for rest pain, load pain, and satisfaction (Tables 20.1 and 20.2).

Table 20.1 Distribution and frequencies of diagnosis

Primary diagnosis	Frequency	Percent
Primary osteoarthrosis	757	85.1
Secondary osteoarthrosis	63	7.1
Inflammatory arthritis	6	0.7
Necrosis	28	3.1
Fracture	22	2.5
Congenital dysplasia	13	1.5
Other	1	0.1

Table 20.2 Distribution and frequencies of surgical approaches

Approach	Frequency	Percent
Anterior	156	17.5
Anterolateral	170	19.1
Transgluteal (lateral)	126	14.2
Posterolateral	432	48.5
Transgluteal with trochanteric osteotomy	6	0.7

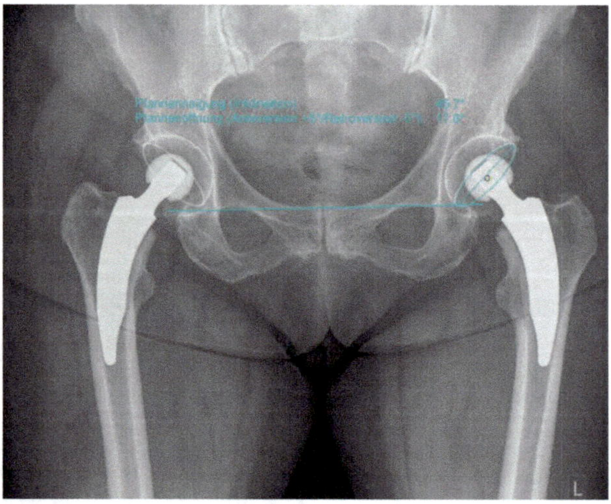

Fig. 20.3 Postoperative position analysis (inclination and anteversion)

The detection and follow-up time points are preoperatively, postoperatively at 6 weeks, the period between 6 and 12 months, after 24 months, and after 36 months. A long-term follow-up is planned for at least 10 years. All adverse events will also be recorded (Fig. 20.3).

20.3 Results

Compared to the preoperative observations ($n=890$ cases), all scores and parameters for the 1-year follow-up ($n=711$) and the 2-year follow-up ($n=440$) could be improved:

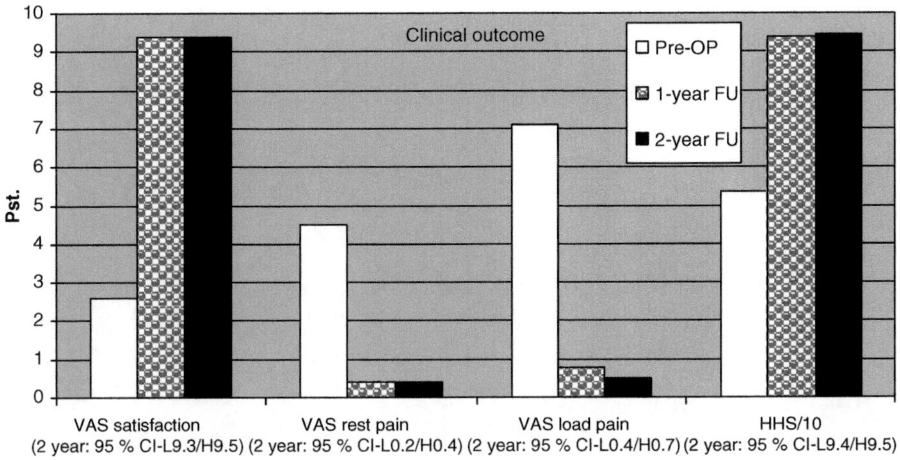

Fig. 20.4 Comparison of clinical outcome (VAS and HHS) preoperatively vs. 1y-FU and 2y-FU

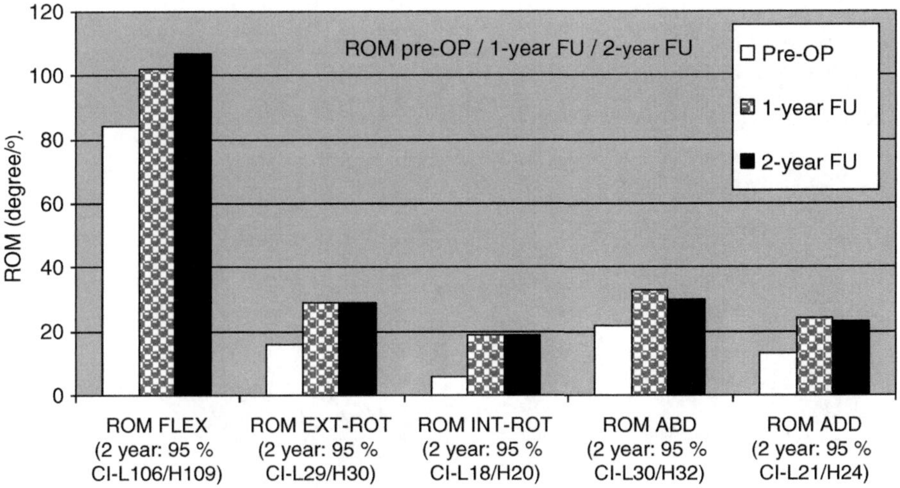

Fig. 20.5 Comparison of range of movement (flexion, external rotation, internal rotation, abduction, and abduction) preoperatively vs. 1-year FU and 2-year FU

Harris hip score (HHS) was preoperatively: 54 points/after 1-year follow-up: 94 points/after 2-year follow-up: 95 points, visual analog scale satisfaction (VAS) was preoperatively: 2.6/after 1-year follow-up: 9.4/after 2-year follow-up: 9.4 points, rest pain visual analog scale (VAS (Fig. 20.4)) was preoperatively: 4.5 points/after 1-year follow-up 0.4 points/after 2-year follow-up: 0.4 points, visual analog scale pain stress (VAS) was preoperatively: 7.1 points/after 1-year follow-up of 0.8 points/after 2-year follow-up: 0.5. Also the amounts for range of movement were able to show an improvement: ROM flexion (preoperative: 84°/1-year follow-up of 102°/2-year follow-up: 107°) (Fig. 20.5).

Table 20.3 Distribution of cup position in inclination

Inclination cup	Frequency	Percent
<35°	76	8.5
35–40°	262	29.5
41–45°	302	34.0
46–50°	158	17.8
>50°	91	10.2

Table 20.4 Distribution of cup position in anteversion

Anteversion cup	Frequency	Percent
Retroversion	0	0.0
<10° anteversion	41	4.6
10°–15° anteversion	343	38.6
>15° anteversion	505	56.8

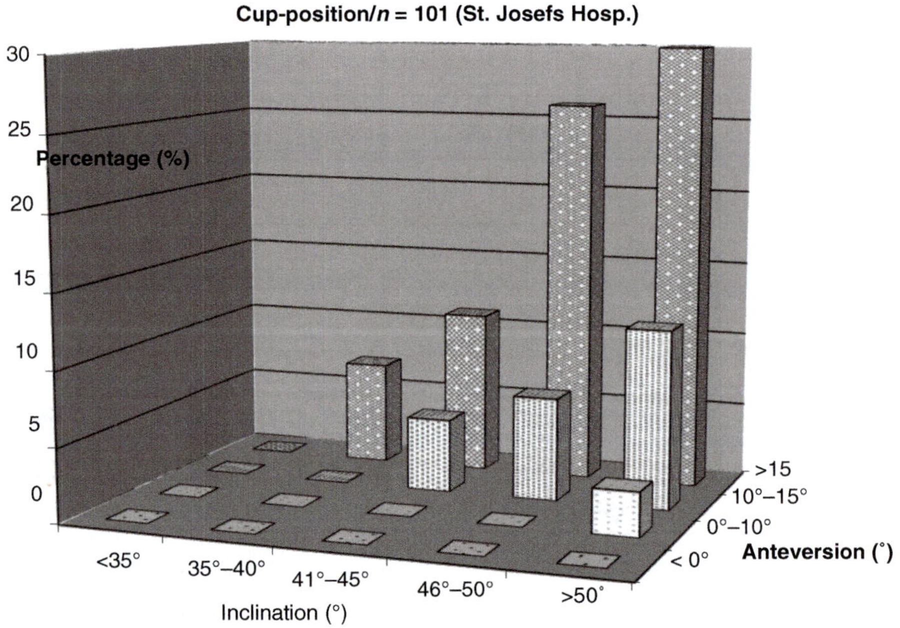

Fig. 20.6 Frequency of combinations for cup position (inclination and anteversion)

The radiological analysis showed that no visible migration was recorded at 1-year follow-up as well as the 2-year follow-up (Tables 20.3 and 20.4; Fig. 20.3 and Fig. 20.6). In a few cases, so-called radiolucent lines occurred, but there was no clinical or radiological correlation detected (1-year follow-up of 6.3 %/2-year follow-up of 7.1 %). However, it was also found that 66 % of radiolucent lines which occurred in 1-year follow-up in the 2-year follow-up were no longer existent. It showed also that in a CT study conducted in this group of authors, radiolucent lines visible in the native X-ray in the CT scans could not be shown.

Table 20.5 Frequencies of intraoperative complications

Intraoperative complication	Frequency
None	868
Proximal fracture of the femur	3
Fissure of the femur	6
Fissure of the trochanter	6
Avulsion of the trochanter	1
Acetabulum perforation	2
Vascular lesion	2
Incorrect implantation	1
Others	2

Table 20.6 Frequencies of local complications during hospital stay

Local complication during hospital stay	Frequency
None	857
Dislocation posterior	1
Deep infection	1
Superficial infection	3
Hematoma/seroma	18
Fracture	1
Trochanter fracture	2
Vascular lesion	1
Femoral nerve palsy	1
Sciatic nerve palsy	2
Others	2

The data collected in intraoperative and early postoperative interval with implant-related complications and adverse events during follow-up were rare (dislocation of the hip, $n=2$; malposition of the cup, $n=1$; acetabular fracture, $n=1$). The standard, non-implant-related complications were infection ($n=9$) and postoperative hematoma ($n=3$) (Tables 20.5 and 20.6).

20.4 Discussion

The clinical application of an isoelastic monoblock pressfit cup manufactured with highly cross-linked polyethylene (HXLPE) and doped with vitamin E for elective hip replacement shows a good clinical and functional behavior. A low rate of so-called radiolucent lines in some cases is without clinical correlation and must be observed.

Taking into consideration the results of a CT scan investigation from this group of authors, it is also possible that these radiolucent lines are visible in native X-ray imaging in the expression of the osseous integration at the interface between the titanium particle coating and bone. For the 3-year follow-up migration tests (EBRA)

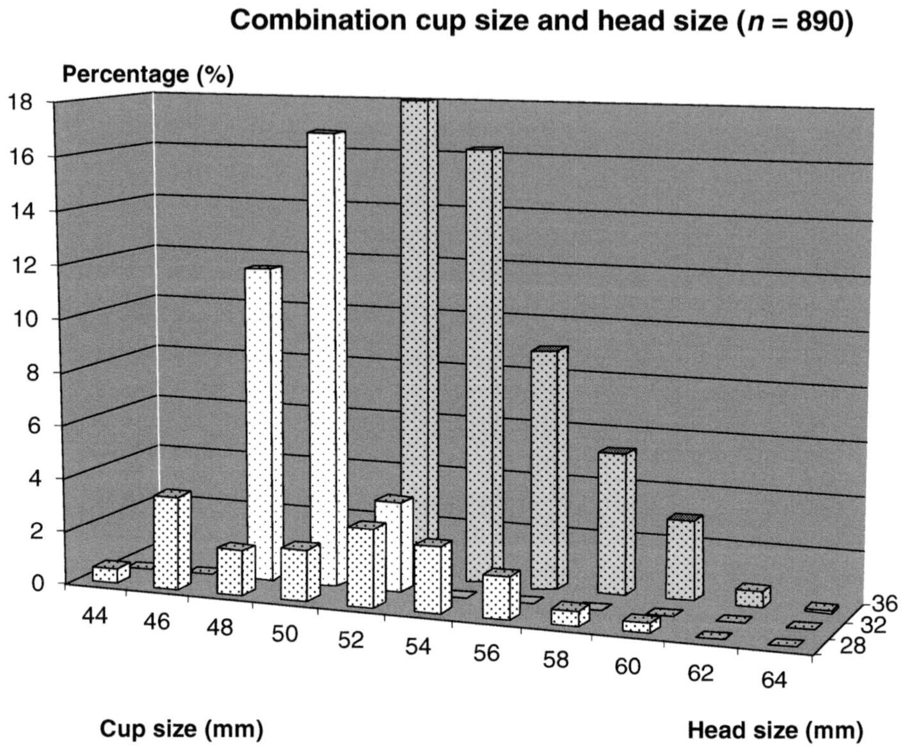

Fig. 20.7 Frequency of cup size (mm) and head diameter (mm) for 28 mm heads, 32 mm heads, and 36 mm heads

are scheduled. For the expected results a particular high importance in view of the radiolucent lines is given. But otherwise in some studies, it could be already demonstrated that migration analysis (Pakvis et al. [4]) and creep behavior (investigated by Vielpeau et al. [6]) with these cementless HXLPE cups enriched with vitamin E have very good results. Since in this study different inner diameters (28, 32, and 36 mm) have been used for the commonly used outside diameter sizes, the following radiological analysis may be able to provide information here if the results shown in the in vitro experiment of a no adverse abrasion behavior can also be confirmed for large heads (e.g., 32 or 36 mm) in the clinical application. However, there were no differences in dislocation and range of motion, so that the smaller head sizes (28 mm) compared with larger head sizes (32 and 36 mm) can be considered as equivalent to the present time (Fig. 20.7).

These early results of this young study indicate that the cementless isoelastic monoblock pressfit cup, which is made of highly cross-linked polyethylene (HXLPE) enriched with vitamin E, is suitable to achieve excellent clinical and functional results besides all variance of the other surgical-related factors (especially different surgical approaches and different used femoral implants). If present results from in vitro studies about better abrasion resistance, reduced material aging, and low adhesion potential for bacteria also confirm clinically, this implant is likely to prove in the future for clinical application (Fig. 20.8).

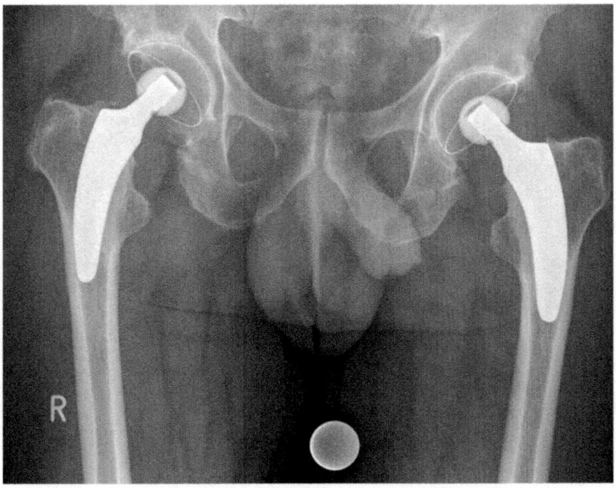

Fig. 20.8 A 3-year follow-up of a 62-year-old male patient after elective simultaneous one-stage bilateral total hip replacement (THR) with RM Pressfit vitamys® cups and short stems

References

1. Banche G, Bracco P, Bistolfi A, Allizond V, Boffano M, Costa L, Cimino A, Cuffini AM, Del Prever EM. Vitamin E blended UHMWPE may have the potential to reduce bacterial adhesive ability. J Orthop Res. 2011;29(11):1662–7.
2. Beck M, Delfosse D, et al. Mechanical properties of UHMWPE and highly cross-linked UHMWPE/vitamin E (ISO 12242 u. ISO 12242-2, ASTM 2003-02) EFORT 2012 tribology book. Heidelberg: Springer Press; 2012.
3. Ihle M, Mai S, Pfluger D, et al. The results of the titanium-coated RM acetabular component at 20 years: a long-term follow-up of an uncemented primary total hip replacement. J Bone Joint Surg Br. 2008;90(10):1284–90.
4. Pakvis D, Luites J, van Hellemondt G, Spruit M. A cementless, elastic press-fit socket with and without screws. Acta Orthop. 2012;83(5):481–7.
5. Rothwell A. The New Zealand Joint Registry – thirteen year report. New Zealand Joint Registry/New Zealand Orthopaedic Association. 2012. http://njr.cdhb.health.nz/reports/A2D65CA3.pdf.
6. Vielpeau C, et al. The creep behavior in vitamin E stabilized highly cross-linked polyethylene. 14th EFORT Congress 2013. Istanbul; 2013.
7. Wyss T, Kägi P, Mayrhofer P, Nötzli H, Pfluger D, Knahr K. Five-year results of the uncemented RM pressfit cup clinical evaluation and migration measurements by EBRA. J Arthroplasty. 2013;28(8):1291–6.

Index

K. Knahr (ed.), *Tribology in Total Hip and Knee Arthroplasty*,
DOI 10.1007/978-3-642-45266-6, © EFORT 2014

GPSR Compliance

The European Union's (EU) General Product Safety Regulation (GPSR) is a set of rules that requires consumer products to be safe and our obligations to ensure this.

If you have any concerns about our products, you can contact us on ProductSafety@springernature.com

In case Publisher is established outside the EU, the EU authorized representative is:

Springer Nature Customer Service Center GmbH
Europaplatz 3
69115 Heidelberg, Germany

Batch number: 10704695

Printed by Printforce, the Netherlands